Design and Analysis of
Group-Randomized Trials

Oxford University Press

Oxford   New York
Athens   Auckland   Bangkok   Bogota
Bombay   Buenos Aires   Calcutta   Cape Town
Dar es Salaam   Delhi   Florence   Hong Kong   Istanbul
Karachi   Kuala Lumpur   Madras   Madrid
Melbourne   Mexico City   Nairobi   Paris
Singapore   Taipei   Tokyo   Toronto   Warsaw

and associated companies in
Berlin   Ibadan

Published by Oxford University Press, Inc.
198 Madison Avenue, New York, New York 10016

Oxford is a registered trademark of Oxford University Press

Library of Congress Cataloging-in-Publication Data
Murray, David M.
Design and analysis of group-randomized trials /
David M. Murray.
p.   cm.—(Monographs in epidemiology and biostatistics)
Includes bibliographical references and index.

ISBN 978-0-19-512036-3

1. Group-randomized trials.
I. Title. II. Series.
R853.G76M87   1998   610'.7'2—dc21   97-20411

Printed in the United States of America
on acid-free paper

Preface

Health-promotion and disease-prevention research is a primary focus of many of the major research-funding agencies, including the National Institutes of Health (NIH) and the Centers for Disease Control and Prevention (CDC). Nonprofit organizations have also provided support for health-promotion and disease-prevention research.

Much of this research involves comparative studies designed to assess the effect of an intervention program on endpoints related to a health problem. Many of these studies involve identifiable groups that are not constituted at random. When such groups serve as the unit of assignment, so that they are randomized to study conditions, these studies are called group-randomized trials. These trials are now widely used to evaluate health-promotion programs based in worksites, schools, hospitals, clinics, neighborhoods, whole towns and cities, and other such groups that are identified by some physical, geographic, social, or other connection among their members, and the issues of design and analysis are the same regardless of the type of group. These issues are not new, nor are they unique to public health, as educators, social scientists, survey statisticians, demographers, and others have struggled with these problems for more than a half century.

While some group-randomized trials have dealt with these issues of design and analysis correctly, most have not. As evidence, consider the report by Donner et al. (1990), who reviewed group-randomized trials that were published between 1979 and 1989. They found that fewer than 20% of the trials dealt with these issues adequately in their sample-size calculations and that less than 50% dealt with them adequately in their analysis. Similarly, Rooney and Murray (1996) reviewed the school-based smoking-prevention literature from 1975 through 1991 and found that only 16% of the published studies had dealt with these issues adequately in their analysis. Finally, Simpson et al. (1995) reviewed primary prevention trials involving the allocation of identifiable groups that were published between 1990 and 1993 in the *American Journal of Public Health* and in *Preventive Medicine.* They reported that fewer than 20% dealt with these issues adequately in their sample-size calculations and that less than 57% dealt with them adequately in their analysis.

The continuing use of poor methods for design and analysis in group-randomized trials is somewhat surprising, because there has been a dramatic increase the number of published papers related to these methods over the last fifteen years. Indeed, there is now a wealth of good information available for those willing to find it. Unfortunately, that information is scattered across a wide variety of journals in several disciplines, and no single volume provides a summary.

The absence of a single text with broad coverage of the issues of design and analysis that face group-randomized trials stands in sharp contrast to the ready availability of well-known texts for other kinds of studies. Examples include clinical trials (e.g., Meinert, 1986), case-control studies (e.g., Schlesselman, 1982), observational studies (e.g., Kelsey et al., 1996), quasi-experimental studies (e.g., Cook and Campbell, 1979), and surveys (e.g., Kish, 1965).

The purpose of this book is to provide the first comprehensive text on the design and analysis of group-randomized trials. It is written to help those involved in group-randomized trials do a better job of planning, reviewing, funding, conducting, analyzing, and interpreting them. The book is aimed primarily at researchers who are involved in group-randomized trials, both academic and non-academic, including statisticians and other data analysts, graduate students, and evaluation staff who participate in the work. That audience is widely distributed in schools of public health, medicine, social work, and liberal arts and in departments of epidemiology, biostatistics, psychology, education, sociology, community health, and related schools and departments, as well as in research centers outside of the university setting. Other members of the primary audience include those who prepare program announcements and participate in the review and management of group-randomized trials. The audience also includes the many scientists and editors who review proposals for group-randomized trials as well as manuscripts based on those trials. Finally, the audience includes faculty in departments of epidemiology and biostatistics who teach research-methods courses, as well as graduate students in those programs. The careful reader should come away with the tools and skills necessary to critique a published group-randomized trial, to design a trial, to power that trial adequately, and to analyze the data from the trial using methods that are valid for the structure of the data.

The book is organized into ten chapters. Chapter 1 provides an introduction to group-randomized trials and an overview of the basic issues of design and analysis common to those trials. It also offers a perspective on the history and future of those trials. Chapter 2 describes the components required to plan a group-randomized trial. Chapter 3 presents the major cross-sectional and cohort designs that are available for those trials. Chapter 4 describes the analytic issues that face group-randomized trials. Chapter 5 presents the major analyses applicable to cross-sectional designs. Chapter 6 presents the major analyses applicable to cohort designs. Chapters 7 and 8 illustrate those analyses using data from the Minnesota Heart Health Program. Chapter 9 presents methods to determine power, detectable difference, and sample size. Chapter 10 provides a series of case studies based on published trials to illustrate these issues of design and analysis.

Most of these chapters are written at a conceptual level. Even for statistical issues, there is no matrix algebra or calculus. Chapters 7 and 8 illustrate the analytic methods presented in Chapters 5 and 6 and so are quite applied. Chapter 9 is also quite applied.

First-time readers and investigators who are not analytically oriented will want to focus on Chapters 1–4 and 10. These chapters provide an overview of the conceptual issues in group-randomized trials as well as case studies. Readers who are analytically oriented will also want to study Chapters 5–9. Those interested in the conceptual aspects of the analysis can focus on Chapters 5 and 6. Those interested in details and examples will also want to study Chapters 7 and 8. The discussion of sample size in Chapter 9 presumes that the reader has studied Chapters 5–8. Because readers interested in Chapters 5–8 are likely to refer to different sections for different studies, some repetition has been built into those sections so that the individual sections can stand alone.

Many colleagues have provided assistance in the preparation of this book. Most notable are Peter Hannan and Bill Baker, two longtime colleagues in the Division of Epidemiology. Peter Hannan helped unravel many of the statistical issues that are presented in the book and was the first to read and critique each section. Bill Baker solved many programming challenges and created all the major databases used for the book. Russell Wolfinger also deserves special mention. He is the statistician at SAS, Inc., who developed the SAS PROC MIXED software and provided feedback both on statistical issues and on the application of SAS PROC MIXED and the GLIMMIX macro. David Zucker, formerly at the National Heart Lung and Blood Institute and now at the Department of Statistics, Hebrew University, Jerusalem, played a critical role in the mid-1980s in helping me to understand the analytic implications of nested designs, as did Allan Donner of the Department of Epidemiology and Biostatistics, University of Western Ontario.

Several colleagues have read one or more preliminary versions of at least some of the chapters, and I am very grateful for their feedback: Allan Donner, Henry Feldman, Patricia Grambsch, Peter Hannan, Tom Louis, Art Peterson, and Russ Wolfinger. Art Peterson and Allan Donner deserve special mention in this regard, as both read an earlier version of the entire book and offered detailed critiques; the final version reflects their many good suggestions. Much is owed, as well, to the students who enrolled in my Community Trials course over the last ten years in the Division of Epidemiology, School of Public Health, University of Minnesota. That course served as the proving ground for many of the ideas and much of the presentation style for this book. I also want to recognize the secretarial support provided by Carol Hansen. Finally, I want to recognize the support of the University of Minnesota and particularly the faculty of the Division of Epidemiology in the School of Public Health. Without my recent sabbatical and the support provided by my colleagues, this book could not have been written.

DMM

Minneapolis, Minnesota
February 28, 1997

Contents

Design and Analysis of
Group-Randomized Trials

1

Introduction

> Randomization by cluster accompanied by an analysis appropriate to randomization by individual is an exercise in self-deception, however, and should be discouraged.
>
> Cornfield (1978), pp. 101–102

Group-randomized trials are comparative studies in which (1) the units of assignment are identifiable groups and (2) the units of observation are members of those groups. In this context, an identifiable group refers quite broadly to any group that is not constituted at random, so that there is some physical, geographic, social, or other connection among its members.

This chapter opens with several examples of group-randomized trials and an enumeration of the distinguishing characteristics of such trials. Those characteristics have implications for both the design and the analysis of group-randomized trials and set the stage for the rest of the book. This chapter also provides some perspective on group-randomized trials by reviewing the many labels that have been used for these trials in different settings, by comparing them to other studies, by reviewing their recent history, by documenting the continuing need for such trials, and by offering thoughts on their future.

Examples

Adolescent-Smoking Prevention

Social influences play an important role in the etiology of adolescent smoking (USDHHS, 1994). Adolescents are more likely to begin to smoke if they live in an environment with many smoking models, believe that smoking is normative for their age group, feel ill-equipped to respond to the social pressure that their peers can create to encourage smoking, and have not been prepared for the commercial appeals from the tobacco industry. The National Cancer Institute has recommended that smoking-prevention programs target these social influences so as to give students opportunities to learn that smoking is not normative, to practice effective methods to resist peer pressures to smoke, and to develop countermessages to tobacco advertising (Glynn, 1989). Schools are a natural setting for such programs, because virtually all young adolescents can be reached through schools and because smoking-prevention curricula are consistent with the schools' educational objectives. Investigators, school officials, and parents want to know if these social-influences programs reduce adolescent smoking.

Evaluation of school-based smoking-prevention programs is complicated by the difficulty of randomly assigning individual students to intervention and control conditions. Not only would that be logistically impossible in many schools, but the mixing that would occur outside of the class used for the intervention would seriously contaminate the study conditions. This would bias any comparison toward the null hypothesis of no intervention effect. As a result, the standard practice in school-based smoking-prevention studies has been to allocate whole schools to study conditions while collecting outcome-evaluation data from individual students. This approach poses no logistical problems for the schools and largely avoids contamination, because all the students in the target grade(s) in a school are in the same condition.

Heart Attack Delay Time

In 1995, the National Heart Lung and Blood Institute began the Rapid Early Action for Coronary Treatment (REACT) trial to evaluate an intervention designed to reduce delay time in seeking medical attention among patients experiencing a heart attack (Simons-Morton et al., under review). Ten cities were assigned at random to the intervention condition and 10 others to the control condition. The intervention has several components, but critical among them is a mass-media campaign that involves the local television and radio stations. The investigators want to know if their intervention reduces delay time among heart attack victims in the intervention cities relative to the control cities.

Even with careful selection of stations and broadcast times, it would not be possible to limit the delivery of the mass-media messages only to those residents in a city who had been randomly assigned to an intervention condition. Instead, virtually all adults resident in the cities whose stations broadcast the messages would be exposed to the intervention. As a result, the investigators had no choice but to allocate whole cities to the two study conditions.

Nutrition Education

The public is generally aware of the need to reduce fat and salt in the diet so as to reduce the risk of cancer and cardiovascular disease. However, many who might want to follow this advice have difficulty when ordering in a restaurant, because it is not always easy to tell which menu items have reduced fat and salt content. One approach to this problem has been to label menu items that are low in fat and salt so that patrons can consider that information as they decide what to order. An evaluation of such a menu-labeling program seeks to determine whether there is an increase in the proportion of patrons who order the reduced-fat and -salt items as a result of the labeling program.

This is another situation where random assignment of members instead of groups to study conditions would be difficult. Such a plan would require that both labeled and unlabeled menus be available in each participating restaurant at the same time, with good control over allocation of menus to patrons, and with careful records of what was ordered on a patron-by-patron basis. In contrast, if whole restaurants are randomized to study conditions, so that all patrons in a given restaurant receive the same menu, no effort is required to monitor or control allocation of menus, nor is it necessary to monitor orders by patrons.

Beverage-Alcohol Service

Bartenders and waiters can play an important role in limiting service to patrons who appear intoxicated. Volunteer efforts have proven difficult to implement, and policy interventions may prove more effective. Counties that pass ordinances requiring training for bartenders and waiters want to determine whether that training is effective in reducing service to patrons who appear intoxicated.

In this case, the unit of observation is not a person but the beverage-alcohol establishment—that is, the bar or restaurant. Those establishments will be observed to determine the rate at which they serve patrons who appear intoxicated. By comparing counties with and without the ordinances requiring training, researchers will be able to provide evidence on the effectiveness of such a public-policy approach to limit service to patrons who appear intoxicated.

Distinguishing Characteristics

As these examples illustrate, there are several characteristics that distinguish a group-randomized trial from the familiar clinical trial. First, the unit of assignment is an identifiable group rather than an individual. Such groups are not formed at random, but rather through some connection among their members. Groups may be defined by their physical structure, as is the case for schools and restaurants; other examples are worksites, hospitals, etc. In other cases, the groups may be defined by geography, as with whole communities and counties; other examples are neighborhoods and states. In still other cases, the groups may be defined by a social connection, as with a church congregation or other social or religious organization.

The second distinguishing characteristic of a group-randomized trial is that different units of assignment are allocated to each study condition. This action nests the assignment units within the study conditions. In each of the examples above, one set of schools, communities, or restaurants was assigned to the intervention condition while another set was assigned to the control condition.

The third characteristic of group-randomized trials is that the units of observation are members of the groups that serve as the units of assignment. The nesting of different units of observation in each unit of assignment and different units of assignment in each condition creates the hierarchical structure characteristic of group-randomized trials. Study conditions are the highest aggregate level, units of assignment form an intermediate level, and the units of observation are the lowest aggregate level. In more complex group-randomized trials, there may be even more layers in the hierarchy.

The fourth distinguishing characteristic is that group-randomized trials typically involve only a limited number of assignment units in each study condition. While there are exceptions, it is uncommon to find a group-randomized trial with more than 15 assignment units allocated to each condition and quite common to observe group-randomized trials with fewer than 10 assignment units allocated to each condition.

The Impact of These Characteristics

These characteristics operate together to set the stage for the special issues of design and analysis that face investigators who wish to conduct a group-randomized trial. These issues must be addressed as the trial is planned to ensure that the trial will provide a valid answer to the research question of interest.

Analysis Issues

Let $Y_{i:k:l}$ represent an observation from the ith member nested within the kth group nested within the lth condition; the nesting is reflected by the colons (:). For now, let all the groups have the same number of members, m, and all the conditions have the same number of groups, g. The $Y_{i:k:l}$ may be continuous or discrete, and their distribution need not be specified. When membership in each group is established by random assignment, it is reasonable to assume that the errors associated with the members of a group are independent. Let the within-group variance be σ_y^2. Then the variance of the group mean is simply:

$$\sigma_{\bar{y}_g}^2 = \frac{\sigma_y^2}{m} \tag{1.1}$$

Given the additional assumption of constant variance across groups, the variance of the condition mean is:

$$\sigma_{\bar{y}_c}^2 = \frac{\sigma_y^2}{mg} \tag{1.2}$$

That variance provides the basis for the standard error for any intervention effect that is defined as a contrast among condition means.

Now consider the situation in a group-randomized trial. Here the units of assignment are identifiable groups, not constituted through random assignment. As described by Kish more than thirty years ago, the members of an identifiable group will have something in common, due to commonalities in selection, exposure, mutual interaction, or some combination of those factors (Kish, 1965). That commonality will be reflected in a measurable degree of intraclass correlation:

$$ICC_{m:g:c} = corr(y_{i:k:l}, y_{i':k:l}) \tag{1.3}$$

The positive intraclass correlation serves to reduce the variation among the members of the same group so that the within-group variance in this simplest of group-randomized trials is:

$$\sigma_e^2 = \sigma_y^2 (1 - ICC_{m:g:c}) \tag{1.4}$$

The intraclass correlation is the fraction of the total variation in the data that is attributable to the unit of assignment:

$$ICC_{m:g:c} = \frac{\sigma_{g:c}^2}{\sigma_e^2 + \sigma_{g:c}^2} \tag{1.5}$$

where $\sigma_{g:c}^2$ is the component of variance attributable to the unit of assignment and $\sigma_y^2 = \sigma_e^2 + \sigma_{g:c}^2$. The variance of the group mean is then:

$$\sigma_{\bar{y}_g}^2 = \frac{\sigma_e^2}{m} + \sigma_{g:c}^2 \tag{1.6}$$

A little algebra will show that: [1]

$$\sigma^2_{\bar{y}_g} = \frac{\sigma^2_y}{m}\left(1 + (m-1)ICC_{m:g:c}\right) \tag{1.7}$$

The variance of the condition mean in a group-randomized trial is then:

$$\sigma^2_{\bar{y}_c} = \frac{\sigma^2_y}{mg}\left(1 + (m-1)ICC_{m:g:c}\right) \tag{1.8}$$

This formulation of the variance of the condition mean in a group-randomized trial has several important implications:

1. The variance of the condition mean in a group-randomized trial is different from the variance of the condition mean that would be expected under the assumption of independent errors. The difference is represented by the factor $(1 + (m-1)ICC_{m:g:c})$. That factor has been called the design effect (*DEFF*) by Kish (1965) and the variance inflation factor (*VIF*) by Donner et al. (1981). In the context of group-randomized trials, *VIF* is a more descriptive label.

2. When $ICC > 0$, as is almost always the case in a group-randomized trial, the *VIF* increases both as the intraclass correlation increases and as the number of observation units in each assignment unit increases. Even for small *ICC*s, the *VIF* will be large when m is large. As a result, the variance of the condition mean is almost always larger in a group-randomized trial than in a study based on random assignment of the same number of individuals to the study conditions.

3. When $ICC > 0$, any test that ignores the variation due to the unit of assignment will have a Type I error rate greater than the nominal level (Zucker, 1990).[2] As a result, the usual analysis methods that assume independent errors are not appropriate for group-randomized trials.

Phrased another way, the intraclass correlation in a group-randomized trial represents a violation of the independence-of-errors assumption that underlies most of the analyses used in clinical trials. Application of those familiar analyses to data from a group-randomized trial will yield a standard error for the intervention effect that is too small and a *p*-value that overstates the significance of the result.

4. When $ICC > 0$, any test that properly recognizes the variation due to the unit of assignment will have reduced power, all other factors constant, compared to a study in which the observations are independent.

5. The degrees of freedom for the test of the intervention effect will depend on the structure of the variance of the condition mean. Because that variance

in a group-randomized trial will always involve a component of variance associated with the unit of assignment, the degrees of freedom for the test of the intervention effect will always be tied to the number of groups allocated to each condition. Because that number is usually limited, the degrees of freedom for the test of the intervention effect are usually limited. This will further reduce the power of a test that employs the proper degrees of freedom compared to a test that uses more degrees of freedom.

6. When the proper degrees of freedom are limited, application of methods that provide too many degrees of freedom will yield a Type I error rate that is greater than the nominal level (e.g., Murray et al., 1996).

Design Issues

Because group-randomized trials often employ only a limited number of identifiable groups as units of assignment, there will rarely be enough assignment units to ensure that randomization has an opportunity to evenly distribute potential sources of bias among the intervention conditions. This makes potential bias the norm in group-randomized trials rather than the exception; absent randomization, bias is almost inevitable. As a result, investigators should employ randomization whenever possible and must anticipate the potential sources of bias as they design their trials and plan their analyses. The potential sources of bias in a group-randomized trial and the defenses that are available to guard against them are the focus of Chapter 2.

Because the variation in the data is usually greater and the degrees of freedom for the effects of interest are usually fewer, there is even more pressure on the investigator to design an efficient study. The familiar methods of matching, stratification, repeated measures, and regression adjustment for covariates can be used to improve the efficiency of the design, but their application is more complex than in a clinical trial. Those issues are discussed further in Chapter 3.

Investigators who wish to conduct a group-randomized trial must anticipate all the sources of random variation and correlation in their data, as well as the magnitude of those variances and correlations, and design a study that is large enough to have adequate power for the tests of interest. They must also select analytic measures appropriate to the design of their study and the nature of their variables so as to maintain the nominal Type I error rate. The threats to the validity of the analysis of a group-randomized trial and the defenses that are available to guard against them are discussed in Chapter 4.

Perspective

Labels Used in Other Disciplines

Group-randomized trials represent a subset of a larger class of designs often labeled *nested, hierarchical, multilevel,* or *clustered* designs. As noted above, units of observation are typically nested within identifiable groups or clusters, which are in turn nested within study conditions. This defines a hierarchy of levels in the design: units of observation, units of assignment, and study conditions. More complex designs may have even more levels.

As used here, the label *group-randomized trial* refers to a design in which identifiable groups are assigned to study conditions for the express purpose of assessing the impact of one or more interventions on one or more endpoints. The terms *nested, hierarchical, multilevel,* and *clustered* designs can be used more broadly to refer to any data set that has a hierarchical structure, and these more general terms are often used to characterize observational studies as well as comparative studies.

Many examples of both observational and comparative hierarchical designs can be found in education, where students are nested within classrooms, which are nested within schools, which are nested within school districts, which are nested within communities, etc. Investigators in education often refer to such designs as hierarchical or multilevel designs (Bryk and Raudenbush, 1992; Goldstein, 1987).

Other examples can be found in survey sampling, and in disciplines that employ surveys, such as epidemiology, sociology, and demography. In these disciplines, cluster sampling is a commonly used technique and the surveys are often said to have cluster-sampling designs (Kish, 1965). Cluster-sampling designs can be a good way to limit cost when the investigator lacks a complete enumeration of the population of interest and does not want to expend the resources required to generate such an enumeration. Because simple random sampling is impossible without a complete enumeration, clusters such as blocks or neighborhoods or other identifiable groups are enumerated and sampled in a first stage, followed by enumeration and sampling of individuals within the selected clusters in a second stage. Applied properly, cluster-sampling methods can yield unbiased estimates of population rates or means at a lower cost than would have been the case with simple random sampling. Unfortunately, cluster sampling invariably leads to increased variation and more limited degrees of freedom. These problems are well known to survey-sampling statisticians (Kish, 1965, 1987; Skinner et al., 1989).

Biostatisticians often use the term *cluster-randomization study* to refer to a group-randomized trial (Donner et al., 1981). This terminology is based on the fact that an identifiable group is a cluster. It borrows from the terminology of survey sampling. With the broad definition given to "group" in this text, the phrases *cluster-randomization study* and *group-randomized trial* are equivalent.

I have long used the term *community trial* to refer to group-randomized trials (e.g., Murray and Hannan, 1990). This term emerged from the community-based heart disease–prevention studies of the 1980s (Farquhar et al., 1990; Luepker et al., 1994; Carleton et al., 1995). None of those studies were randomized trials, but all involved whole communities as the unit of assignment with collection of data from individuals within those communities. Community trial is an attractive label, because it includes both randomized and nonrandomized designs. However, it is often thought to refer only to studies that involve whole communities (e.g., Lilienfeld and Stolley, 1994), and so creates confusion when applied to studies involving other identifiable groups. The term *group-randomized trial* is more general.

Contrast With Other Types Of Research

Research studies can be positioned on a continuum from tightly controlled experiments, to quasi-experiments, to controlled observational studies, to surveys (Kish, 1987). In public health and medicine, the gold standard design for assessing the efficacy of an intervention has long been the randomized clinical trial, a tightly controlled experiment designed to maximize the investigator's ability to draw a causal inference about the effect of the treatment(s) on the endpoint(s). The clinical trial is well known and there are whole volumes devoted to it (e.g., Meinert, 1986). Clinical trials are characterized by randomization of individuals to study conditions, often after extensive screening for eligibility, and by careful monitoring over time to ascertain the results. As such, they often are quite strong on internal validity, which is the validity of causal inference, but weak on external validity, which is the validity of generalization to other populations, settings, and times. The participants may or may not represent any identifiable population or subpopulation, but they are always randomized as individuals to the study conditions. The study conditions may not reflect the real world well, but clinical trials are characterized by good experimental control.

Quasi-experiments have many of the characteristics of experiments, including those related to the interventions, endpoints, and allocation rules, but do not employ randomization. Like clinical trials, quasi-experimental designs have been in use for some time, and there are excellent texts on this family of designs (e.g., Cook and Campbell, 1979). Study conditions are constituted by self-selection, by historical accident, or often through the purposeful action of the investigator, but without randomization of individuals to study conditions.

In fact, many quasi-experiments could also be characterized as nonrandomized group trials, as data are often collected from individuals nested within identifiable groups that have been nonrandomly assigned to study conditions. Quasi-experiments may employ the same level of rigor as experiments with regard to screening, measurement, and quality of interventions, but do not include randomization as part of their protocol. Quasi-experiments are not as strong as true experiments on internal validity but are often stronger on external validity because they take place outside of the clinical or laboratory setting.

Controlled observational studies are much less structured than experiments or quasi-experiments, but still have much in common with those designs. Measurement of exposures, confounders, endpoints, and other variables still requires as much rigor as possible. In these studies, the investigator has no control over which participants receive the intervention or other exposure of interest and which participants remain unexposed. Case-control and cohort studies are classic examples of observational studies and contribute important knowledge to epidemiology, public health, and medicine. A number of excellent texts describe these study designs (e.g., Kelsey et al., 1996; Schlesselman, 1982). Proper specification and measurement of potential confounding variables are especially important in observational studies, for the investigator cannot rely on randomization of participants to conditions to evenly distribute potential sources of bias. Instead, the investigator must rely on techniques of design and analysis in an effort to minimize bias and allow insight into the true relationships among the variables under study.

Surveys represent the end of the continuum opposite controlled experiments. The investigator can control what is measured, from whom the measurements are taken, and how the measurements are taken, but has little control otherwise. As such, surveys are uncontrolled observational studies (Kish, 1987). They often provide the highest levels of external validity but the lowest levels of internal validity. They are appropriate when the investigator wants to estimate the population level of one or more variables, describe the joint distribution of those variables, or provide data to allow comparison of one population to another. They are not designed to provide information on causal relationships, regardless of the manipulations that may be applied to the data after they are collected. Surveys have been in use much longer than the other methods, and many excellent texts are available (e.g., Kish, 1965).

Group-randomized trials employ random allocation of identifiable groups to study conditions; as a result, they are true experiments. Randomization provides a statistical basis for the assumption of independence of errors at the level of the unit of assignment and serves to distribute potential sources of bias evenly across the study conditions. If a sufficient number of groups are randomized to each condition, inferences based on a valid analysis can be as strong as those obtained from a randomized clinical trial. For this reason, the group-randomized trial is the gold standard for design in public health and medicine when allocation of identifiable groups is required.

Nonrandomized group trials employ identifiable groups as the unit of assignment but do not employ randomization. As such, they represent a form of quasi-experiment. Nonrandomized group trials face substantially greater threats to internal validity than do group-randomized trials, and for this reason group-randomized trials are clearly preferred. At the same time, if circumstances prevent randomization, a nonrandomized group trial may be the only design alternative. However, as with any quasi-experiment, special care must be taken both in the design and analysis of the trial and especially in the interpretation of the data.

Recent Progress

The last 25 years has witnessed dramatic improvements in the quality of the design and analysis of trials based on the allocation of identifiable groups to study conditions. In the 1970s, it was quite common to see studies in which a single identifiable group was assigned to each study condition. The literature from the 1970s and 1980s on school-based programs to prevent use of tobacco, alcohol, and other drugs included many such studies. The first community trial for prevention of coronary heart disease used exactly that design (Puska et al., 1983). Quite independently, developments in these two areas inspired developments that led to steady improvements in the design and analysis of group-randomized trials.

Cornfield's (1978) paper in the *American Journal of Epidemiology* symposium on coronary heart disease prevention trials defined the two basic issues of analysis that face group-randomized trials. He noted that the variance between assignment units is larger than the variance within assignment units. He also noted that there will generally be many fewer degrees of freedom available to estimate that between-unit variance than to estimate the within-unit variance. Those two issues were discussed earlier and lie at the heart of the design and analytic challenges that face group-randomized trials.

Flay's (1985) review of the adolescent smoking–prevention literature in *Health Psychology* documented the design and analytic weaknesses of what he termed the "early generations" of smoking-prevention studies. All were based on one or two schools per condition, often without random assignment. His critique was pointed but fair, and pushed an entire field to improve the design and analysis of their studies.

Responding directly to Cornfield's (1978) warning, Donner and colleagues at the University of Western Ontario published a steady stream of papers on the issues of analysis facing group-randomized trials through the 1980s and

1990s. Responding in part to Flay's criticism and in part to the issues raised by Cornfield's warning, the author and colleagues from the University of Minnesota began their examination of the issues of design and analysis in group-randomized trials in the mid-1980s. Other investigators from the National Institutes of Health, the University of Washington, the New England Research Institute, and elsewhere added to this growing literature, especially in the 1990s.

By the late 1980s and early 1990s, many group-randomized trials were under way that were of very high quality in terms of their methods of design and analysis. Examples include the Community Intervention Trial for Smoking Cessation (COMMIT) (Gail et al., 1992) and the Child and Adolescent Trial for Cardiovascular Health (CATCH) (Zucker et al., 1995). These improvements occurred as investigators and reviewers alike gradually came to understand the special issues of design and analysis that face group-randomized trials and the methods required to address them.

Unfortunately, the improvements have not been represented in all group-randomized trials. Even in the 1990s, grants were funded and papers were published based on poor designs and poor analyses. Simpson et al. (1995) reviewed group-randomized trials that were published between 1990 and 1993 in the *American Journal of Public Health* and in *Preventive Medicine*. They reported that fewer than 20% dealt with the design and analytic issues adequately in their sample size or power analysis and that only 57% dealt with them adequately in their analysis.

Even today, it is still common to hear investigators argue that their study was not designed to be analyzed at the level of the unit of assignment, and so they should not be held to that standard. Others argue that their intervention was designed to change the behavior of individuals, and so their analysis should be based on individuals. Such arguments ignore the methodological realities of the group-randomized trial and represent exactly the kind of self-deception that Cornfield (1978) warned against two decades ago. They also ignore the reality that analyses of these trials can be based on individuals yet still reflect the extra variation due to the nested design.

As investigators began asking for articles and books that they could read to become better informed on these issues, I had to tell them that there was no single volume available that brought together both the issues and the solutions for the design and analysis of group-randomized trials. That became the driving force behind this book; I saw an opportunity to draw together the considerable information that was available but scattered across a variety of journals and books. As the book evolved, the gaps in knowledge concerning analytic methods became ever more apparent and sparked new work in a variety of areas, both by the team at Minnesota and by colleagues elsewhere. As a result, this book includes much new material. The purpose of the book remained constant however—to help students and investigators understand the design and analytic issues that face group-randomized trials as well as the strategies available to address them.

The Continuing Need

Disappointing results have been published recently for several large trials based on allocation of identifiable groups to study conditions. In particular, the results of the Stanford Five City Project (FCP) (Farquhar et al., 1990), the Minnesota Heart Health Program (MHHP) (Luepker et al., 1994), the Pawtucket Heart Health Program (PHHP) (Carleton et al., 1995), and COMMIT (COMMIT Research Group, 1995a, b) were all less than their sponsors had hoped. Their results led some to question the value of group-randomized trials in general and of community trials in particular.

To question group-randomized trials in general based on these results is not only shortsighted but also completely impractical. Whenever the investigator wants to evaluate an intervention that operates at a group level, manipulates the social or physical environment, or cannot be delivered to individuals, a group-randomized trial design is the best comparative design available. However, as is clear from the preceding discussion, there are many challenges to the design of these trials. As a result, the investigator must take care to understand those challenges and the strategies that are available to meet them.

The questions raised about community trials in particular have considerable merit. There can be no question that it is harder to change the health behavior and risk profile of a whole community than it is to make similar changes in smaller identifiable groups such as those at worksites, physician practices, schools, and churches. And while no quantitative analysis has been published, it seems that the magnitude of the intervention effects reported for group-randomized trials has been greater for trials that involved smaller groups than for trials involving such large aggregates as whole communities. With smaller groups, it is possible to include more groups in the design, thereby improving the validity of the design and the power of the trial. With smaller groups, it is easier to focus intervention activities on the target population. With smaller groups, the cost and difficulty of the implementation of the study generally are reduced. For these and similar reasons, future group-randomized trials would do well to focus on smaller identifiable groups rather than on whole cities or larger aggregates.

In an editorial that accompanied the COMMIT findings, the editor of the *American Journal of Public Health* responded directly to those who had questioned the utility of the group-randomized trial:

[W]e should not abandon community trials but should gather the knowledge necessary to refine them. (Susser, 1995, p. 158)

The question is not whether to conduct group-randomized trials, but how to construct a trial so that it is (1) sufficiently rigorous to avoid the pitfalls common to all comparative trials as well as those peculiar to group-randomized trials, (2) powerful enough to provide an answer to the question of interest, and (3) inexpensive enough to be practical. The question is not whether to conduct group-randomized trials, but rather how to do them well. That is the central question addressed in this book.

The Future

The issues of design and analysis of group-randomized trials are now actively under investigation, and new information is appearing at a rapid rate. The *American Journal of Epidemiology* recently published the second symposium on community intervention trials (Donner, 1995; Murray, 1995; Fortmann et al., 1995; Koepsell et al., 1995; Green et al., 1995). *Evaluation Review* devoted a recent issue entirely to methods for evaluation of group-randomized trials (McKinlay, 1996; Feldman et al., 1996; Harrow et al., 1996; McGraw et al., 1996; Murray et al., 1996; Hannan and Murray, 1996). *The Journal of Educational and Behavioral Statistics* devoted a recent issue entirely to the problems and prospects of hierarchical linear models, which have direct relevance for group-randomized trials (Kreft, 1995; Draper, 1995; Rogosa and Saner, 1995; DeLeeuw and Kreft, 1995; Morris, 1995; Goldstein, 1995; Longford, 1995; Raudenbush, 1995). *Sociological Methods and Research* devoted a recent issue to the methods of multilevel analysis, another term for hierarchical linear models (Hox and Kreft, 1994; Hox, 1994; Kreft and DeLeeuw, 1994; Snijders and Bosker, 1994; Goldstein, 1994; Muthén, 1994; McDonald, 1994). The *Journal of Community Psychology* devoted a special issue to the methods for evaluation of group-randomized trials (Kaftarian and Hansen, 1994; Goodman and Wandersman, 1994; Pentz, 1994; Hunt, 1994; Kim et al., 1994; Wagenaar et al., 1994; Ellickson, 1994; Springer and Phillips, 1994; Murray and Wolfinger, 1994; Cook et al., 1994; Hansen and Kaftarian, 1994; Braithwaite, 1994). *Annals of Epidemiology* will publish a series of papers from the September 1996 National Heart Lung and Blood Institute (NHLBI) conference on Community Trials for Cardiopulmonary Health (Resnicow and Robinson, 1997; Ockene et al., 1997; Lasater et al., 1997; Schooler et al., 1997; Murray, 1997; Feldman, 1997; Baranowski, et al., 1997; Flora and Saphir, 1997; Winkleby, 1997). There are still many methodological areas in need of further investigation.

For example, additional research is needed on the use of continuous surveillance as a method that would allow monitoring of trends in the endpoints, the use of community-level indicators as endpoints in lieu of more expensive individual-level measurements, the use of frequent but small surveys in lieu of infrequent but large surveys as another method that would allow careful monitoring of trends in the endpoints, analysis methods for non-Gaussian data, and the comparison of model-based and randomization-based methods in order to identify the conditions under which one approach is favored over the other. These are only a few of the areas in need of additional work.

There is every reason to expect that continuing methodological improvements will lead to better trials. There is also evidence that better trials will have more satisfactory results. For example, Rooney and Murray (1996) recently presented the results of a meta-analysis of group-randomized trials in the smoking-prevention field. One of the findings was that stronger intervention effects were associated with greater methodological rigor. Stronger intervention effects were reported for studies that planned from the beginning to employ the unit of assignment as the unit of analysis, that randomized a sufficient number of assignment units to each condition, that adjusted for baseline differences in important confounding variables, that had extended follow-up, and that had limited attrition. One hopes that such findings will encourage use of good design and analytic methods.

At the same time, improvements in methodological rigor alone will not be enough. No matter how well designed and evaluated a group-randomized trial may be, strengths in design and analysis cannot overcome a weak intervention. As Susser noted in his editorial,

> Future trials will need to draw on a deeper understanding, now lacking, of methods for bringing about social change. (Susser, 1995, p. 158)

The message here is that we still have much to learn about changing ingrained behaviors in whole populations.

Evidence of the need for stronger intervention programs also comes from the recent large group-randomized trials that reported disappointing results. This is particularly true for studies such as COMMIT (COMMIT Working Group, 1995a, b) and for CATCH (Luepker, Perry et al., 1996). Both COMMIT and CATCH had very strong design and analytic plans (Gail et al., 1992; Zucker et al., 1995). Both COMMIT and CATCH reported favorable results for some endpoints, but neither achieved the intervention effects postulated for other endpoints. The same can be said for MHHP, FCP, and PHHP. A recent pooled analysis of those three programs demonstrated clearly that the results were well below expectations even when adequate power was available in the pooled analysis (Winkleby et al., 1997).

Another source of evidence on the need for better intervention programs comes from group-randomized trials that have reported positive intervention effects. For example, the meta-analysis of more than 100 group-randomized trials in the adolescent-smoking field concluded that social-influences smoking-prevention programs are effective and should be widely disseminated (Rooney and Murray, 1996). A recent review also reported numerous positive findings in health-promotion trials based on the allocation of physicians' practices (Ockene et al., in press) to study conditions.

Future trials will be stronger and more likely to report satisfactory results if they (1) address an important research question, (2) employ an intervention that has a strong theoretical base and preliminary evidence of feasibility and efficacy, (3) randomize a sufficient number of assignment units to each study condition so as to have good power, (4) are designed in recognition of the major threats to the validity of the design and analysis of group-randomized trials, (5) employ good quality-control measures to monitor fidelity of implementation of intervention and measurement protocols, (6) are well executed, (7) employ good process-evaluation measures to assess effects on intermediate endpoints, (8) employ reliable and valid endpoint measures, (9) are analyzed using methods appropriate to the design of the study and the nature of the primary endpoints, and (10) are interpreted in light of the strengths and weaknesses of the study.

Endnotes

1.

$$\sigma_{\bar{y}_g}^2 = \frac{\sigma_e^2}{m} + \sigma_{g:c}^2$$

$$= \frac{\sigma_e^2 + m\sigma_{g:c}^2}{m}$$

$$= \frac{(\sigma_e^2 + \sigma_{g:c}^2) + (m\sigma_{g:c}^2 - \sigma_{g:c}^2)}{m}$$

$$= \frac{(\sigma_e^2 + \sigma_{g:c}^2) + (m-1)\sigma_{g:c}^2}{m}$$

$$= \frac{(\sigma_e^2 + \sigma_{g:c}^2) + \frac{(\sigma_e^2 + \sigma_{g:c}^2)(m-1)\sigma_{g:c}^2}{\sigma_e^2 + \sigma_{g:c}^2}}{m}$$

$$= \frac{(\sigma_e^2 + \sigma_{g:c}^2)\left(1 + (m-1)\frac{\sigma_{g:c}^2}{\sigma_e^2 + \sigma_{g:c}^2}\right)}{m}$$

$$= \frac{\sigma_y^2}{m}\left(1 + (m-1)ICC_{m:g:c}\right)$$

2. The Type I error rate is the probability that the effect will be observed to be statistically significant simply by chance. For most applications, that rate is set at 5%.

2

Planning the Trial

> If we compare a cluster sample with an element sample comprised of the same number of elements, typically we will find that in cluster sampling: (1) the cost per element is lower . . . ; (2) the element variance is higher . . . ; (3) the costs and problems of statistical analysis are greater.
>
> Kish (1965), pp. 149–150

Planning a group-randomized trial is a complex process. Because it involves many of the same steps that are required to plan other types of research, the familiar resources for the design and conduct of clinical trials and observational studies will be of help to those who want to plan a group-randomized trial (e.g., Meinert, 1986; Kelsey et al., 1996; Schlesselman, 1982). This chapter will focus on the adaptations that must be made to accommodate group-randomized trials. It will review each of the major components of the planning process and outline the development of a formal proposal for the study.

The Research Question

The driving force behind any group-randomized trial must be the research question. The question will be based on the problem of interest and will identify the target population, the setting, the endpoints, and the intervention. In turn, those factors will shape the design and analytic plan.

Given the importance of the research question, the investigators must take care to articulate it clearly. Unfortunately, that doesn't always happen. Investigators may have ideas about the theoretical or conceptual basis for the intervention, and often even clearer ideas about the conceptual basis for the endpoints. They may even have ideas about intermediate processes. However, without very clear thinking about each of these issues, the investigators may find themselves at the end of the trial unable to answer the question of interest.

To put themselves in a position to articulate their research question clearly, the investigators should first document thoroughly the nature and extent of the underlying problem and the strategies and results of previous efforts to remedy that problem. A literature review and correspondence with others working in the field are ingredients essential to that process, as the investigators should know as much as possible about the problem before they plan their trial.

Having become experts in the field, the investigators will be able to pose not just one question but a whole series of questions. They should choose from among that series the single question that will drive their group-randomized trial. The primary criteria for choosing that question should be: (1) Is it important enough to do?, and (2) Is this the right time to do it? Reviewers will ask both questions, and the investigators must be able to provide well-documented answers.

Most group-randomized trials seek to prevent a health problem, so that the importance of the question is linked to the seriousness of that problem. The investigators should document the extent of the problem and the potential benefit from a reduction in that problem.

The question of timing is also important. The investigators should document that the question has not been answered already and that the intervention has a good chance to improve the primary endpoint in the target population. That is most easily done when the investigators are thoroughly familiar with previous research in the area; when the etiology of the problem is well known; when there is a theoretical basis for the proposed intervention; when there is preliminary evidence on the feasibility and efficacy of the intervention; when the measures for the dependent and mediating variables are well-developed; when the sources of variation and correlation as well as the trends in the endpoints are well understood; and when the investigators have created the research team to carry out the study. If that is not the state of affairs, then the investigators must either invest the time and energy to reach that state or choose another question.

Once the question is selected, it is very important to put it down on paper. The research question is easily lost in the day-to-day details of the planning and execution of the study, and because much time can be wasted in pursuit of issues that are not really central to the research question, the investigators should take care to keep that question in mind.

The Research Team

Having defined the question, the investigators should determine whether they have expertise sufficient to deal with all the challenges that are likely to arise as they plan and execute the trial. They should identify the skills that they do not have and expand the research team to ensure that those skills are available. The nature of the skills needed will depend on the research question. Even so, all group-randomized trials will need expertise in research design, data collection, data processing and analysis, intervention development, intervention implementation, and project administration. Because those skills are rarely found in a single investigator, most trials will require a team, with responsibilities shared among its members.

Because the team usually will need to convince a funding agency that they are appropriate for the trial, it is important to include experienced and senior investigators in key roles. There is simply no substitute for experience with similar interventions, in similar populations and settings, using similar measures, and similar methods of data collection and analysis.

Most teams will remember the familiar academic issues (e.g., statistics, data management, intervention theory), but some may forget the very important practical side of trials involving identifiable groups. However, to forget the practical side is a sure way to get into trouble. For example, a school-based trial that doesn't include on its team someone who is very familiar with school operations is almost certain to get into trouble with the schools. A hospital-based trial that doesn't include on its team someone who is very familiar with hospital operations is almost certain to get into trouble with the hospitals. A trial planned for a special population that doesn't include on its team someone who is very familiar with that population is almost certain to get into trouble with that population. And the same can be said for every other type of identifiable group, population, or setting that might be used.

In most cases, it is not be possible to assemble the entire team before the plan is put together. However, the core group should be aware of the skills and experience they need and draw people with the right skills and experience into the planning process as they are needed.

The Research Design

Fundamentals

The fundamentals of research design apply to group-randomized trials as well as to other comparative designs. Because they are discussed in many familiar textbooks (e.g., Cook and Campbell, 1979; Kirk, 1982; Kish, 1987; Meinert, 1986; Winer et al., 1991), they will be reviewed only briefly here.

The goal in the design of any comparative trial is to provide the basis for valid inference that the intervention as implemented caused the result(s) as observed. To meet that goal, three elements are required: (1) there must be control observations, (2) there must be a minimum of bias in the estimate of the intervention effect, and (3) there must be sufficient precision for that estimate.

Without control observations, the investigator cannot know what would have happened had the intervention not been delivered. Lacking that standard, the investigator cannot know what effect the intervention had when it was delivered. As a result, control observations are essential.

Even so, control observations can come in many forms. They can be made between members, within members, in similar groups, in different groups, etc. The nature of the control observations and the way in which the groups are allocated to treatment conditions will determine in large measure the level of bias in the estimate of the intervention effect. Bias exists whenever the estimate of the intervention effect is different from its true value. If that bias is substantial, the investigators will be misled about the effect of their intervention, as will the other scientists and policy makers who use their work.

Sources of bias are sometimes called threats to the internal and construct validity of the trial, because they threaten the ability of the investigators to draw the causal inference between the intervention as delivered and the outcome as measured (Cook and Campbell, 1979). They are sometimes called alternative, rival, or competing explanations, for they can stand as alternatives, rivals, or competitors to the intervention as an explanation for the study's results. A review of potential sources of bias is given in the next section, together with a discussion of strategies to limit bias.

Even if adequate control observations are available so that the estimate of the intervention effect is unbiased, the investigator should know whether the effect is greater than would be expected by chance, given the level of variation in the data. Statistical tests can provide such evidence, but their power to do so will depend heavily on the precision of the intervention effect estimate. As the precision improves, it will be easier to distinguish true effects from the underlying variation in the data. There are a number of factors that can reduce precision in a group-randomized trial. Those factors, together with strategies available to improve precision, are presented later in this chapter.

Though a more detailed discussion follows, it is important to identify from the outset the three most important methods to limit bias and improve precision in any comparative trial, including a group-randomized trial. Those are randomization, replication, and variance reduction. Randomization of groups to study conditions is the single most effective strategy to limit bias in the estimate of the intervention effect. Sufficient replication will provide enough groups so that randomization can be effective. Replication also serves to improve precision, as the standard error for the intervention effect will decline as the number of groups and members increases. Finally, a number of variance-reduction strategies are available to improve precision further, including selecting measures with low natural variation, matching or stratification of groups prior to randomization, regression adjustment for nuisance variables that are related to the endpoints, and repeated measures of the same groups and members. Each will be discussed later in this chapter.

Potential Sources of Bias

What are the potential sources of bias in a group-randomized trial? This will vary from study to study, because what is a potential source of bias in one context might not be in another. The investigators must look at each study carefully, consider which of the potential sources of bias might apply, and then develop strategies to defend against those sources in the context of their study. Fortunately, many of these sources of bias are well understood and defenses have been developed (e.g., Cook and Campbell, 1979; Kish, 1987; Meinert, 1986).

For group-randomized trials, the four sources of bias that are particularly problematic are selection, differential history, differential maturation, and contamination. Each of these sources is discussed and illustrated below, together with other potential sources of bias.

Selection

Bias due to selection refers to differences between participants existing before the intervention is carried out that might explain the differences observed among the study conditions after intervention occurs. Randomization of a large number of groups to each condition increases the probability that potential sources of bias will be distributed evenly and reduces any threat they might pose to the validity of the design. Randomization of a limited number of groups to each condition may not achieve this goal, so that trials that involve only a few groups may still face measurable bias due to selection. Trials that do not employ randomization may face considerable bias due to selection.

Consider a worksite intervention in which four divisions of a utility company are recruited to participate. Two are randomized to the intervention condition and the other two are randomized to the control condition. The individuals in the two divisions assigned to the intervention condition will be different, somehow, from those in the divisions assigned to the control condition. The differences might not be large, but they will exist. Without accounting for those differences, the investigators might misinterpret posttest differences as an intervention effect when they represent nothing more than selection bias.

History and Differential History

One of the most challenging aspects of group-randomized trials is that they occur in the real world, beyond the careful control of the investigators. Because group-randomized trials occur in dynamic settings like schools, worksites, neighborhoods, and whole communities, there are many forces that can affect the results of the study. Some of those may be local, while others may arrive from a distance, such as messages on television or radio. Any external influence other than the intervention that can affect the results of the study is a potential source of bias; such influences are often grouped together under the general label of history.

Consider a clinic-based intervention to encourage nurses to check the immunization status of all children who have appointments so that they can alert the physician to order missing immunizations (Harper and Murray, 1994). The evaluation plan for such an intervention might involve checking the appointment records before and after the intervention to determine whether the number of immunizations increased.

History can be a source of bias in this study in a number of ways. For example, suppose that the local health department introduced a new series of public-service announcements encouraging parents to check the immunization status of their children. Or suppose that there was an outbreak of a particular childhood infectious disease, and that the media attention associated with it caused parents or physicians to be more attentive to the general immunization status of children. Or suppose that the local schools introduced a new policy requiring proof of immunization for selected childhood diseases. Any of these external influences could increase the number of childhood visits at the study clinics in which the child received an immunization. It would be impossible to determine how much of the observed change in the number of immunizations was due to the intervention and how much was due to one of the external influences.

Whereas history refers to an external influence that affects the entire population under investigation, differential history refers to an external influence that affects one study condition more than another. It is generally the more serious concern for group-randomized trials.

Any external influence that affects primarily one condition and causes a change consistent with an intervention effect could lead the investigators to conclude erroneously that the intervention had caused the effect. In the same way, any external influence that affects primarily one condition and causes a change that is inconsistent with an intervention could lead the investigators to conclude that the intervention had failed. Either way, it may prove difficult to disentangle bias due to differential history from true intervention effects, especially if the investigators are unaware of the external influence.

Differential history is all too common in group-randomized trials. Such trials occur in the real world and usually involve important issues that may be the target of other activities. Those activities may affect one condition more than another, especially if there are only a few groups in each condition.

Consider as an example a community-based heart disease–prevention program in which only two communities are assigned to each condition, with perhaps thousands of observations taken at baseline and follow-up in each community. Unknown to the investigators, the major medical clinic servicing one of the control communities has decided to launch a major effort to treat hypertension, reduce smoking, and improve exercise in its patient population. Such a program could clearly improve risk factors related to heart disease in that control community and could bias the intervention effect toward zero. In this case, a finding of no effect could very well be due to the external influence in one control community that masked a real intervention effect. In the absence of other information, the investigators may never know the truth.

Maturation and Differential Maturation

Bias due to maturation occurs when natural growth or development affects the results of the study. In group-randomized trials, a broad definition of maturation is required, because maturation can occur not only among members but also among groups. For example, if persons are the members, maturation often manifests itself in the gradual physical and cognitive changes that are observed as a natural result of aging. At a group level, such gradual changes are reflected in secular trends.

Consider a study designed to reduce alcohol use among college students. All entering freshmen are surveyed for their alcohol consumption, receive the intervention over the course of their four-year program, and complete an exit survey just prior to graduation. A decline in drinking is observed between the entering freshman and graduating senior surveys. How might bias due to maturation stand as a plausible alternative explanation for the results of this study?

There are at least two possibilities. The first is maturation at the level of the member, here the student. It is well known that drinking behavior peaks during college and then declines (Kandel and Logan, 1984). Thus, it is possible that the decline reflected the natural decline in the alcohol consumption by young adults as they mature out of the heavy drinking common among college freshmen and sophomores. The second is maturation at the group level, here the college. It may be that the drinking patterns among students attending the intervention colleges were declining as part of a downward secular trend in alcohol consumption in that area. Either of these forms of maturation offers a plausible alternative explanation for the observed decline and so threatens the validity of the study.

Differential maturation is often the more serious concern in group-randomized trials. It reflects growth or development that affects one study condition more than another. Differential maturation can masquerade as an intervention effect or mask an intervention effect.

Consider a trial in which two towns are selected for an intervention program to reduce coronary heart disease (CHD) and two other towns are selected for the control condition. Unknown to the investigators, the CHD risk factors are on a favorable trajectory in the intervention communities compared to the control communities, but the absolute levels of those risk factors are similar in the four communities when measured during the baseline survey. As long as the trajectories hold, the two conditions will move apart over time, with the intervention communities evidencing lower risk over time. In the absence of other information, the investigators may never know that their "intervention effect" was simply the natural result of the different secular trends operating in their study communities.

Contamination

Bias due to contamination exists when important components of the intervention program find their way into the control condition. Contamination may occur passively or actively. Either form can be a serious source of bias.

Consider a study designed to evaluate the impact of a cancer-prevention program. Two intervention towns are compared to two control towns located in a different state. Over the course of the study, the investigators are surprised at the appearance in the control towns of intervention programs that bear a remarkable similarity to the programs they are delivering in the intervention towns. At some point, they discover a number of unanticipated "connections" between the towns. Teachers from the towns may meet periodically at educational conventions and discuss their health-promotion programs. Hospital and clinic administrators may serve on the same regional boards and exchange information on their health-promotion activities. Leaders in one community may have relatives or close friends in leadership positions in another community. These and other similar "connections" can often provide conduits through which interventions supposed to be under the control of the investigators are transmitted to the control sites, only to appear there in a somewhat modified form.

If the investigators fail to monitor the level of "intervention-like" activity in their control sites, they may not realize that contamination has occurred. All too often, investigators will assume that the control condition cannot possibly have the same sort of intervention program that the investigators have developed, and not bother to test their assumption. The Minnesota Heart Health Program was fortunate to monitor the control communities and the investigators were quite surprised at the level of exposure to intervention-like programs in those communities. Indeed, contamination is one of the reasons suggested for the limited effects observed in that trial (Luepker et al., 1994).

Testing and Differential Testing

When familiarity with the measurement procedure changes a respondent's performance, bias may be introduced in the form of a testing effect. Testing effects are as common among the endpoints included in group-randomized trials as in other studies, and care must be taken to limit their potential to bias the estimate of the intervention effect.

Consider a program designed to improve physical fitness among sedentary adults. Participants complete a treadmill test at baseline, receive the intervention, and are tested again after six weeks. Even in the absence of an effective intervention, the participants will do better at the second assessment because of their prior experience with the treadmill. In the absence of adequate control observations, such an improvement might be attributed mistakenly to the intervention.

Bias due to differential testing exists if the testing effect observed in the groups assigned to one condition is different from the testing effect observed in the groups assigned to another condition. Suppose that the groups involved in the physical fitness study were in different locations; the intervention groups might be in one town and the control groups might be in another town. The investigators might rely on local equipment to avoid the expense of transporting a treadmill to both towns or of bringing all the participants to a central location. To the extent that the treadmill in one town was easier to use than the treadmill in the other town, one would expect less of a testing effect among the participants in the town with the simpler treadmill. Without adequate control observations, the investigators might misinterpret their results as evidence for or against an intervention effect.

Instrumentation and Differential Instrumentation

Bias due to instrumentation occurs when there is an effect on the results of the study due to a change in the measurement instrument or protocol. Instrumentation may also appear when there is differential sensitivity across the range observed in the study.

Consider a self-report measure for smoking among younger and older adolescents. Simple wording changes between the seventh-grade survey and the tenth-grade survey could create what would appear to be large changes in the level of smoking among the respondents, due merely to the unintended change in the meaning of the survey items.

Alternatively, an instrument that is sensitive to change in the lower end of the distribution of smoking self-reports, but not terribly sensitive to change in the upper end of the distribution, might suggest differential change in respondents or groups who start at different points on the scale. For example, if the question was originally worded to be sensitive to low levels of smoking, but wasn't as sensitive to higher levels of smoking, then respondents who didn't smoke much at baseline might appear to change more than respondents who smoked more at baseline. This would occur not because those respondents differed in the amount of change, but simply because of a ceiling effect in the instrument.

Bias due to differential instrumentation exists when the instrumentation effect observed in one condition is different from that observed in another condition. Suppose, for example, that the adolescent-smoking study had a local survey coordinator in each of two participating schools. Suppose further that the coordinator in one school believed that the survey instrument contained some confusing language and decided to "fix" that problem prior to the follow-up survey, but failed to advise the investigators of the change. This well-intended act might result in a greater or lesser change in that school compared to the other school, due only to the differential change in the language of the instrument.

Regression to the Mean and Differential Regression to the Mean

Respondents who score well above or below their true score on a given test tend to score closer to their true score on a subsequent administration of that test. This regression to the mean phenomenon is most likely to become a problem when participants are selected on the basis of a high or low score that includes some measurement error.

Consider an intervention program designed to reduce domestic violence. The investigators want to work in a population where domestic violence is particularly high, and so conduct a survey of four nearby communities to find the two with the highest level of domestic violence. They then deliver their intervention program in the two communities with the highest reported levels, and conduct a follow-up survey six months later. The results indicate that the violence levels measured at the follow-up survey are lower than those measured as part of the screening survey. Should the investigators conclude that their intervention was effective? Given the unreliability attached to many indicators of domestic violence, regression to the mean must be considered as a plausible alternative explanation in this example. If the high levels observed in the screening survey simply represented random inflation from the true level, one would expect that the level would be lower at the follow-up, even in the absence of an intervention effect. In the absence of adequate control observations, the investigators may be unable to rule out regression to the mean as an alternative explanation for their findings.

Differential regression to the mean will exist as a potential source of bias whenever the direction and/or degree of regression to the mean varies among the conditions. Suppose the investigators in the domestic-violence study included the two other communities from their screening survey as control sites. This might seem reasonable since they were in the same area but didn't "need" the intervention as badly as the two communities with the highest reported violence rates in the screening survey. To the extent that the two control communities had reported low levels of violence due to random deflation from their true level, those communities would be expected to have higher violence levels in the follow-up survey. Should the investigators conclude that violence went up in the absence of their intervention and down as a result of their intervention? Clearly, regression to the mean could explain the pattern observed in both the intervention and the control communities.

Mortality and Differential Mortality

In research design, mortality refers to the loss of participants for any reason. In group-randomized trials, this may be a loss of either groups or members. Loss of some participants in a large field trial is unavoidable, and so long as that loss is not related to intervention, it may not bias the estimate of the intervention effect. However, because it is often difficult to know why losses occur, it is best to minimize losses of any kind.

Mortality is most often considered at the member level. In epidemiologic cohort studies, respondents are tracked until they experience the event of interest or until the end of the study. Missing data rates as low as a few percent are common. In population surveys, participation rates of 80% and higher are common. In group-randomized trials, follow-up rates are more varied, and sometimes drop to dangerous levels. As the proportion of respondents lost to follow-up increases, the threat of mortality as a source of bias increases. Mortality rates greater than 20% are of considerable concern, and mortality rates greater than 40% often render the results ungeneralizable.

In group-randomized trials, mortality can also occur at the group level. It is not uncommon for a worksite, school, hospital, or other identifiable group to choose to discontinue participation in a study. This can happen when the survey methods are onerous or, when the intervention is unpopular; or it may have nothing to do with the study, such as when a new management team chooses to discontinue a program approved by the previous management. As the proportion of the groups lost to the study increases, there is increased potential for mortality to bias the estimate of the intervention effect.

Differential mortality exists when the mortality differs among the study conditions. Even if the investigators limit mortality, the same rate of mortality across all the study conditions provides no guarantee that differential mortality is absent. It is possible that the type of group or member lost from the study varies across the conditions. This is the true source of differential mortality. As long as the type of group or member lost is the same across all conditions, uneven mortality rates need not be a concern as a potential source of bias.[1] Unfortunately, it is quite common for investigators to focus on the mortality rates rather than on the nature of the mortality.

As an example, consider a school-based smoking-prevention program. Two schools are randomized to an intervention condition and two to a control condition. Students are measured at baseline in the seventh grade and again two years later in the ninth grade. In the intervention schools, the students participate in a prevention program as seventh- and eighth-graders. If the mortality rate is 15% in both conditions, some would conclude that differential mortality is not a source of bias in the estimate of the intervention effect. However, if smokers were more likely to leave the intervention schools and nonsmokers were more likely to leave the control schools, the bias due to differential mortality could create what looked like a substantial and favorable intervention effect when in fact there was none.

Compensatory Equalization of Interventions

Bias due to compensatory equalization of interventions requires that some authority act to distribute components of the intervention program in the control condition. It is more likely to occur when the divisions of a larger entity are allocated to different study conditions.

Consider the worksite study conducted in the four divisions of the utility. If the head of the personnel department was persuaded that the intervention program was very helpful and should be made available companywide, that administrator might ruin the study by arbitrarily sending employees from other divisions to the intervention sessions or by distributing the materials companywide.

Compensatory Rivalry

Bias due to compensatory rivalry exists when the groups or members assigned to the control condition react to their assignment by launching their own effort to improve the outcome of interest. Suppose, for example, that one hospital was assigned to an intervention program to reduce employee sick days and another hospital was assigned to a control condition. If the administrator of the control hospital reacts to the assignment by developing his or her own program to reduce sick days, the investigators may fail to observe an intervention effect not because the intervention was ineffective, but because this compensatory rivalry biased the estimate toward zero.

Resentful Demoralization

The opposite response is often called resentful demoralization. It has been a concern to investigators planning a group-randomized trial who might fear that the groups assigned to the control condition will reduce their efforts to improve the outcomes of interest. If the control groups reduce their effort, this could bias the estimate of the intervention effect away from zero.

Mono-operation Bias

One of the common problems in group-randomized trials is the use of a single operation to measure the endpoint. The use of a single operation to represent the intervention is even more common. Both can create what is called mono-operation bias. This bias exists when the cause-effect relationship is due at least in part to the particular operations employed. Unless the trial includes multiple operationalizations of both the intervention and endpoint, the investigator will not know how much of the finding is generalizable to the constructs and how much is particular to the operations.

Mono-method Bias

A related bias is based on the methodology used in the trial. Even if multiple operations are used to measure the endpoint, if all are based on the same general methodology—for example, self-report—then all may suffer from some bias associated with that methodology. Similarly, even if multiple operations are used to represent the intervention construct, if all are based on the same general methodology—for example, CD-ROM technology—then all may suffer from some bias associated with that methodology.

Hypothesis Guessing

If the participants in the trial think they know what the trial is about, this may influence their responses. The investigator may not know how much the observed result is due to the intervention and how much is due to such hypothesis guessing.

Evaluation Apprehension

Sometimes responses are influenced by the participants' desire to present a good image to the investigators. This can be a particular problem in public health, where healthy lifestyles are often perceived as good and desirable qualities. In order to appear to have those qualities, the respondents may exaggerate their physical activity; underreport their smoking, weight, and drinking; or exaggerate their consumption of fruits and vegetables and underreport their consumption of foods high in fat and salt. Whenever the respondent perceives social pressure to report in a particular way, evaluation apprehension is a potential source of bias.

Experimenter Expectancies

Sometimes the measurement staff convey subtle messages to the participants that affect the responses of the participants. Sometimes the measurement staff's own expectations affect the way that they observe and record the data. Both are examples of the threat of experimenter expectancies. An excellent example of the former might occur when the intervention staff later collects the outcome evaluation data. It may be hard for the participants who have not made the desired changes to be honest during their interview. It also may be hard for the experimenter not to look more closely for good responses in the intervention condition than in the control condition.

Strategies to Limit Bias

There are a number of strategies that can be used in a group-randomized trial to limit bias in the estimate of the intervention effect.

Randomization

Randomization of a large number of groups to each condition offers the best protection against many of the sources of bias that can appear in group-randomized trials, including history, maturation, testing, instrumentation, and regression, both as simple threats and as differential threats. As the number of groups randomized to each condition increases, it will become increasingly implausible to attribute any observed result to any influence other than the intervention.

While randomization can be helpful in limiting a number of potential sources of bias, it must be done properly. Improper randomization often will result in bias, though the investigator may not look for it, believing that the randomization was effective. Meinert (1986) provides an excellent discussion of the mechanics of randomization, and the reader is referred to that and other texts on clinical trials for details.

There are some sources of bias for which randomization is simply not effective. Randomization often provides no protection against mortality or differential mortality, as mortality often occurs after randomization and may be related to the intervention. Randomization affords no protection from contamination, from compensatory reactions, or from resentful demoralization.

Despite these limitations, randomization offers the best defense against many of the most important sources of bias in group-randomized trials. For this reason, randomization should be included in the design whenever possible.

A Priori *Matching or Stratification of Groups*

While randomization of even a small number of groups to each study condition ensures equal probability of assignment for each group to a given condition, it cannot ensure that all potential sources of bias will be equally distributed. Where the number of groups is limited, and especially when the groups are heterogeneous, matching or stratification prior to randomization can make randomization much more effective. Consider a study with five identifiable groups to be assigned to each of two conditions, for a total of ten groups in the trial. If simple random assignment of groups is used, there are $10!/(5!(10-5)!) = 252$ different combinations of 5 groups that could be randomized to the intervention condition, with the remaining 5 groups assigned to the control condition. If those groups were quite homogeneous, the investigator might be willing to accept any of the 252 combinations and settle for simple random assignment. Indeed, with simple random assignment, each of those 252 combinations would be equally likely, and each would have a probability of $1/252 = 0.004$. But what if those groups are heterogeneous with respect to the endpoint? If those groups can be rank ordered on the endpoint, or some proxy for the endpoint, and the groups adjacent in rank are paired, there will be 25 different ways to assign groups from within pairs, and each of those is likely to provide a set of study conditions that is reasonably balanced with respect to the endpoint. Assume any of those 25 combinations is acceptable and none of the other 227 combinations is acceptable. Randomization from within matched pairs can guarantee an acceptable result. Simple random assignment would provide only a $25/252 = 10\%$ chance of an acceptable result. Clearly the odds favor randomization from within matched pairs.

Matching or *a priori* stratification without randomization is not as strong, but if the factors are chosen carefully, it may be the best alternative to randomization. Consider the Community Partnership Program funded by the Center for Substance Abuse Prevention. Under that program, grants were awarded to intervention communities on the basis of merit and other considerations (Cook et al., 1994). The evaluator then sought to find control communities that would provide close matches at baseline on the endpoint and on other factors related to the endpoint. In this case, randomization was not possible, so that matching was the only viable strategy to limit selection and the differential threats to the validity of the design. Given a sufficient number of very well-matched sets, the degree of protection may be quite good, though it will never be as good as in a randomized trial.

Avoid the Pitfalls That Invite Bias

Many of the potential sources of bias can be defended in part by avoiding the pitfalls that invite those particular sources.

To limit the bias due to history and differential history, the groups should be selected such that all would be expected to experience the same history over the full duration of the study. This can often be accomplished by choosing groups from the same geographic area and by ensuring that the data schedule is the same in all conditions. Historical controls, controls from an older or younger cohort, or controls from a different geographic area will increase the risk of differential history.

To limit bias due to maturation and differential maturation, the groups should be selected such that all would be expected to experience the same maturation over the duration of the study. This can often be accomplished by choosing groups that have memberships with similar age distributions, since age is a good proxy for most individual maturational processes. Choosing groups in such a way that all are from the same geographic area can help ensure that they will be part of the same secular trend.

Investigators must take special care with any measurements that may be subject to testing effects. Any measure that shows improvement in performance with experience should be viewed with caution. This problem can be avoided by choosing measures that do not show this kind of experience-based response, but there will be many circumstances in which such accommodation is unavoidable. Under those conditions, a good defense is to ensure that the participants are brought to a stable level of performance before baseline measures are taken, so as to eliminate such testing effects. Differential testing can be avoided by bringing respondents in all conditions to the same stable level of performance.

Investigators can guard against instrumentation threats by not changing the instrument after the baseline administration. If a question must be changed, the investigator should retain the original item as well as the "improved" item, so that parallel analyses of the two items can provide some measure of the impact of the wording change. Further protection can be provided by ensuring that all participating organizations agree to use of the study's "standard" instruments.

Regression to the mean can be minimized by selection of measurement procedures that have very good reliability, as it is the unreliability of the instrument that allows regression to the mean to occur. Differential regression to the mean can be minimized by using the same criteria for selecting the groups and members in all conditions. Where the measures are known to have only modest reliability, multiple screening assessments will help to establish the respondent's true score. This is a common practice in studies that focus on individual levels of cholesterol, diet, or blood pressure, for example, since all three are subject to substantial intra-individual variation.

Investigators can limit mortality by carefully explaining all the implications of participation to the eligible organizations in advance. Many organizations do not like to agree to participate in a study only to be surprised by the appearance of new requirements along the way. Mortality can be limited by taking steps to ensure that all contacts with the participating organizations are conducted in a professional and unobtrusive manner, by covering all costs incurred as part of the research, and through use of a cross-sectional design instead of a cohort design, especially if the measurements are burdensome. Differential mortality can be reduced by requiring all participating organizations to agree to participate in any of the study conditions, prior to randomization. In general, as fears about mortality increase, the randomization to conditions should be delayed so that most of the mortality occurs prior to that critical stage of the trial. Finally, a written agreement between the investigators and the participating organization that spells out clearly the expectations and obligations of both parties can be very helpful. The agreement should be between the organizations involved and not just the individuals, as this will help avoid discontinuation by new management at some future date.

Investigators should control the distribution of the components of the intervention program to limit contamination. Investigators can control the distribution of their own intervention materials, participation in workshops, and other training programs, and include in the participation agreement a promise from the participating organizations not to disseminate any of the program components.

Compensatory reactions and resentful demoralization can be limited by providing the control condition with something that is seen as valuable. In group-randomized trials, a "no intervention" control condition is rarely possible. A "usual care" control condition is the norm in group-randomized trials, but it is not the only alternative. Control groups may be assured that they will receive training and materials for the intervention program after the study is over, and so become a "delayed-intervention" control condition. Control groups may be given an "alternative intervention" judged not likely to affect the endpoint but still aimed at a problem considered to be important by the participating organizations in the control condition. Control groups may be offered ongoing consultation on issues of importance to them as they arise over the course of the study; often the availability of the kind of expertise to which the investigators have access can be an important attraction for participating organizations.

Employ Objective Measures

Objective measures can sharply limit hypothesis guessing, evaluation apprehension, and experimenter expectancies. For example, consider adolescent smoking as an endpoint. Reliance on self-report data could fool the investigators into thinking that their intervention worked, due to evaluation apprehension or hypothesis guessing that affects only self-report measures (Murray et al., 1987). By adding biochemical measures, investigators avoid these sources of bias. A finding of no effect based on the biochemical measures would outweigh a favorable finding based on the self-report data. Similarly, observations of food eaten at school lunch could be used in addition to recall methods. The latter would be subject to a variety of recall biases, evaluation apprehension, and demand characteristics, whereas the observations, if sufficiently unobtrusive, would be free of these threats (Lytle et al., 1993). Where the more objective measures are more expensive or difficult, they may be applied in a subsample, either to provide data to confirm the validity of the simpler measures or to calibrate those measures against a better standard.

Employ Independent Evaluation Personnel Who Are Blind to Conditions

Blinding the evaluation personnel to study conditions can reduce the threats of evaluation apprehension and experimenter expectancies. If it is not possible to blind the evaluation personnel, they should be recruited apart from the intervention personnel and have no involvement in the intervention program nor any interest in the outcome.

Employ Different Methodologies

Mono-operation and mono-method bias may be avoided by using multiple operations based on different methodologies. This is usually difficult in group-randomized trials due to their size, complexity, and cost. Indeed, most such trials are two-condition designs, with a single intervention condition and a single control condition. As a result, it may not be possible to have multiple operations to represent intervention. As an alternative, process data may be useful to assess whether change occurred in both the endpoint and the intermediate variables as predicted by the theory underlying the intervention. If the pattern of change is confirmed, there would be greater confidence in generalizing from the operations to the constructs. It is generally easier to employ multiple operations and methods to assess endpoints. This is recommended unless there is good agreement on a single measure as a "gold standard."

Analytic Strategies

Even if the investigator employs many of the defense strategies described here, it is possible that threats to the validity of the design will emerge over the course of the study. The investigator has no absolute control over any of the differential threats, especially those associated with history, maturation, and mortality. In addition, contamination can be a problem even in the best-designed studies. For these reasons, it is generally recommended that investigators put in place measurement mechanisms to detect these sources of bias as they emerge. This way, they will have data available at the time of the analysis that may be used to try to limit their effect.

To detect potential selection bias, investigators should measure potential confounders when they gather data from the groups and members. Those data can be analyzed at baseline to assess the degree to which the conditions differ in their distribution of those factors. Where potential confounding is observed, regression adjustment for the confounders can serve to limit the bias that those factors would otherwise introduce into the estimate of the intervention effect.[2]

To detect bias due to differential history, maturation, and contamination, the investigators should put in place a monitoring system that will record any external influence that might affect the endpoint, any secular trend related to the endpoints or to the intervention, and any "intervention-like" activity in any of the intervention and control sites. Local staff may be helpful in this regard, as they can monitor school or worksite newsletters, local newspapers, and other media outlets for information on local or regional activity related to the outcomes of interest. Abstracting services for the local newspapers in the participating sites may be used for this review if local staff are not available. Periodic population surveys also may be used to assess such exposures. The most dangerous course would be to assume that nothing related to the intervention or the endpoint will happen in the control sites over the course of the study and that the only activity in the intervention sites is what is being delivered by the investigator.

Many of these data may be collected during the normal course of the study. However, to assess secular trends accurately, it may be necessary to gather these data for a period of time prior to the intervention. The precision of the estimates will obviously depend on the size and frequency of the surveys. In general, it may be better to conduct more surveys, each based on a smaller sample, than to conduct only a few surveys, each based on a larger sample.

Once the data are available, they may be analyzed to determine whether there are differences among the conditions and whether those differences are patterned in time as the investigators would expect given the time course of their study. These measures may also be used as time-varying covariates in analyses aimed at testing intervention effects. Such covariates may help the investigators determine whether the results are attributable to the intervention program.

Exposure data also may be analyzed to determine whether there is evidence of a dose-response relationship. If the average effect of the intervention is limited, the dose-response analysis may indicate whether a large dose of the intervention might be effective. In the same way, lack of evidence of a dose-response relationship would suggest that future investigations not pursue the same type of intervention.

Factors That Can Reduce Precision

Equation 1.8 defined the variance of the condition mean in a group-randomized trial as:

$$\sigma_{\bar{y}_c}^2 = \frac{\sigma_y^2}{mg}\left(1 + (m-1)ICC_{m:g:c}\right)$$

When the intervention effect is a function of the condition means, its precision will be directly related to the components in this formula.

Insufficient Replication

Insufficient replication will limit the precision of the estimate of the intervention effect in any comparative trial. Because the number of groups (g) and the number of members (m) appear in the denominator of this formula, insufficient replication of either will reduce the precision of the estimate of the intervention effect. The deleterious effect will be greater for insufficient replication of the groups than for insufficient replication of the members, because the number of members also contributes to the VIF, $(1 + (m-1)ICC_{m:g:c})$.

High Variation in Measures

Endpoints that have large variances (σ_y^2) will reduce precision relative to endpoints with small variances. Thus, precision will be better for a measure like body mass index, with a variance of about 36, than for diastolic blood pressure, with a variance of about 100, which will be better than for serum cholesterol, with a variance of about 1000.

High Intraclass Correlation in Measures

Endpoints that have high intraclass correlations will reduce precision relative to endpoints that have small intraclass correlations. Hannan et al. (1994) reported intraclass correlations for a variety of variables related to coronary heart disease measured at a community level. Physiologic risk factors tended to have lower intraclass correlations at that level than did behavioral measures, which in turn had lower intraclass correlations than did psychosocial variables such as attitudes or beliefs. Given that pattern, the precision of the intervention effect estimate could be expected to be better for physiological measures than for psychosocial measures.

Random Heterogeneity of Participants

As long as the pattern is unrelated to condition, the variance will be smaller if the participants are homogeneous than if they are heterogeneous. As a result, precision will be limited with increasing random heterogeneity of respondents.

As an example, consider two group-randomized trials in which age eligibility is much more restricted in one trial than the other. The trial with the less restrictive age-eligibility criteria will have a more heterogeneous sample and so the endpoint may have a larger variance.

Reliability of Intervention Implementation

Any factor that reduces the reliability of the implementation of the intervention will also increase variance and limit precision. Group-randomized trials are especially susceptible to this threat, since it is more difficult to standardize delivery of an intervention to identifiable groups than to individual participants seen in a clinic or laboratory.

The Minnesota Heart Health Program provides an example (Luepker et al., 1994). Here, three communities received a 5–6 year intensive intervention that targeted four CHD risk factors and employed eight outreach strategies (community analysis, community organization, health professional education, mass and select media, risk factor screening and education, adult education, youth education, and environmental programs). Each community had a field staff of 10–30, and the intervention program was managed by a core faculty and staff of 75+ at the University of Minnesota. While conceptually the intervention programs delivered in the three sites were quite similar, there were significant differences from community to community based on personalities, opportunities, resources, etc. It was thought that such "tailoring" of the intervention would be helpful, though it certainly served to increase the unreliability of the intervention implementation. Any trial that involves multiple and geographically disparate groups may have difficulty delivering the same intervention in the same way over time in each site.

Random Irrelevancies in the Experimental Setting

Random irrelevancies in the experimental setting are random events that affect the values on the endpoint for participating groups and members. Ideally, the only event that would affect the endpoint would be the intervention program. Other factors that affect participants at random serve only to increase variance and limit precision.

Consider a trial conducted in a series of small rural communities and a second trial conducted in a series of neighborhoods in a large urban area. There would likely be more random irrelevancies in the experimental setting in the urban area than in the rural communities. If so, the precision would be greater, all other factors constant, in the trial involving the rural communities.

Strategies to Improve Precision

There are several strategies that can improve precision in any comparative trial: increased replications, endpoints with low variability, matching or stratification in the design and/or in the analysis, repeat observations on the same groups and members, modeling trends, and regression adjustment for nuisance variables. Each of these may have application in a group-randomized trial. This section provides an overview for these strategies. Many are developed further in Chapters 5 and 6 and are illustrated in Chapters 7 and 8.

Increased Replication

Just as insufficient replication of either groups or members reduces precision, increased replication will improve precision. The improvement per unit increase will be greater for groups than for members, as the otherwise beneficial effect of increasing the number of members (m) is offset by the adverse effect that same increase has on the VIF, $(1 + (m - 1)ICC_{m:g:c})$.

Figure 2.1 illustrates the relative impact of increases in the number of groups per condition and the number of members per group on the detectable difference based on a t-test, with ICC fixed at 0.10 and the variance fixed at 1.0. The y-axis is the detectable difference in standard deviation units. The x-axis is the number of members per group. As that number increases from left to right, the detectable difference decreases, reflecting modest improvement in precision. The separate lines in the figure represent different numbers of

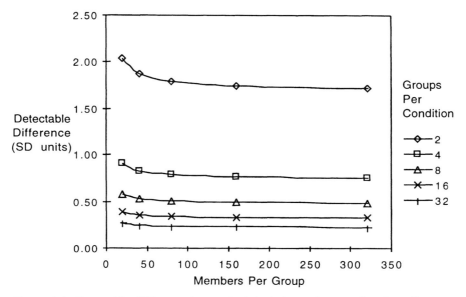

Figure 2.1. Detectable difference in standard-deviation units as a function of groups per condition and members per group when *ICC* is 0.10.

groups per condition. As that number increases from top to bottom, the detectable difference drops rapidly, marking a sharp improvement in precision. The law of diminishing returns operates for both groups and members, such that the benefit added from each additional unit declines as the total number of units grows.

Choose Endpoints Carefully

Given endpoints that are otherwise similarly regarded, it will be advantageous to choose the one with the highest reliability, the lowest variance, and the lowest intraclass correlation. Figure 2.2 illustrates the relative impact of reductions in the magnitude of the *ICC*, here fixed at 0.01, which is an order of magnitude smaller than in Figure 2.1. Compared to the initial *ICC* of 0.10, all the detectable differences are reduced, reflecting further improvements in precision, when the *ICC* is reduced to 0.01.

The effects are most substantial when there are few groups per condition and many members per group, as would be expected given the formula for the *VIF*, $(1 + (m-1)ICC_{m:g:c})$.

The law of diminishing returns also operates for the *ICC*, such that the relative gain declines as the *ICC* gets ever smaller. Figure 2.3 provides the parallel analysis when the *ICC* is fixed at 0.001, yet another order of magni-

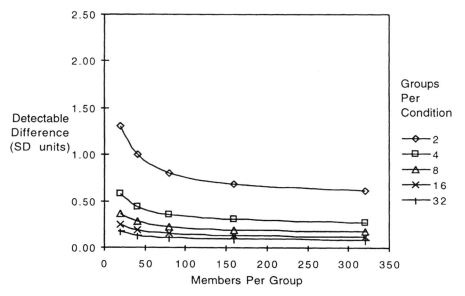

Figure 2.2. Detectable difference in standard-deviation units as a function of groups per condition and members per group when the *ICC* is 0.01.

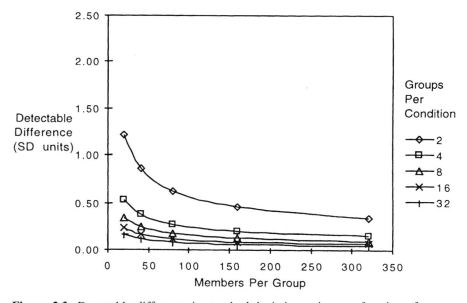

Figure 2.3. Detectable difference in standard-deviation units as a function of groups per condition and members per group when the *ICC* is 0.001.

tude smaller: Reducing the *ICC* to zero would result in little appreciable improvement beyond this pattern.

A Priori *Matching and Stratification in the Analysis*

Earlier in this chapter, *a priori* matching and stratification were discussed as strategies to defend against many potential sources of bias, including selection, differential maturation, and differential history. *A priori* matching or stratification can provide protection against bias whether or not either is reflected in the analysis by helping to balance the distribution of potential confounding influences.

A priori matching and stratification may improve precision if those design features are reflected in the analysis. Precision is improved when there is measurable reduction in the standard error for the intervention effect due to the correlation between the matching or stratification variable(s) and the endpoint. If that reduction makes up for the reduced denominator degrees of freedom (*ddf*) in the matched or stratified analysis, power will also be improved. Until recently, this issue had not been examined in the context of group-randomized trials, and it was not clear whether the benefits of matching and stratification observed in clinical trials would apply to group-randomized trials.

Martin et al. (1993) showed that a matched analysis was more powerful than an unmatched analysis in a group-randomized trial, but only if the matching correlation was above 0.30 or the number of groups per condition was above 10. An unmatched analysis was more powerful than a matched analysis when the number of groups available for a study was less than 10 or the matching correlation was less than about 0.30. Certainly the number of groups is quite small in many trials, often less than 10 per condition. The matching correlation is also usually small, as it is the correlation between the endpoint and the matching factor when both are measured at the group level, not the member level. As a result, Martin et al. (1993) suggested that matching might not provide as much benefit in group-randomized trials as it does in clinical trials.

Diehr et al. (1995a) extended this work in a simulation study to assess the Type I error rate for an unmatched analysis of matched data based on a group-randomized trial design. They varied the intraclass correlation, number of communities, and sample size per community. Both their algebra and their simulation show than an unmatched analysis of data from a matched design provided an analysis with a Type I error rate at or just below the nominal level. The matched analysis of the same data always gave a Type I error rate at the nominal level and so was preferred from that standpoint. However, when the matching correlation or the number of groups per condition was small, Diehr et al. (1995a) confirmed Martin et al.'s (1993) finding that the unmatched analysis provided more power. Given the magnitude of matching correlations likely to obtain in a group-randomized trial ($r<0.30$), the matched analysis will generally be favored when there are 10 or more groups assigned to each condition, and the unmatched analysis will generally be favored when there are fewer than 10 groups assigned to each condition. The critical number of groups will vary as a function of the matching correlation and readers are referred to the tables in Diehr et al. (1995a) for more specific cases.

Post Hoc Stratification

Post hoc stratification offers advantages similar to those from *a priori* matching or stratification. The investigator may be able to reduce selection bias as well as to increase within-stratum homogeneity, and so increase precision. *Post hoc* stratification does not reduce the *ddf* for the main effects, since the strata are crossed with the groups, and will provide more *ddf* for the interactions than would be available for the main effects. As a result, *post hoc* stratification will improve power whenever it serves to improve precision. However, if the data are stratified too thinly, cell means will be unstable and the added *ddf* will not compensate for the greater variability, such that power may be reduced.[3]

Repeat Observations on the Same Groups or Members

One way to improve precision in clinical trials is to take repeat observations on each participant. That can be done in the context of giving each participant each treatment, usually in a different random order for each participant, or in the context of simply following participants over time to observe the effect of their assigned treatment over time. Because observations taken on the same participant will be correlated over time, the precision of the analysis will be improved as the correlation serves to reduce the residual error.

This strategy may also be used in a group-randomized trial. Here, repeat observations may be taken on the groups alone, or on both the groups and the members. To the extent that the observations on the same groups or members are correlated over time, that correlation will reduce the components of variance used to assess the effect of the intervention, and so improve precision.

Modeling Time

Repeat observations provide an opportunity to model time in a variety of ways. For a simple pretest-posttest design, time may be omitted entirely from the analysis in an analysis of posttest data. Alternatively, the pretest data may be included as a covariate in an adjusted analysis of posttest data. Finally, both rounds may be included explicitly in a repeated-measures analysis, with or without adjustment for concurrent covariates. Where additional observations are available either before and/or after the intervention, a more precise analysis may be available if the investigator can specify a particular pattern over time for the expected treatment effect (e.g., Dwyer et al., 1989; Koepsell et al., 1991; Murray, Hannan et al., 1994).

Regression Adjustment for Covariates

Regression adjustment for covariates is a common part of many familiar analyses. These include multiple linear, Poisson, and logistic regression, and the analysis of covariance.

As discussed above, regression adjustment for covariates that are confounders may be employed to limit bias due to selection or other factors. Regression adjustment for covariates can also serve to reduce within-group and between-group variance, even if there is no evidence of confounding. In this context, the process is often termed regression adjustment for nuisance variables.

In clinical trials and in many observational studies, adjustment is made only for covariates at the member level. In group-randomized trials, covariates may be measured either at the group or member level.

Any regression adjustment that reduces the within-group variance or the intraclass correlation without increasing the other term will reduce the between-group variance and so improve precision. Factors that may reduce the within-group variance are often well known to investigators familiar with the endpoint. For example, investigators familiar with blood pressure would know that height, weight, arm circumference, and room temperature will explain variation in blood pressure and may be useful as covariates to improve precision. To the extent that there are systematic differences among the groups in any of these factors, their use as covariates may also reduce the intraclass correlation and further improve precision.

Several recent papers have demonstrated the use of regression adjustment for covariates to reduce both intraclass correlation and within-group variance in data from group-randomized trials (Murray and Short, 1995, 1996, 1997). Those papers reported benefits from adjustment for covariates measured at the level of the member and at the level of the group. They also demonstrated that regression adjustment for some covariates may serve to increase the intraclass correlation, so investigators must be mindful of that possibility. If such an adjustment has a measurable effect on the estimate of the intervention effect, it will be appropriate to retain that covariate to limit confounding in spite of its adverse effect on precision. Investigators should be thoughtful in the selection and use of covariates in group-randomized trials, just as they would be in other studies. Inclusion of unnecessary covariates in the regression model will serve only to reduce the precision of the estimate of the intervention effect.

Variables of Interest and Their Measures

The research question will identify the primary and secondary endpoints of the trial. The question may also identify potential effect modifiers. It will then be up to the investigators to anticipate potential confounders and nuisance variables. All these variables must be measured if they are to be used in the analysis of the trial.

Primary and Secondary Endpoints

In a clinical trial, the primary endpoint is a clinical event, chosen because it is easy to measure with limited error and is clinically relevant (Meinert, 1986). In a group-randomized trial, the primary endpoint need not be a clinical event, but it should be easy to measure with limited error and be relevant to public health. In both clinical and group-randomized trials, the primary endpoint, together with its method of measurement, must be defined in writing before the start of the trial. The endpoint and its method of measurement can not be changed after the start of the trial without risking the validity of the trial and the credibility of the research team. Secondary endpoints should have similar characteristics and also should be identified prior to the start of the trial.

Effect Modifiers

In a group-randomized trial, an effect modifier is a variable whose level influences the effect of the intervention. For example, if the effect of a school-based drug use–prevention program depends on the baseline risk level of the student, then baseline risk is an effect modifier. Effect modification can be seen intuitively by looking at separate intervention effect estimates for the levels of the effect modifier. If they differ to a meaningful degree, then the investigator has evidence of possible effect modification. A more formal assessment is provided by a statistical test for effect modification. That is accomplished by including an interaction term between the effect modifier and condition in the analysis and testing the statistical significance of that term. If the interaction is significant, then the investigator should present the results separately for the levels of the effect modifier. If not, the interaction term is deleted and the investigator can continue with the analysis.

Proper identification of potential effect modifiers comes through a careful review of the literature and from an examination of the theory of the intervention. Potential effect modifiers must be measured as part of the data-collection process so that their role can later be assessed.

Confounders

A confounder is related to the endpoint, not on the causal pathway, and unevenly distributed among the conditions; it serves to bias the estimate of the
intervention effect. There is no statistical test for confounding; instead, it is
assessed by comparing the unadjusted estimate of the intervention effect to the
adjusted estimate of that effect. If, in the investigator's opinion, there is a
meaningful difference between the adjusted and unadjusted estimates, then the
investigator has an obligation to report the adjusted value. It may also be
appropriate to report the unadjusted value to allow the reader to assess the
degree of confounding.

The adjusted analysis will not be possible unless the potential confounders
are measured. Proper identification of potential confounders also comes
through a careful review of the literature and from an understanding of the
endpoints and the study population.

The investigators must take care in the selection of potential confounders to
select only confounders and not mediating variables. A confounder is related
to the endpoint and unevenly distributed in the conditions, but is not on the
causal pathway between the intervention and the outcome. A mediating variable has all the characteristics of a confounder, but is on the causal pathway.
Adjustment for a mediating variable, in the false belief that it is a confounder,
will bias the estimate of the intervention effect toward the null hypothesis.

Similarly, the investigator must take care to avoid selecting as potential
confounders variables that may be affected by the intervention even if they
are not on the causal pathway linking the intervention and the outcome. Such
variables will be proxies for the intervention itself, and adjustment for them
will also bias the estimate of the intervention effect toward the null hypothesis.

An effective strategy to avoid these problems is to restrict confounders to
variables measured at baseline. Such factors cannot be on the causal pathway,
nor can their values be influenced by an intervention that hasn't been delivered. Investigators may also want to include variables measured after the intervention has begun, but will need to take care to avoid the problems described
above.

Nuisance Variables

Nuisance variables are related to the endpoint, not on the causal pathway, but
evenly distributed among the conditions. They cannot bias the estimate of the
intervention effect but they can be used to improve precision in the analysis.
A common method is to make regression adjustment for these factors during

the analysis so as to reduce the standard error of the estimate of the intervention effect, thereby improving the precision of the analysis.

Such adjustment will not be possible unless the nuisance variables are measured. Proper identification of potential nuisance variables also comes from a careful review of the literature and from an understanding of the endpoint. The cautions described above for the selection of potential confounding variables apply equally well to the selection of potential nuisance variables.

The Intervention

No matter how well designed and evaluated a group-randomized trial may be, strengths in design and analysis cannot overcome a weak intervention. While the designs and analyses employed in group-randomized trials were fair targets for criticism during the 1970s and 1980s, the designs and analyses employed more recently have improved, with many examples of very well-designed and carefully analyzed trials. Where intervention effects are modest or short-lived even in the presence of good design and analytic strategies, investigators must take a hard look at the intervention and question whether it was strong enough.

The Etiology of the Problem

One of the first suggestions for developing the research question was that the investigators become experts on the problem that they seek to remedy. If the primary endpoint is cigarette smoking among ninth-graders, then the team should seek to learn as much as possible about the etiology of smoking among young adolescents. If the primary endpoint is obesity among Native American children, then the team should seek to learn as much as possible about the etiology of obesity among those young children. If the primary endpoint is delay time in reporting heart attack symptoms, then the team should seek to learn as much as possible about the factors that influence delay time. And the same can be said for any other endpoint.

One of the goals of developing expertise in the etiology of the problem is to identify points in that etiology that are amenable to intervention. There may be critical developmental stages, or critical events or influences that trigger the next step in the progression, or it may be possible to identify critical players in the form of parents, friends, coworkers, or others who can influence the development of that problem. Without careful study of the etiology, the team will largely be guessing and hoping that their intervention is designed properly. Unfortunately, guessing and hoping rarely lead to effective interventions.

Theoretical Basis

Powerful interventions are guided by good theory on the process for change, combined with a good understanding of the etiology of the problem of interest. Poor theory will produce poor interventions and poor results. This was one of the primary messages from the community-based heart disease–prevention studies, where the intervention effects were modest, generally of limited duration, and often within chance levels. Fortmann et al. (1995) noted that one of the major lessons learned was how much was not known about how to intervene in whole communities.

Theory that describes the process of change in individuals may not apply to the process of change in identifiable groups. If it does, it may not apply in exactly the same way. Good intervention for a group-randomized trial will likely need to combine theory about individual change with theory about group processes and group change.

A good theoretical exposition will also help identify channels for the intervention program. For example, there is strong evidence that recent immigrants often look to long-term immigrants of the same cultural group for information on health issues. This has led investigators to try to use those long-term immigrants as change agents for the more recent immigrants.

A good theoretical exposition will often indicate that the phenomenon is the product of multiple influences and so suggest that the intervention operate at several different levels. For example, obesity among schoolchildren appears to be influenced most proximally by their physical activity levels and by their dietary intake. In turn, their dietary intake is influenced by what is served at home and at school and their physical activity is influenced by the nature of their physical activity and recess programs at school and at home. The models provided by teachers and parents are important both for diet and physical activity. This multilevel etiology suggests that interventions be directed at the school food-service, physical education, and recess programs; at parents; and possibly at the larger community.

Preliminary Evidence

Group-randomized trials would benefit by following the example of clinical trials, where some evidence of feasibility and efficacy of the intervention is usually required prior to launching the trial. When a study takes several years to complete and costs hundreds of thousands of dollars or more, that seems a very fair expectation. Even shorter and less expensive group-randomized trials would do well to follow that advice.

What defines preliminary evidence of feasibility? It is not reasonable to ask that the investigators prove that all intervention and evaluation protocols can be implemented in the population and setting of interest in advance of their trial. However, it is reasonable to ask that they demonstrate that the major components of the proposed intervention can be implemented in the target population; that can be done in a pilot study. It is also reasonable to ask that the major components of the proposed evaluation are feasible and acceptable in the setting and population proposed for the trial; that, too, can be done in a pilot study.

What defines preliminary evidence of efficacy? It is not fair to ask that the investigators prove that their intervention will work in the population and setting of interest in advance of their trial. However, it is fair to ask that they provide evidence that the theory supporting the intervention has been supported in other situations. It is also fair to ask that the investigators demonstrate that similar interventions applied to other problems have been effective. Finally, it is reasonable to ask that the investigators demonstrate that the proposed intervention generates short-term effects for intermediate outcomes related to the primary and secondary endpoints and postulated by the theoretical model guiding the intervention. Such evidence provides reassurance that the intervention will be effective if it is properly implemented.

Preparing a Proposal

Having thought through all these issues, the team will be ready to put their plans down on paper in the form of a proposal. A good proposal will include all of the information needed by a review panel to determine whether the research question is important, whether the intervention and evaluation methods proposed are appropriate to the question, and whether the team of investigators is up to the task. Putting the proposal together also will help the investigators identify gaps in their planning.

One outline for a grant application for NIH support for a group-randomized trial is shown in Figure 2.4. The first two levels of the outline are required, but beyond that the order represents but one of many possible approaches to organizing the material. In addition, other agencies may require other formats, though the essential ingredients will be the same. Furthermore, the written plan will be useful as a work plan even if it is never submitted as a grant application.

Face Page

The Face Page provides the title of the application, identifies the request for proposals to which the application is responding (if any), defines the total cost

Face Page
Abstract
Budget and Justification
Biographical Sketches
Resources and Environment
Research Plan
    Specific Aims
    Background and Significance
    Preliminary Studies
        Experience of the Investigators
        Development and Testing of the Intervention Methods
        Development and Testing of the Evaluation Methods
    Methods
        Overview
        Hypotheses
        Design
            Research Design
            Sampling Scheme
            Recruitment
            Assignment to Conditions
        Intervention Program
            Theoretical Model
            Development
            Implementation
        Evaluation Program
            Outcome Evaluation
                Endpoints and Their Measures
                Data-Collection Methods
                Analysis Methods
                Power Analysis
            Process Evaluation
                Variables of Interest and Their Measures
                Data-Collection Methods
                Analysis Methods
        Timeline
        Critique
            Strengths
            Weaknesses
Human Subjects
    Subject Population
    Sources of Data
    Recruitment and Consent
    Risks and Benefits
    Other Ethical Issues
Consultants
Management and Administration
Literature Cited
Appendixes

Figure 2.4. Outline for a grant application.

of the proposed project, and identifies the Principal Investigator and his/her institution.

Abstract

The Abstract provides a brief summary of the proposed research. It should identify the purpose of the research, point toward the significance of the work, and outline the methods to be used.

Budget and Justification

This is a critical section and serves two purposes. It gives the investigators an opportunity to lay out the details of their work plan in the form of itemized costs for each year of the study, and to justify those costs. It also gives the investigators an opportunity to define the role to be played by each of the personnel to be involved in the project, to document their expertise and qualifications for their role, and to justify their cost. Smart investigators will take advantage of these opportunities. As competition for scarce research support increases, budgets and their justification will become increasingly important as a tool to persuade the reviewers that the proposed research provides good value for the cost. As competition for writing space within the portion of the application reserved for the research plan increases, the justification section provides an opportunity to give details on methods and personnel that might otherwise be hard to include in the application.

One of the benefits of preparing the budget is that it forces the investigators to cost out their research plan. Smart investigators will actually cost out several alternatives and provide evidence that they have done so. Different designs will have different costs (e.g., cohort vs. cross-sectional samples), and these costs should be worked out during the planning process. Spreadsheets have become a valuable tool in this regard, as they allow investigators to rapidly cost out a number of design, intervention, survey, and staffing alternatives. There are several recent papers that address the relative costs of some of the important design features common to group-randomized trials, and investigators are encouraged to study those (McKinlay, 1994; Raudenbush, 1997). Kish (1987) also provides a good discussion of the relative costs associated with different design alternatives.

There is no better instruction for developing budgets for a research project than to work closely with more experienced investigators as the budget is put together. Of particular importance is to have input from people who have experience with the type of design, the type of analysis, the type of interventions, the type of measures, and the type of identifiable groups that will be involved in the proposed study. Each organizational system has its own quirks, and investigators experienced in worksite studies, school-based studies, community-based studies, church-based studies, etc., will prove invaluable in guiding less experienced investigators who want to work in those systems.

Biographical Sketches

This section gives the investigators an opportunity to highlight the strengths of their research team. Smart investigators will use this space to demonstrate that the research team includes the mix of skills required for the proposed research, as described above. The general rule is to include in the research team at least one person who has experience in each of the activities proposed in the application.

If the organization that will sponsor the proposal cannot provide all the skills required for the study, consultants should be recruited who can fill those needs. What kind of consultants, if any, are required will of course depend on the proposed study and on the skills available within the sponsoring organization. Whenever possible, the consultants should participate in the development of the proposal, in a visible way, so that the reviewers can be satisfied that the investigators and consultants can and will work together on the study.

Resources and Environment

The Resources and Environment section provides an opportunity to describe the organization that will sponsor the application; the space, equipment, and other resources available to the investigators through that organization; and any deficits in resources and environment that the investigators will seek to satisfy through the application itself. Where investigators from multiple organizations have come together to develop an application, each should provide a description of the resources and environment for its organization.

Research Plan

The Research Plan is the most important section of any proposal. It should describe the aims of the study, provide sufficient background information to persuade the reviewers that the study is important, summarize the relevant experience of the research team, describe all the methods proposed for the study, present a timeline, and offer a critique of the study's strengths and weaknesses. A top-quality research plan will generate excitement for the study on the part of the reviewers.

Specific Aims

In a standard NIH grant application, the research question is found in the Specific Aims section. This section is generally limited to a page which can help force the investigators to be clear in their thinking. The aims may be phrased in terms of a question or as a list of specific goals, objectives, or hypotheses. They should identify the research question, the problem, the population, the setting, the primary and secondary endpoints, and the intervention. Well-written aims will be clear, connected, and will lead naturally to the research plan.

Background and Significance

The Background and Significance section should include a brief but complete review of the literature and a clear statement of the significance of the proposed trial. In this section, investigators should persuade the reviewers that the research question is important, that the answer is not yet known, and that the next logical step in the progression of research in the area is the proposed study. This section should be written both for experts in the field and for informed nonexperts as well, as it is likely that the review committee will include representatives from both factions. Importantly, this section should generate enthusiasm in the reviewers for the significance of the work proposed.

As the reviewers read this section, they will be looking for an answer to the questions "Why is this important?" and "Why should this study be done now?" The investigators need to provide answers to those two questions, but they need to do more than that. Only the most important, most timely, and most exciting proposals will be funded in an era of increasing competition and limited resources. As a result, the investigators need not only to provide answers to those questions, but to generate excitement for their ideas.

Preliminary Studies

This section should be used to show the reviewers that the team is ready to conduct the trial. Ideally, the investigators should describe their efforts to recruit the identifiable groups that will participate in the study, to develop and test the proposed intervention program, and to develop and test the proposed evaluation procedures. Of course, in order to do that, the investigators must have done that preliminary work, and that is the more important point.

Given their cost and complexity, it will be difficult to persuade anyone to support a trial that exists only as an idea, however well written the application. Reviewers will need to be convinced that the applicants can do what they propose, and that is best done by documenting that each of the proposed activities has actually been done, albeit not altogether, in sequence, or on the scale of the proposed trial. This should lead to the development of protocols and materials for all major intervention and evaluation activities, to be included in an appendix to the application. Having such protocols and materials available for the reviewers to examine will prove very helpful if they are well developed. Failure to provide them or provision of poorly developed materials will indicate that the investigators are not yet ready to conduct the proposed trial.

One of the most important products of the preliminary studies should be the development of good estimates of reliability and variance for the major endpoints; their intraclass correlation; any variance reduction expected from regression adjustment for covariates, stratification, or matching; and the magnitude of the expected intervention effect. These estimates are essential for the power analysis, which is the focus of Chapter 9.

Methods

The Methods section should describe the methods in sufficient detail to allow the reviewers to judge whether those methods will answer the research question if they are properly implemented.

Overview. An Overview is not required, but it is helpful for complex applications. A good overview is a capsule summary of the design and expected outcomes of the study. It is helpful when there are multiple studies embedded in a single trial, when the research will progress through a series of stages, or when there are multiple levels of intervention and evaluation. Orientation to these complexities in advance of the detailed presentation will make it easier for the reader to grasp the details as they are presented.

Hypotheses. A brief presentation of the hypotheses of the study is a good way to lead into the proposed design. Investigators who don't want to be held to a specific set of outcomes may want to be general in their statement of their hypotheses, suggesting that their intervention will result in a "significant improvement" in some endpoint. However, many reviewers prefer to see a clearly delineated statement of expectations, such as a statement that the intervention is expected to result in a "3.0 mm Hg net decline (pretest to posttest) in diastolic blood pressure in the intervention condition relative to the control condition."

Design. The Design section should include a narrative description of the research design; in addition, a graphical presentation will be helpful for more complex designs. If there are multiple studies embedded in the trial, or if there are multiple layers in the design, each study and layer should be described. This description should clearly identify the units of assignment, intervention, observation, and analysis for each study and for each layer. It should convey the timing of the measurements relative to each other and to the intervention.

Selection of a design is one of the most important decisions to be taken in the planning of any study, including a group-randomized trial. There are many factors to be considered and many options. Fortunately, the research question will provide guidance, as will the costs associated with the various options. Generally, investigators should consider several options, compare their strengths, weaknesses, and costs, and select the design that optimizes these factors. That design will vary from situation to situation, and the choice will often depend upon the nature of the intervention and the nature of the units of assignment, intervention, and observation.

Information on the relative strengths and weaknesses of various designs may be found in traditional texts on experimental design (e.g., Winer et al., 1991; Kirk, 1982). Those strengths will generally hold for nested designs even if presented for non-nested designs. Chapter 3 focuses on the selection of a specific design for a group-randomized trial and on the strengths and weaknesses of the many alternatives.

The timing and size of the surveys should be presented in the Design section. Many trials are built around a simple Pretest-Posttest Control Group Design, often with large surveys conducted at pretest and posttest in each group. This is the perfect structure for intervention effects that are properly described as following a step function, but many intervention effects may follow a different pattern. Other factors aside, investigators should time their collection of data so as to capture change when it occurs in their study population, especially when it is differential change in the study conditions; the former may represent a secular or maturational trend, whereas the latter may represent an intervention effect. To the extent that the investigators can predict when those changes will occur, they will want to concentrate their collection of data at those times.

An alternative strategy is to employ continuous surveillance or plan frequent but small surveys. Some endpoints will lend themselves to surveillance methods. Examples include incidence rates for specific cancers, records of events that can be abstracted from hospital admissions records, or statistics that are kept by existing authorities. Other endpoints will require surveys. Frequent small surveys will often offer advantages in the ability to model control and intervention patterns without necessarily increasing cost.

The Design section should describe how the groups and members are to be selected and recruited for the study. The selection procedures are best presented in terms of the eligibility criteria, since those criteria will also define the populations about which inferences are to be made. The procedures will vary according to the nature of the groups, but should always include a summary of the information provided to the selected groups and a specification of the conditions under which they have agreed to participate in the trial. The case will be stronger if the groups have heard the details of the design; had an opportunity to discuss them with the investigators; understand the procedures for randomization, intervention, and data collection; and have signed an agreement that specifies what is expected from them and from the investigators over the course of the study. Much of this process is required for informed consent, but it also can serve to increase the probability that groups will not be lost to the study after it begins as a result of incomplete or inaccurate information provided during the recruitment phase.

The Design section should describe how the groups are to be allocated to study conditions. Lacking a clear statement on this issue, reviewers will suspect nonrandom assignment, and that will work against the investigators. If a nonrandom allocation procedure is planned, it should be described and defended.[4] If randomization is proposed, the description should include not only how the groups are to be randomized, but also the timing of the randomization. Early randomization—that is, prior to recruitment—will generally serve to increase the representativeness of the groups, but only if they are successfully recruited. Early randomization may lead to attrition, and especially to differential attrition if the groups are not persuaded that the study is worthwhile; for that reason, early randomization is not recommended. Late randomization— that is, after the groups have agreed to participate regardless of the outcome of the randomization—may serve to reduce the representativeness of the groups in the study, as some may not be willing to agree to participate regardless of the outcome of the randomization. Late randomization will generally result in less attrition, because the groups likely to drop out will usually do so early rather than late; for that reason, it is the recommended approach to timing the randomization.

Intervention Program. The Intervention section of the proposal should describe not only the theoretical basis for the intervention but also the practical issues of how the intervention will be delivered, how its delivery will be monitored, and how its quality will be assured. Here group-randomized trials will often depart substantially from clinical trials, because the interventions in group-randomized trials tend to be far more complex and behaviorally oriented, and sometimes involve powerful exogenous forces such as the mass media. It is far easier to get into trouble trying to deliver a complex social intervention than it is trying to deliver a simple medication. As a result, considerable attention needs to be given to developing the specific messages, materials, and procedures for the intervention; to testing them; and to presenting them and the results of those tests as part of the proposal.

Evaluation Program. The Evaluation section of a proposal often will be divided into two major sections, one dealing with outcome evaluation and one dealing with process evaluation. Within each section, the investigators should describe the variables of interest, how they are to be measured, and how they are to be analyzed. For the major endpoints, the investigators should present the methods and results of their power analysis.

Generally speaking, accepted measures are preferred over new measures, and tested measures are preferred over untried measures. Measures that can be shown to have good reliability and validity will be preferred over measures lower in these attributes. There can be no substitute for experience in the selection of measures, and if the research team is not well experienced, they should supplement their number with consultants who are.

In some fields, there are measurement methods that are well established and accepted. For example, in adolescent smoking–prevention studies, it is well established that simple self-report measures may well underestimate smoking rates in the target population, especially if the data are not anonymous (Murray, O'Connell et al., 1987; Murray and Perry, 1987). Biochemical validation is a widely used method in this field to enhance the validity of the self-report data; if the population is old enough, the biochemical measures themselves may be used as measures of smoking. Applications proposing to measure adolescent smoking that do not discuss these issues will be at a disadvantage.

The investigators must take care to ensure that their proposed measurement methods will be acceptable not only to the scientists who will review the application but also to the study population to whom those methods are to be applied. Even if a method exists that has the full support of the research community, it will not be possible to use it if it is not acceptable to the study population.

Measures for process evaluation must be included as well as for outcome evaluation. Process-evaluation measures should document what happened over the course of the study in both the intervention and control conditions so that the investigators will be able to plausibly claim at the end of the study that whatever intervention effects were observed are properly attributed to the intervention and not to some alternative explanation. Especially in group-randomized trials, it is dangerous to assume that the study's intervention is the only "intervention-like" activity that is taking place in the intervention condition or to assume that no "intervention-like" activities are occurring in the control communities. Monitoring systems should be put in place in both conditions to document the level of "intervention-like" activity that does occur.

Process-evaluation data can also be invaluable during the study as program-management tools. Such data can be used to push the intervention team to repair some component that does not appear to be working as intended.

Having described the variables of interest and their measures, and having provided as much documentation as possible as to the reliability and validity of those measures, the investigators will need to include a discussion of the logistics of how those measures are to be collected. Surveillance systems or surveys will often be required, and the application should include a description of the timing and staffing of those systems or surveys. Here, too, there is no better instruction than working with a more experienced investigator who understands the common pitfalls that can spoil the data-collection operation in the systems that are targeted by the proposed study. School surveys, worksite surveys, abstraction of hospital and physician records, etc., all have their special peculiarities, and the investigators will be well advised to include a person familiar with these issues on their team, either as a member or as a consultant.

The section on the Evaluation Program must also include a discussion of how those measures are to be analyzed. This will be true both for outcome-evaluation and process-evaluation measures, though the analytic methods are likely to vary considerably between those two sections.

The analytic plan for any measure must reflect its scale of measurement and its role in the conceptual model of the phenomenon of interest. The analytic plan should consider the coding schemes to be applied to the data, and also the major comparisons of interest, including subgroup analyses if any. The analytic plan should include a discussion of the assumptions that come with the proposed analyses and of the appropriateness of those assumptions. The analytic plan should identify the software and computers to be used for the analysis and the person or persons who will direct the analysis. Chapters 4–8 provide an extensive discussion of the analytic methods appropriate to continuous and categorical measures. There are also many examples of how to include categorical and continuous covariates in the analysis and how to reflect matching and stratification in the analysis.

The analytic plan should be written specifically for the primary and secondary endpoints in the proposed study and reflect the design of the study. Too often, applications include only general statements such as "The data will be analyzed via multiple regression." Statements such as that can mean anything, and so effectively mean nothing.

The analytic plan should also include a discussion of how dropouts and missing data are to be handled, since they are inevitable in a group-randomized trial. Strategies range from ignoring these problems to sophisticated procedures for imputation of missing data and analysis according to the intention-to-treat principle. Whatever strategies are proposed, the investigators should take care to ensure that they protect the validity of the design. At minimum, investigators should describe their plans to identify missing data and dropouts, to compare what information they have on those observations to the observations with complete data, and to assess the likely impact that the missing data and dropouts will have on the proposed analyses. Where that impact is measurable and negative, additional steps should be specified that will limit the negative impact of missing data.

The section on the Evaluation Program must include a power analysis for the primary endpoint. It should include both the methods used and the results, given in enough detail that a reviewer could check the calculations. The analytically inclined reviewers will want to see the formulae and parameter estimates employed and will want to know how those estimates were derived. Smart investigators will compute detectable differences across some range for each important parameter and present the results of all those calculations. This will allow the reviewers to gauge how much damage would be done if one or more groups dropped out of the study, or if the parameters turned out to be different from what was projected. Smart investigators will also take expected attrition into account in their power analysis, so that the reviewers can be satisfied that the study will have sufficient power even given a realistic level of attrition. Chapter 9 is devoted entirely to methods for power analysis, and the reader is referred there for examples.

Finally, the section on the Evaluation Program should include a presentation of the plans for quality control for the data collection and analysis and for data management. Standard references for clinical trials can provide useful guidelines (e.g., Meinert, 1986).

Timeline. The investigators should develop a timeline, noting all important events and activities over the course of the study. This will help them think through the various activities, to develop adequate staffing plans, to budget accurately, and to manage the study once it is under way. An abbreviated version of the timeline, noting all major milestones and activities, should be included as part of the application.

Critique. Once submitted, the proposal will be subject to review and critique by a team of experienced scientists. Therefore, it is to the investigators' advantage to conduct their own review and critique of their proposal prior to submission of their application. A critical review of the plan, once the plan is written down, can help the investigators to identify weaknesses and repair them. They can also include in the application a brief but thoughtful critique that lists any weaknesses that remain, and the alternative solutions that have been considered and rejected. That critique will help assure the reviewers that the investigators have considered their plan carefully and done everything that they can to address any remaining weaknesses.

The critique should review the design and clarify its exposition. Is the basic design clearly described? Have the sources of and selection and recruitment procedures for groups and members been described? Has the assignment rule been presented? Does the Design section include a clear presentation of the timing and sequence of observations and interventions? Have the investigators discussed alternative designs and given the reasons for choosing the design proposed?

The investigators should consider each potential source of bias in their design. The write-up of the critique need not discuss each of those sources, but should address the major potential sources of bias for group-randomized trials. As noted above, these include selection, differential history and maturation, and contamination. Investigators should assess the extent to which their plan adequately defends against these threats and summarize their case in their critique.

Once the critique of the design is completed, the investigators should critique the intervention plan. Is the theoretical basis for the intervention clear? Are the intervention components described in sufficient detail? Is the implementation plan clear? Are the training program and staffing plan well described? Are the methods for monitoring the quality of the intervention implementation adequate? Have representative copies of materials been included in the Appendix?

Once the critique of the intervention plan is completed, the investigators should critique the evaluation plan. Are the variables of interest and their measures well described? Have data on their reliability and validity been included? Is the plan for collection of data and staffing for that data collection clear? Have methods for quality assurance for the data and for management of the data been presented? Is it clear who will have responsibility for management of the data? For editing? For analysis? Has sufficient time been allocated to edit and analyze data? Has an analysis plan been described for each major endpoint? Has a power analysis been presented for each major endpoint? Have the investigators described their method to deal with missing and incomplete data? Are the proposed intervention effects plausible based on previous research? Are they of public-health importance or clinical significance?

The investigators should consider the assumptions underlying their analysis. The write-up need not discuss each assumption in detail, but it must make note of the fact that those assumptions will or will not be met. Does the analysis plan match the design? Does the analysis plan match the scale of the data?

The investigators should provide an assessment of the significance of the products to be expected from the research. How will the results be presented? What will the major products be? How will those be available for use in the future?

Often it will be helpful to have someone outside the team read the application and offer critical comments. For major projects, the team may want to arrange a mock review, or even practice site visits.

Human Subjects

The Human Subjects section will be governed by the sponsoring agency's Internal Review Board and by the funding agency's requirements. In general, this section should document the steps proposed to ensure that participants will provide informed consent and that adequate precautions are planned to protect the safety and the privacy of the participants.

Consultants

Letters from consultants documenting the specific work that they have agreed to do and the time allotted for that work should be included. Biographical sketches for consultants should also be included.

Management and Administration

Complex applications in particular will need to include a presentation on how the many components and staff will be organized and managed to ensure that the project will be completed successfully. Where multiple organizations or multiple sites are involved, this section will need to address issues of communication and monitoring of activities.

Literature Cited

The application should include a complete listing of all references cited in the text. All references should be accurate and complete.

Appendixes

The length and content of the Appendixes will depend on the nature of the application. In general, the Appendix provides an opportunity to present protocols, intervention manuals and materials, measurement instruments, and other detail that won't fit within the space limitations of the text of the application.

Investigators should understand, however, that reviewers are not required to look at anything left to the Appendix, and that many of the reviewers won't even receive the Appendixes. As a general rule, nothing of importance should be left to the Appendix other than stand-alone documents that augment what is presented in the text. In addition, investigators should take care not to include too much material in the Appendix, as that will only frustrate the reviewers; it will do nothing to improve their review. In particular, reviewers are not likely to read an extensive set of manuscripts, books, or papers included in the Appendix; to watch videotapes or experiment with software included in the appendix; to review scores of brochures, handouts, or other intervention materials; to wade through dozens of manuals; etc. Investigators should include only essential and representative components of their proposed intervention and evaluation programs.

Summary

Group-randomized trials are often complex studies, with greater challenges in design, analysis, and intervention than what is seen in other studies. As a result, much care and effort is required for good planning. This chapter has described that planning process. Subsequent chapters will present alternative designs, the analyses appropriate for those designs, and the methods for power analysis for those analyses.

Endnotes

1. Analysis of attrition patterns is important in any group-randomized trial. The extent that investigators can show that those lost to follow-up in the two conditions were similar both in their current status and in their risk status will provide important evidence that differential mortality was not a source of bias for the estimate of the intervention effect.

2. Regression adjustment for confounders is often not considered in randomized clinical trials, as many analysts would rather trust that the randomization has evenly distributed the potential sources of bias. However, when the number of groups allocated to each condition is small, as in most group-randomized trials, such trust may not be well placed. As in any study, the investigator has a responsibility to assess potential confounding, and if it is found, to take steps to limit its effect.

One of the arguments often made against regression adjustment for confounding in a randomized trial is that the analyst would rather not have to depend on a statistical model to correct for confounding. That argument has always seemed hollow, because the same analyst is already relying on a statistical model, simply one that presumes no confounding. In other words, whether the analyst adjusts or not, there is still a model. The prudent course would seem to be to limit bias as much as possible in the design of the study, to check to see whether that effort has been successful, and if not, to take additional steps to limit its influence in the analysis.

Having made that argument, regression adjustment for confounders is not a risk-free proposition. As documented in Cook and Campbell's (1979) excellent text on quasi-experimental design, regression adjustment for multiple covariates can not only reduce bias but can also introduce bias. Indeed, this is one of the reasons that some statisticians are reluctant to make regression adjustments for covariates in a randomized trial. However, the danger comes largely from the use of confounders that are not reliably measured, so that if adjustment is limited to variables with good reliability, that risk will be small.

3. It is important to note that power for an interaction is always less than power for a main effect. If that is not taken into account in the planning stage, there may be inadequate power for interactions at the time of the analysis.

4. Some would argue that nonrandom assignment cannot be defended. However, there will be situations in which random assignment is not possible. The investigators should take care to show why random assignment is not possible, why the study is still worth doing, and why the reviewers can have confidence that the data will be interpretable even without random assignment.

3

Research Designs

> Science is concerned with understanding variability in nature, statistics is concerned with making decisions about nature in the presence of variability, and experimental design is concerned with reducing and controlling variability in ways that make statistical theory applicable to decisions made about nature.
>
> Winer et al. (1991), p. 1

There are four major features that combine to differentiate the designs commonly used in group-randomized trials. The first is whether the design is a main-effects or factorial design. The second is the schedule for data collection. The third is whether the design is a cohort or a cross-sectional design. The fourth is whether or not the design will include *a priori* matching or stratification. Decisions related to these features will be strongly influenced by the research question, but also by other considerations. This chapter will review the alternatives available for each of these features and the factors that can influence the investigators' decisions.

Main-Effect and Factorial Designs

Main-Effect Designs

The simplest group-randomized trial has a main-effect design with only two levels. This arrangement is chosen when the research question involves the effect of a single intervention.

In some cases the investigators are interested in several different levels of intervention, with each compared to a common control. This will also require a main-effect design, but with more than two levels. For example, in the Child and Adolescent Trial for Cardiovascular Health (CATCH), students were randomized to a usual-care control condition, to a school-only intervention condition, or to a school-plus-family intervention condition (Luepker, Perry et al., 1996). This design allowed the investigators to address the question of the effect of the school-only intervention against a usual-care control group, and then to address the question of the added benefit of the family intervention by comparing the school-plus-family condition to the school-only condition.

Factorial Designs

Some questions require two or more independent variables. For example, the CATCH investigators might have been interested in the school and family interventions separately. In this case, a factorial design would be used, as shown in Figure 3.1. With this design, the investigators would be able to assess the main effect of each of the two interventions as well as their joint effect.

More complex designs are rarely employed in group-randomized trials, because they would substantially expand the size and cost of the trial. For example, incomplete factorial and latin squares designs have not been used in the context of group-randomized trials in public health, nor have factorial designs involving more than two independent variables.

The Data-Collection Schedule

Quite apart from the question of main effect vs. factorial designs, the investigators must consider whether data collection will be organized around discrete time intervals, and if so, how many such intervals will be included. Alternatively, the investigators may choose to establish a continuous surveillance operation.

Posttest-Only Control Group Design

When each of the groups and members is measured only once, after the intervention has been delivered in the intervention condition, the design is often

School Intervention	Family Intervention	
	No	Yes
No	Usual Care	Family Only
Yes	School Only	School Plus Family

Figure 3.1. Layout of a factorial-design alternative to the main-effect design employed in CATCH.

called a Posttest-Only Control Group Design. This can be a very weak design for a trial based on allocation of identifiable groups to study conditions, especially if a nonrandom assignment rule is used or if only a few groups are randomized to each condition. Cook and Campbell (1979) went so far as to call the nonrandomized Posttest-Only Control Group Design "generally uninterpretable." On the other hand, if a large number of groups are randomized to each study condition, then the Posttest-Only Control Group Design can be a very strong design.

One need only consider the sources of bias presented in Chapter 2 to see how this design can be both weak and strong, depending on the circumstances. Consider just the four major sources of bias in a group-randomized trial: selection, differential maturation and history, and contamination. Without baseline measurements, the investigators cannot know whether the conditions were comparable prior to the introduction of the intervention; as a result, the investigators cannot know whether selection bias exists. If a large number of identifiable groups had been randomized to each condition, the investigators could rely on the randomization procedure to distribute evenly factors that otherwise might create selection bias. Absent those conditions, such protection is completely lacking.

With only a single measurement on each group and member, the investigators cannot know whether the maturational patterns in the study conditions were the same prior to the intervention. As above, if a large number of identifiable groups had been randomized to each condition, the investigators could rely on the randomization procedure to distribute the maturational patterns evenly among the study conditions. Absent those conditions, differential maturation will remain a potential source of bias.

For the threats of differential history and contamination, it is not simply the number of time intervals that is important, but instead the type of information that is gathered over the course of the study. If adequate exposure measures are not included, it may be difficult to rule out bias due to contamination and differential history. If such measures are included, but only at the end of the study, it may still be difficult to rule out bias due to those factors, unless the measures are structured to measure the timing and source of the exposures as well as the simple presence or absence of such exposures. These threats will be exacerbated if only a few identifiable groups are allocated to each study condition. However, if a large number of groups is randomly assigned to each condition, then local history and contamination may become less plausible.

Pretest-Posttest Control Group Design

The Pretest-Posttest Control Group Design expands upon the Posttest-Only Control Group Design by adding a baseline or pretest survey to the design.

For example, the CATCH design included a baseline survey and a follow-up survey, as diagrammed in Figure 3.2. This design allows the investigators to assess the comparability of the conditions on measured variables prior to the introduction of the intervention to assess the extent of any selection bias. If selection bias is observed, the investigators can try to limit it in the analysis.

With only one baseline observation, it is impossible to measure differential maturation or secular trends directly. An indirect method is to look for evidence of any difference in the age of the members measured in each condition. Age is often a good proxy for maturation, so that differences in age give suggestive evidence that there may be differences in maturation. Similarly, comparability in age gives suggestive evidence against differential maturation. Proxy measures also may be available with which to build a case for or against differential secular trends. Data on the primary endpoint may not be available, but if data are available over time for variables related to the primary endpoint, those may be used to assess the danger of different secular trends in the study conditions.

The Pretest-Posttest Control Group design provides a greater measure of protection against bias due to local history and contamination, but only if the investigators include exposure measures as part of their data-collection protocol. In addition, the ability to detect local history or contamination effects will depend on the nature and timing of those exposure measures. Baseline data can provide evidence of local history or contamination that occurs prior to the baseline survey. Follow-up data can provide evidence of local history or contamination that occurs between the baseline and follow-up surveys. As noted above, those data will be more useful if they assess both the timing and source of these exposures, not simply their presence or absence.

The Pretest-Posttest Control Group design may provide protection against bias due to differential instrumentation, depending on the pattern of the results of the study. If the study conditions have similar levels on the primary endpoint at pretest, then differential instrumentation cannot stand as a plausible alternative explanation for greater change in one condition than another. However, if the conditions have rather different levels at baseline, differential instrumentation will remain a threat, unless the investigators can provide other

	Time Interval	
Condition	Pretest	Posttest
Intervention		
Control		

Figure 3.2. Layout of the Pretest-Posttest Control Group Design.

evidence against it. For example, if one condition has a lower level than another at baseline, and "catches up" while the second condition does not change, the lack of change may reflect a ceiling effect in the instrument rather than a lack of true change. The best defense given such situations is to have data from other sources to show that the instrument is sensitive to change beyond the levels achieved in the present study.

Additional Discrete Time Intervals

With additional baseline time intervals for data collection, the investigators can measure the trends in the groups in their study, in terms of the endpoints, in terms of important sources of bias, and in terms of competing exposures. It then becomes possible to stratify or match on those trends, or, alternatively, to make adjustment for differences in trends during the analysis. It is also possible to present evidence to indicate that no differential trends were present in the data, if the data so suggest. Used well, additional baseline or follow-up intervals can provide considerably greater evidence for or against bias due to local history, contamination, selection, and differential maturation. However, the best way to avoid or minimize these sources of bias from the outset will always be to randomly assign a sufficient number of groups to each condition, so that chance has an opportunity to evenly distribute all sources of bias.

With additional follow-up time intervals for data collection, the investigators can examine the pattern of the intervention effect over time. Given enough intervals, they may be able to specify a model for that pattern and substantially improve the precision of the analysis. Examples are provided in Chapters 5–8.

These advantages naturally come with a price. Not only must the additional time intervals be included in the design, often at considerable expense, but with more than two time intervals in the design, the possibilities that exist for the structure of the covariance matrix increase substantially. As will be discussed in Chapter 4, the investigators will want to take care to properly specify that structure in order to ensure a valid analysis.

Continuous Surveillance

Continuous surveillance extends the strategy of having additional discrete time intervals. Instead of collecting data in discrete surveys conducted during discrete time intervals, data are collected continuously as endpoints occur in the target population. For example, the REACT study introduced in Chapter 1 involves continuous surveillance of heart attacks in each of the 20 participating communities (Simons-Morton et al., under review). Those data will be used to model time trends in delay time in each community, so that the average trend in the intervention condition can be compared to the average trend in the control condition (Feldman et al., under review). Here, too, the analyst will be able to take advantage of the precision afforded an analysis based on a comparison of regression slopes.

Cross-Sectional and Cohort Designs

The third feature that differentiates among the designs commonly employed in group-randomized trials is whether the design is a nested cross-sectional design or a nested cohort design. In the nested cross-sectional design, identifiable groups are assigned to the study conditions, and members within those conditions are measured to assess the impact of the intervention. In the simplest nested cross-sectional design, each group and member is measured once. In nested cross-sectional designs that extend over time, each group may be measured more than once, but each member is still measured only once. As such, the essential feature of the nested cross-sectional design is that different members are measured during each time interval included in the design.

In the nested cohort design, identifiable groups are assigned to the study conditions, and members within those conditions are followed over time to assess the impact of the intervention. The essential feature of the nested cohort design is that the same members are measured at each time interval included in the design.

Several recent papers have reviewed the relative costs and benefits of cohort vs. cross-sectional designs in the context of group-randomized trials (Feldman and McKinlay, 1994; Gail et al., 1996; Diehr et al., 1995b; Koepsell et al., 1992; McKinlay, 1994). There is general agreement that the primary consideration should be the research question.

The primary reason for choosing a cross-sectional design over a cohort design should be that the research question involves change within an entire population. If this is the case, the investigators will want to represent that population at each time interval when data are collected. That often requires a nested cross-sectional design.

The primary reason for choosing a nested cohort design should be that the research question involves change within specific members of the population. Such change cannot be assessed without repeated measurements on those members, and it is the repeated measurements on the same members that define the nested cohort design.

Nested cross-sectional and nested cohort designs carry a number of strengths and weaknesses relative to each other. These will often play a role in guiding the investigators to choose one over the other, even beyond the primary influence of the research question.

In studies with a short follow-up time, for example, a nested cohort design may provide data that are just as representative of the population as a nested cross-sectional design. This will be true if in-migration, out-migration, and attrition are limited. If the cost of following the cohort is similar to the cost of recruiting a new cross-sectional sample, then the nested cohort design will usually be preferred, as it will usually provide greater precision for the estimate of the intervention effect.

In studies that have a long follow-up time, nested cross-sectional designs usually will provide data that are more representative of the underlying population. At the same time, such designs cannot assess change within the specific members of the population. In contrast, a cohort sample may represent the population when it is first drawn, but gradually lose its representation due to changes in the population (in-migration and out-migration). However, cohort designs can be used to assess change within specific members of that population.

Even if in-migration and out-migration are not a problem, the nested cohort design may become less representative of the original cohort over time due to nonrandom attrition. Attrition can be high if the measurements are burdensome or if the follow-up time is long. Attrition at the member level is not an issue in a nested cross-sectional design, as each member of the population is observed only once.

Which of the two designs will be less expensive will depend on a number of factors. In a cohort study, there will be some expense associated with tracking and locating participants, as well as obtaining data from remote locations once the participants are located. In a cross-sectional study, there will be some expense associated with recruiting a new cross-sectional sample. Investigators will need to examine the relative impact of these costs to determine which of the designs will be less expensive (Kish, 1987; McKinlay, 1994).

Many investigators think of cohort designs as more powerful than cross-sectional designs. That is often true because the over-time correlation within members can be substantial and serve to improve the precision of the estimate of the intervention effect. Other factors constant, this will improve the power of the cohort design. However, the magnitude of the over-time correlation is likely to decline as the length of the study increases; that will reduce the efficiency advantage usually given to the cohort design.

Another advantage often attributed to the cohort design is that it allows the investigators to better estimate the intervention effect in a population that received the "full dose" of the intervention. That assumption is made because the cohort members who have remained in the community throughout the study at least had the opportunity to have been fully exposed. However, to the extent that the cohort members, through differential attrition, do not represent all those who had that opportunity, the intervention-effect estimate derived from the cohort may be biased and the nature of that bias may be hard to assess.

It is also quite possible to estimate the intervention effect in a population that received the "full dose" of the intervention even when the study is based on a cross-sectional design, as long as that design is planned properly (Diehr et al., 1995b). A baseline sample would be surveyed, then screened at follow-up to determine who was still resident in the community; only those "stayers" would be retained for analysis. A separate posttest sample would be drawn and screened to determine who had been resident in the community from the beginning of the study; only those "stayers" would be surveyed and included in the analysis. This hybrid design could provide independent representative samples of "stayers," the subpopulation of interest, with both lower cost and less bias than would a more traditional nested cohort design.

As this last example illustrates, many kinds of cross-sectional and cohort designs are available, and the variations are limited only by the creativity of the investigator. Each of these designs will have advantages and disadvantages. Chapters 5 and 6 review the major types of cross-sectional and cohort designs, with a focus on the advantages and disadvantages for each.

A Priori Matching and Stratification

The last feature that differentiates among the designs employed in group-randomized trials is whether they include *a priori* matching or stratification. *A priori* matching and stratification in the context of a group-randomized trial are quite different from *a priori* matching and stratification in a clinical trial. In a clinical trial, individual patients or participants are matched or stratified prior to randomization to conditions from within matched sets or strata. In a group-randomized trial, it is the groups that are matched or stratified prior to randomization to conditions from within matched sets or strata. As a result, it requires information on the matching or stratification factors for each group in advance of the randomization.

There are three quite different reasons to employ *a priori* stratification or matching in the design. First, an *a priori* stratified or matched design will be preferred whenever the investigators want to ensure balance across conditions on an important potential source of bias. As discussed in Chapter 2, when the investigators anticipate or observe considerable heterogeneity among the groups at baseline, simple random assignment is an unreliable method to achieve baseline comparability among the study conditions if the total number of groups is quite small. Under those conditions, it is far safer to match or stratify the groups on the factors related to the primary endpoint and then to randomize the groups from within the matched sets or strata. This will ensure that the conditions are reasonably comparable at least on the matching or stratification factors. If those factors are selected carefully, the design will be strengthened considerably against the most common sources of bias. This is exactly why so many of the major group-randomized trials conducted in recent years have matched or stratified their groups prior to allocation to study conditions (e.g., Gail et al., 1992; Zucker et al., 1995; Davis et al., under review; Feldman et al., under review). This procedure is highly recommended for group-randomized trials with a limited number of groups. This would include any study with fewer than 20 groups per condition.

Second, an *a priori* stratified design will be preferred whenever the investigators have an *a priori* interest in testing whether the intervention effect is different across strata defined by characteristics of the groups. A *priori* stratification can also ensure balance in the number of groups in each condition $\times$ stratum cell, and estimation of stratum-specific effects will be easier when such balance exists. Absent *a priori* stratification, some of the condition $\times$ stratum cells may be so thin as to make it quite difficult to assess stratum-specific effects.

Third, an *a priori* matched design will improve the precision of the analysis for the main effect of condition to the extent that the matching factors are well correlated with the primary endpoints. As noted in Chapter 2, if that correlation is above 0.30, or if there are more than 10 groups per condition, the increased efficiency of the matched analysis will usually offset the reduced degrees of freedom and make it more powerful than an unmatched analysis. A *priori* stratification will improve the precision of the analysis for the main effect of condition for any positive value of the correlation between the stratification factor(s) and the endpoint, because stratification does not reduce the degrees of freedom for that main effect test. However, the main-effect analysis for condition is interpretable only if the stratum-specific effects are homogeneous. If that is established, the analysis proceeds absent the condition $\times$ stratum term and the stratification factors are treated like the other covariates in the model. These issues are discussed further in Chapters 5 and 6.

The choice of matching vs. stratification will often depend on the number of groups available, on the expected accuracy of the matches, and on the analytic plan. If the investigator is interested in testing the null hypothesis of homogeneity of the stratum-specific intervention effects, then the stratified design should be used. If not, then the choice can be guided by the expectations about the quality of the matching. If the investigator believes that very close matching is possible, then matching and a matched analysis will be preferred, as the improved precision will make up for the lost degrees of freedom relative to a stratified or unmatched analysis. If moderate matches are possible, then stratification will be preferred, as it will still offer better precision over an unmatched analysis but won't exact as high a price in degrees of freedom as the matched analysis. If only modest matches are possible, the prudent course may be to employ matching in the design to limit bias but to ignore the matching in the analysis (Martin et al., 1993; Diehr et al., 1995a).

The choice of matching or stratification factors is critical to the success of the procedure. Too often investigators match or stratify on factors because they are easily measured. This can be a wasted effort, because matching or stratification on factors unrelated to the primary endpoint will provide no benefit to the study and may instead lull the investigators into a false sense of security. The best factors are those that are highly related to the level and slope of the primary endpoint and yet simple enough to be measured and available before the groups are randomized to study conditions.

Often the best matching or stratification factor is the primary endpoint itself, assessed at baseline. For example, consider the college-drinking study from Chapter 2. If a baseline survey could be administered in each of the participating colleges prior to randomization to conditions, then the colleges could be matched or stratified on the prevalence of drinking. If such data are not available, a proxy measure may be adequate, especially if it is well correlated to the primary endpoint. Another alternative is to match or stratify on risk factors for the primary endpoint, especially if their predictive value is good. The critical factor is that the matching or stratification variables predict the level and slope of the primary endpoint. As the precision of that prediction increases, the benefits from matching or stratification will increase.

Where the matching or stratification factors are measured at the group level, matching or stratification can be based on those measures. Where the matching or stratification factors are measured at the member level, mean values must be computed for each group so that they are available as the basis for the matching or stratification.

Summary

The research question will guide the team in selecting the alternatives that are available for each of the four major features that differentiate among the designs commonly employed in group-randomized trials. Main-effect designs are appropriate when the question is focused on the evaluation of a single intervention or on several levels of intervention that fall along a continuum in one dimension. Factorial designs are appropriate when the question is focused on the independent and joint effects of interventions that operate in two or more dimensions. Multiple time intervals for data collection provide many benefits related to reducing bias and improving precision in the analysis. Nested cross-sectional designs are most appropriate when the investigators are interested in the effects of the intervention on an entire population. The cross-sectional design will often be less expensive, less burdensome for the participants, better protected against threats to validity, and easier to analyze. Nested cohort designs are most appropriate when the investigators are interested in the effect of the intervention in specific members of the population. They are often chosen because investigators assume that they offer more power than their nested cross-sectional counterparts, or because they assume that these designs provide better defenses against bias. Certainly nested cohort studies can be very powerful under the right conditions, and they can provide good defenses bias if they are well designed. At the same time, if they are poorly designed or are employed under conditions for which they are poorly suited, the investigator is not likely to realize the benefits that the nested cohort design can offer. *A priori* matching and stratification offer tools available in the design of the study to limit bias and improve precision. Stratification makes it possible to study effect modification where that is a focus of the investigation.

Regardless of the decisions on the data-collection schedule and nested cross-sectional vs. nested cohort designs, the best protection against bias in a group-randomized trial will come from random assignment of a sufficient number of groups to each study condition. Where the number of groups is limited, the protection against bias will be substantially enhanced if the groups are matched or stratified prior to randomization.

4

Planning the Analysis

The first step in the outline of the experiment's analysis is usually to deduce a mathematical model appropriate to the experimental situation. This model should contain terms representing all of the sources of variation present in the experiment. . . . Where there are several observational units per experimental unit, both the experimental unit error and the observational unit error should be included in the model. Since both types of errors include variability due to factors unknown to or beyond the control of the experimenter, neither should be deleted from the model at the whim of the experimenter or statistician.

Addelman (1970), pp. 1096, 1097–98.

Because group-randomized trials have complex designs, their analysis is usually more complex than that of studies based on simpler designs. Thus, careful planning is required for a valid analysis of the data. Following a review of the fundamentals of data analysis, this chapter will address each of the components of the planning process. The analyst must review the research question, the design, and the endpoints; specify a method for the analysis that is well matched to the question, the design, and the endpoints; conduct the analysis; and assess the appropriateness of the method employed. Because software packages are useful in analyzing data from a group-randomized trial, this chapter also discusses many of those packages that are available.

Fundamentals

Factors That Influence the Analytic Strategy

The Research Question

The research question determines the design and the primary and secondary endpoints. Thus, it will also largely determine the analytic strategy, for that will flow directly from the nature of the design and the endpoints of the trial. If at any point the analyst or investigator loses his or her sense of direction during the analysis, the best remedy is often to review the research question.

The Design

The design will specify the number of conditions, the number of levels of each condition, and whether those conditions are completely crossed or not. It will specify whether the data are from discrete time intervals or represent continuous surveillance. It will specify whether each group and member was measured only once or more than once. It will specify whether the groups were matched or stratified *a priori.* Finally, it will specify the selection and allocation schemes employed for the groups and members.

A single independent variable will suggest what is often termed a *main effects analysis.* Two or more independent variables that are completely crossed form a factorial design and so suggest a *factorial analysis.*

Data that are from discrete time intervals are usually analyzed by treating time as a categorical variable in the analysis. However, given only two time intervals, time may be reflected only indirectly in an analysis of posttest data that makes a regression adjustment for baseline values. Given more than two time intervals, time may be treated as a continuous variable. Given sufficient time intervals or continuous surveillance, the analyst may have many options for how to treat time.

If each member is observed only once, the analysis will be chosen from among those appropriate for nested cross-sectional designs. There is no covariation within members, so that alternate structures for that covariation need not be considered. At the same time, alternate structures for the covariation within or between the groups may need to be considered. If each member was observed more than once, the analysis will be chosen from among those appropriate for nested cohort designs, and alternate structures for the structure of the covariation within and between both groups and members may need to be considered.

If the groups are matched or stratified *a priori,* the analyst will need to consider whether or not to reflect those features in the analysis.

Together, these factors will suggest one or more analysis strategies appropriate for the data. The team will want to specify one analysis as their primary analysis *a priori,* but it will often be helpful to specify secondary analyses as well.

The Endpoint

Many familiar endpoints are continuous; examples include body mass index, blood cholesterol, blood pressure, etc. Others will be dichotomous, representing the presence or absence of a characteristic or symptom of interest; examples include smoking status (smoker vs. nonsmoker), immunization status (yes vs. no), history of illicit drug use (yes vs. no), etc. Some will represent the time between enrollment in the study and the occurrence of an event of interest; such data are often called time-to-event data or survival-time data. Still others will represent counts, such as the number of servings of fruits and vegetables usually eaten each day, or the number of alcoholic beverages consumed at the last drinking occasion. The nature of the endpoint will suggest a distribution for the errors associated with the observations, and this will also help to guide the selection of the analysis strategy.

Bias and Precision

Where the investigator anticipates bias, *a priori* stratification or matching may be helpful, as discussed in Chapter 2. Where the investigator discovers evidence suggesting bias, despite steps taken to prevent it, analytic strategies such as regression adjustment for covariates and *post hoc* stratification may be helpful.

Chapter 2 also identified a number of steps that can be taken in the analysis to improve precision. These include regression adjustment for extraneous variables, stratification or matching, modeling of time, etc. Given the substantial and negative effect that measurable variation due to groups and members can have on the power of the trial, these procedures may be very important methods to reduce that variation and thereby enhance the power of the trial. Care must be used, of course, as application of these methods carries additional assumptions, and the analyst will want to assess the validity of those assumptions as well as the validity of the assumptions that underlie the initial analysis.

Threats to the Validity of the Analysis

The two major threats to the validity of the analysis of data from a group-randomized trial are misspecification of the analytic model and low power.

Misspecification of the Analytic Model

Misspecification of the analytic model can come about in a variety of ways. Most often, it occurs because the analyst has ignored a measurable source of random variation, misrepresented a measurable source of random variation, or misrepresented the pattern of over-time correlation in the data. Such errors result in a random-effects covariance matrix that does not reflect the underlying structure of the data.[1]

In a group-randomized trial, both the groups and the members represent measurable sources of random variation. An example of the first kind of model misspecification occurs when the analyst ignores variation due to the groups.

An example of the second kind of model misspecification occurs when the groups are included in the analysis but not treated as a source of random variation. Another example of the second kind of model misspecification occurs when the component of variance for the groups is assumed constant over levels of a grouping factor when, in fact, that component is heterogeneous with respect to the levels of that grouping factor. An example of the third kind of model misspecification occurs when the over-time correlation in the data is assumed constant when it actually declines in some systematic way.

Misspecification of the model can also be thought of as violating one or more of the assumptions underlying the statistical test used to evaluate the intervention effect. Such tests are valid only when their underlying assumptions are met in the data for which the test is computed. To the extent that one or more of the underlying assumptions is not appropriate for the data, then that assumption is considered to have been violated and the model misspecified.

Consider methods based on the General Linear Model (Searle, 1971). Those methods include multiple linear regression and analysis of variance (ANOVA) and covariance (ANCOVA), with or without matching or stratification, and have been used widely in the analysis of data from group-randomized trials. Good discussions of the assumptions that underlie the General Linear Model and the consequences of their violation are available in many textbooks on statistics for experimental designs (e.g., Snedecor and Cochran, 1989; Winer et al., 1991).

Three of the main assumptions that underlie methods based on the General Linear Model are normality and homogeneity of errors across conditions, and independence of errors. Even substantial violations of the normality assumption are not serious if the sample sizes are equal in all the conditions, but the standard errors can be substantially underestimated if the sample sizes vary. Modest heterogeneity of variance is also not a serious concern if the sample sizes are equal, but the standard errors can be under- or overestimated when the sample sizes are unequal. It is also important to remember that the tests for heterogeneity themselves lose sensitivity with increasing non-normality. Violations of the independence-of-errors assumption can be quite serious, especially when the errors are positively related, as this will always deflate the standard errors. The situation is particularly troublesome for group-randomized trials, where equal sample sizes are almost unknown, where non-Gaussian error distributions are quite common, and where dependence of errors within groups is guaranteed by the allocation of identifiable groups to conditions.

The identifiable groups that are the units of assignment in a group-randomized trial will usually vary in size. As a result, the conditions also will usually vary in size. Careful planning may result in sample sizes that are similar across groups and conditions, but it is highly unlikely that they will be equal in all groups and all conditions. Even if the investigator is fortunate enough to structure such balance by design, attrition can spoil the balance of the data at the time of the analysis. As a result, the protection afforded by equal sample sizes is rarely available in group-randomized trials.

Many group-randomized trials have as their primary endpoints dichotomous variables that represent the presence or absence of some characteristic. Examples include current smoker vs. nonsmoker, any binge drinking in the last two weeks vs. none, incident CHD case vs. noncase, etc. Other trials have as their primary endpoint data that are continuous but decidedly non-normal, such as delay time in reporting a heart attack, which is sharply skewed to the left and has a long right tail in its distribution. As a result, group-randomized trials often cannot meet the assumption of Gaussian errors.

The most severe problem facing group-randomized trials in terms of the assumptions underlying the usual analyses is that the observations from the same group show positive intraclass correlation. As shown in Chapter 1, this positive intraclass correlation reflects a component of variance attributable to the group. Unless it is accounted for in the analysis, the Type I error rate for the test of the intervention effect will be inflated, often badly (Zucker, 1990).

Consider school-based health-promotion studies, a common class of group-randomized trials. Intraclass correlation coefficients in the range of 0.02 are fairly common in these studies (Murray and Hannan, 1990; Murray, Rooney et al., 1994; Siddiqui et al., 1996). The naive reader might view a coefficient of this magnitude as too small to warrant concern. However, given 200 students observed per school, the *VIF* will be 4.98. Suppose the investigator relies on an analytic method that assumes independence of errors at the level of the units of observation, such as fixed-effects analysis of variance. Suppose further that there is no variation attributable to the intervention. Under these conditions, the expected value of the *F*-test for intervention will be 4.98, not 1.0, but the critical value will remain 3.84. The investigator will run a very real risk of falsely interpreting that test as support for an intervention effect. Zucker (1990) has shown that the Type I error rate can easily exceed 50% under these conditions, even though the nominal rate is set at 5%.

This discussion has focused on the potential for data from group-randomized trials to fail several key assumptions underlying the General Linear Model. While that is an accurate characterization, readers should not lose sight of the more general nature of this threat to the validity of the analysis. Whatever analysis is being considered, investigators should take care that the assumptions underlying that analysis are appropriate for the design and the data at hand. Failure to do so may lead to serious problems in any study, not just in a group-randomized trial, and with any analysis, not just those based on the General Linear Model.

Low Statistical Power

The second major threat to the validity of the analysis of data from a group-randomized trial is low power. The power of a test is the probability that an effect of a given magnitude will be found to be statistically significant. In other words, it is the probability of detecting an intervention effect when the intervention has caused an effect of a given magnitude. Chapter 9 reviews statistical power and methods to estimate power. This section is concerned with low power as a threat to the validity of the analysis.

If the other threats to the validity of the analysis are addressed, group-randomized trials are often faced with low statistical power. The main reason is that the intervention effect must be assessed against an error term based on the between-group variance in order to protect the nominal Type I error rate. As noted in Chapter 1, the between-group variance is usually larger when based on identifiable groups than when based on randomly constituted groups. In addition, the precision available to estimate the between-group variance is usually less than that for the within-group variance, because there are usually many fewer groups per condition than there are members per condition. These factors often combine to reduce power so that it can be almost impossible to detect important intervention effects in an otherwise well-designed and properly executed trial.

Strategies to Protect the Validity of the Analysis

There are a number of strategies available to defend against these threats to the validity of the analysis.

Identify All Possible Sources of Random Variation in the Data

Given the risk associated with ignoring measurable sources of random variation, it is important for the analyst to seek to identify all possible sources of such variation. The units of assignment and observation are always sources of random variation. Whether there are other sources will depend on the selection and allocation schemes employed in a given design, as well as on the design itself. Many examples are provided in Chapters 5–8.

Check All Assumptions Concerning the Structure of the Random-Effects Covariance Matrix

Given the risk associated with misrepresenting a measurable source of random variation or the structure of over-time correlation in the data, it is important for the analyst to check the assumptions made about the structure of each source of random variation and each correlation that contributes to the random-effects covariance matrix. For example, if a source is assumed to be distributed Gaussian, it will be important to check to see if that assumption is correct.

Another approach is to fit alternative models and compare their goodness of fit. This strategy will apply particularly to designs in which alternative models for the covariance matrix are possible. In the simplest of group-randomized trial designs, there will be only one structure for the covariance matrix. However, in more complex designs, and particularly for designs with continuous surveillance or multiple time intervals, there will be plausible alternative models for the covariance matrix. Examples of such a design, and the methods for choosing among alternative structures for the covariance matrix, are provided in Chapter 8.[2]

Avoid Assumptions or Employ Robust Methods

The first two strategies to limit threats to statistical validity would help the analyst match the analytic model to the structure of the data. An alternative strategy is to choose an analytic method that avoids those statistical models (e.g., randomization tests, discussed below) or that is robust to violation of the assumptions underlying those models (e.g., empirical-sandwich estimation of standard errors, also discussed below). These strategies are intuitively attractive and may be quite effective under the proper conditions.

Develop the Plan for Design and the Analysis Concurrently

Because the design and the primary endpoints will always substantially determine the analytic plan, it is important that the design and analytic plan be developed concurrently. If the analytic plan presents serious problems for the design, the design may have to be modified. One of the worst mistakes possible is to develop the analytic plan only after the study design is set and the study is under way. Sadly, there won't always be a satisfactory analysis available for every design, and it can be very expensive to discover that after the study is under way.

Plan the Analysis Around the Primary Endpoint

Many group-randomized trials have a variety of endpoints. Treating each of them equally will guarantee an inflated Type I error rate unless special steps are taken. In addition, this approach may not focus enough attention on the primary endpoint to ensure that a valid analytic plan has been developed for that measure. Investigators should take a lesson from clinical trials, where one endpoint is designated as the primary endpoint. Considerable attention is then focused on developing a valid analytic plan for that endpoint. This planning serves to ensure that the trial will have sufficient power for that analysis and that the Type I error rate for the primary analyses is at or below a predetermined level. Other variables are identified as secondary and analyzed and presented separately. The conclusions are based on the results for the primary endpoint, with assistance in the interpretation of those results coming from the analysis of the secondary endpoints.

Statistical Models

Most analytic methods are based on a statistical model. A statistical model is a mathematical expression that attempts to characterize the relationship between a set of independent variables and a single dependent variable. A statistical model will usually include as terms both the independent variables and one or more sources of random variation. Each term in the model must be designated as a fixed or a random effect.

A term is a fixed effect if the investigators are interested in drawing inferences only about the specific levels of the term that are included in the study. Condition is a fixed effect if the investigators are interested only in the levels of condition that are included in the study (e.g., intervention, control). Similarly, time is a fixed effect if the investigators are interested only in the levels of time that are included in the study (e.g., pretest, posttest). Covariates and stratification factors are fixed effects if the investigators are interested only in the levels of those factors that are included in the study (e.g., age, gender, education level, field center in some multicenter trials).

A term is a random effect if the investigators are interested in drawing inferences about some larger population of levels that are only represented by the specific levels included in the study. Group and member are random effects if the investigators are interested in generalizing to other groups and members like those included in the study. Matched pairs or sets are random effects if the investigators are interested in generalizing to other pairs or sets like those included in the study. A stratification factor is a random effect if the investigators are interested in generalizing to other strata like those included in the study (e.g., field centers in other multicenter trials).

As will be seen in this section, the designation of terms as fixed or random effects has important implications for the model, the analysis, and the interpretation of the results. While those implications can't be ignored, the primary factor in determining whether a term is a fixed or random effect must be the intended inference space. Broad inference to other levels like those included in the study is justified only when the term is a random effect. Narrow inference to the particular levels included in the study is justified when the term is a fixed effect. The proper designation of effects as fixed or random will ensure that the Type I and II error rates are at their nominal levels (Zucker, 1990).

It is convenient to organize statistical models along two dimensions. The first dimension distinguishes between models that involve only a single random effect and those that involve two or more random effects. Throughout this book, models that include only one random effect will be classified as Fixed Effect Models, while those that include two or more random effects will be classified as Mixed Effect Models or more simply as Mixed Models.[3] The second dimension distinguishes among models that assume that the errors associated with the units of observation are Gaussian and those that do not. Together these two dimensions define four general models, shown in Figure 4.1.

General Linear Model

The General Linear Model (Searle, 1971) is appropriate for endpoints that are related to one or more fixed-effect independent variables when all remaining variation is appropriately allocated to a single residual error that has a Gaussian distribution. It is the most widely employed statistical model of any kind, and most methods and software for continuous data are built around it.

Let Y_i represent the response from the ith unit of observation. Assume that all levels of each of the independent variables to which inferences are to be made are included in the design so that all independent variables are fixed effects. Assume that the units of observation included in the study represent some larger population to which inferences are to be made so that the unit of observation is a random effect.

For example, suppose that a group of investigators is interested in the relationship between diastolic blood pressure and age, sex, and body mass index.

	Gaussian Distribution	Non-Gaussian Distribution
One Random Effect	General Linear Model	Generalized Linear Model
Two or More Random Effects	General Linear Mixed Model	Generalized Linear Mixed Model

Figure 4.1. A classification scheme for the four major statistical models.

The dependent variable is diastolic blood pressure, which is a continuous variable. The independent variables are age, sex, and body mass index. Let the units of observation be adults aged 24–75 drawn at random from a list of registered voters in the community.

In this situation, it is appropriate to assume that there is only one source of random variation and that the errors are distributed Gaussian. The General Linear Model assumes that each response is the sum of three components:

$$Y_i = \beta_0 + \sum_{l=1}^{c} \beta_l X_{il} + \varepsilon_i \qquad (4.1)$$

The first component is the intercept. The second component is a weighted sum of the fixed effects; the β_l are unknown parameters that must be estimated from the data, and X_{il} is the value of the lth fixed effect for the ith unit of observation. All remaining variation is attributed to the residual error (ε_i).

The expected value of the response Y_i is:

$$E(Y_i) = \mu_i = \beta_0 + \sum_{l=1}^{c} \beta_l X_{il} \qquad (4.2)$$

Under the General Linear Model, the expected value is assumed to be a linear function of the unknown parameters, here the $\beta_l (l = 1 \ldots c)$. The errors are assumed to be independently and identically distributed Gaussian with a mean of zero and a constant variance, σ_e^2.

Generalized Linear Model

The General Linear Model is not appropriate when the expected values cannot be assumed to be a linear function of the unknown parameters, as is often the case for data that have a non-Gaussian error distribution. Traditionally, such data have been dealt with via transformations (e.g., Snedecor and Cochran, 1989; Winer et al., 1991), so that the General Linear Model could be applied to the transformed data. However, that approach is not entirely satisfactory. It gives results in the transformed scale rather than in the original scale; while inverse transformations to the original scale give interpretable results in some instances, there are exceptions.[4] In addition, the transformations often don't work on the boundaries of the sample range.

The Generalized Linear Model stands as a more natural and so more satisfactory approach to the analysis of data that have a non-Gaussian error distribution. The Generalized Linear Model extends the General Linear Model in two ways. First, it expands the possible error distributions to include any distribution in the exponential family. Second, it allows the fixed-effect independent variables to be related to the expected values under any monotonic differentiable function, called the link function. Details are provided in McCullagh and Nelder (1983, 1989), and a good summary is provided in Diggle et al. (1994).

Consider the diastolic blood pressure example again. Suppose that the investigators want to study the relationship between hypertension and age, sex, and body mass index. Persons with a diastolic blood pressure at or above 90 mm Hg are classified as hypertensive and persons with a diastolic blood pressure below 90 mm Hg are classified as normotensive. The dependent variable is now a dichotomous variable, hypertension status. The independent variables are the same, as is the sampling scheme for the units of observation.

In a situation like this, it is inappropriate to assume that the residual error is distributed Gaussian or that μ_i is a linear function of the unknown parameters. The Generalized Linear Model solves this problem by assuming instead that η_i is a linear function of those parameters:

$$\eta_i = \beta_0 + \sum_{l=1}^{c} \beta_l X_{il} \tag{4.3}$$

The linear predictor η_i is connected to the expected value μ_i through some link function $g()$ so that:

$$\eta_i = g(\mu_i)$$

The inverse link function $g^{-1}()$ returns the expected value of the linear predictor to the original scale:[5]

$$\mu_i = g^{-1}(\eta_i)$$

Any monotonically differentiable function may be used to link η_i and μ_i; however, the most widely used links include the identity, log, logit, probit, reciprocal, and power links. For example, the identity link is:

$$\eta_i = \mu_i$$

This link is called the identity link because the result of the link function is identical to the operand of that function. Given this link, and the Gaussian distribution for residual error, the results from the Generalized Linear Model will be equivalent to those from the General Linear Model.

Under the General Linear Model, the variance of the Y_i was given simply as σ_e^2. The variance of any member of the exponential family of distributions can be written quite generally as:

$$\text{Var}(Y_i) = V(\mu_i)\left(\frac{\phi}{\omega_i}\right) \qquad (4.4)$$

Here $V(\mu_i)$ is a variance function that defines the residual error variance as a function of the mean. The function is chosen by selecting a distribution for the residual error from the exponential family. That family includes the binomial, Poisson, gamma, inverse Gaussian, and the Gaussian distributions. The parameter ϕ is a dispersion factor that is assumed constant over all observations; it is determined by the distribution chosen for the residual error. The weighting factor ω_i is included if appropriate; it will have a well-recognized form and take on a value that is specific for each observation.[6]

To illustrate, consider the General Linear Model. Here, the analyst would select the Gaussian distribution for the residual error. Because the variance is constant in the Gaussian distribution, it is not a function of the mean and so the variance function is defined as $V(\mu_i) = 1$. Because the measure of dispersion in the Gaussian distribution is σ_e^2, the dispersion factor is defined as $\phi = \sigma_e^2$.

For each of the distributions in the exponential family, there exists a particular link, called the canonical link, that offers desirable properties (McCullagh and Nelder, 1989). As a result, the canonical links are used as the default links in many computer programs. As McCullagh and Nelder (1989) point out, the canonical links won't always provide the best-fitting model, but they often do.

The canonical link for the Gaussian distribution is the identity link. Under the Generalized Linear Model, this combination performs linear regression that is equivalent to that provided under the General Linear Model. The canonical link for the binomial distribution is the logit link. This combination is often appropriate for dichotomous data and performs logistic regression. The canonical link for the Poisson distribution is the log link. This combination is often appropriate for count data where the mean and variance are equal and performs Poisson regression.

General Linear Mixed Model

Neither the General nor the Generalized Linear Model is appropriate when there are multiple sources of random variation. The General Linear Mixed Model (Donner, 1984a, 1985; Harville, 1977; Laird and Ware, 1982; Laird et al., 1987; Stiratelli et al., 1984; Ware, 1985) provides a natural solution by extending the General Linear Model to allow multiple random effects. Littell et al. (1996) provide a good overview of the General Linear Mixed Model and review many of its general applications.

Consider the diastolic blood pressure example again. Suppose that the sample had not been drawn using a simple random sample from the voter registration list. Suppose instead that the community had been divided into blocks, and that a simple random sample of blocks had been chosen in a first stage. Suppose then that a simple random sample of adults aged 25–74 years had been chosen from each of the selected blocks. Persons drawn from the same block will be more similar to one another than to persons from other blocks. This positive intraclass correlation reflects the presence of two sources of random variation in the data: the blocks and residual error.

In a situation such as this, it is inappropriate to assume that there is only a single source of random variation. The General Linear Mixed Model solves this problem by assuming that each observation is the sum of four components:

$$Y_i = \beta_0 + \sum_{l=1}^{c} \beta_l X_{il} + \sum_{j=1}^{g} b_j Z_{ij} + \varepsilon_i \tag{4.5}$$

The first component is the intercept. The second component is a weighted sum of the fixed effects; the β_l are unknown parameters that must be estimated from the data, and X_{il} is the value of the lth fixed effect for the ith unit of observation. The third is a weighted sum of the random effects; the b_j are unknown parameters that must be estimated from the data, and Z_{ij} is the value of the jth random effect for the ith unit of observation. The final component, ε_i, is the residual error.

The expected value of the response Y_i is conditional on the random effects. Given b_j, the expected value is:

$$E(Y_i|b_j) = \mu_i = \beta_0 + \sum_{l=1}^{c} \beta_l X_{il} + \sum_{j=1}^{g} b_j Z_{ij} \tag{4.6}$$

Under the General Linear Mixed Model, the expected value is assumed to be a linear function of the unknown parameters, here the fixed effects $\beta_l (l=1 \ldots c)$ and the random effects $b_j (j=1 \ldots g)$.

The random effects, including residual error, are assumed to be independently and identically distributed Gaussian with means of zero and constant variance. As in the General Linear Model, the residual-error variance is not a function of the mean.

Generalized Linear Mixed Model

None of the previous models is appropriate when the data have a non-Gaussian error distribution and multiple sources of random variation. The Generalized Linear Mixed Model (Breslow and Clayton, 1993; Wolfinger and O'Connell, 1993) provides a solution by combining the extensions of the General Linear Model that define the Generalized Linear Model and the General Linear Mixed Model.

Suppose that the investigators have drawn the sample for the blood pressure study using the two-stage sampling scheme. This would mean that there were two sources of random variation in the data: block and residual error. But now suppose that they want to examine the relationship between hypertension status and age, sex, and body mass index.

In a situation such as this, it is inappropriate to assume that there is a single source or random variation, that the residual error distribution is Gaussian, or that μ_i is a linear function of the parameters. The Generalized Linear Mixed Model solves this problem by assuming that η_i is a linear function of both the fixed- and random-effect parameters:

$$\eta_i = \beta_0 + \sum_{l=1}^{c} \beta_l X_{il} + \sum_{j=1}^{g} b_j Z_{ij} \qquad (4.7)$$

As in the Generalized Linear Model, the linear predictor η_i is connected to the expected value μ_i through some link function $g()$ so that:

$$\eta_i = g(\mu_i)$$

The inverse link function $g^{-1}()$ returns the expected value of the linear predictor to the original scale:

$$\mu_i = g^{-1}(\eta_i)$$

As in the Generalized Linear Model, any monotonically differentiable function may be used to link η_i and μ_i.

The general form of the variance of Y_i is written as:

$$\mathrm{Var}(Y_i|b_j) = V(\mu_i|b_j)\left(\frac{\phi}{\omega_i}\right) \qquad (4.8)$$

Here $V(\mu_i|b_j)$ is the variance function for the residual error; it is conditional on the other random effects in the model. In the Generalized Linear Model, the variance function was selected by specifying an error distribution for the data. That model was appropriate only for data with an error distribution from the exponential family and only for data with a single random effect. Wedderburn (1974) observed that the estimating equations used to fit the Generalized Linear Model could be solved even without specifying the entire distribution. Instead, all that was required was specification of the link and variance functions. This offered the opportunity to extend the Generalized Linear Model to a broader set of problems involving data whose error distribution could not be specified or that did not match a distribution from the exponential family, including problems involving multiple random effects. Thus, in the Generalized Linear Mixed Model, the analyst specifies link and variance functions but does not specify the entire distribution for the residual error.

The parameters ϕ and ω_i are interpreted as in the Generalized Linear Model. The parameter ϕ is a dispersion factor that is assumed constant over all observations; it is determined by the variance function chosen for the residual error. The weighting factor ω_i is included if appropriate; it will have a well-recognized form and take on a value that is specific for each observation.

Under the Generalized Linear Mixed Model, the identity link combined with the variance function for the Gaussian distribution performs linear mixed-model regression identical to that provided under the General Linear Mixed Model. The logit link combined with the variance function for the binomial distribution performs logistic mixed-model regression. The log link combined with the variance function for the Poisson distribution performs Poisson mixed-model regression. Additional details are provided in Littell et al. (1996).

Models Appropriate for Group-Randomized Trials

Given the assumptions underlying the four general models presented above, single-stage analyses based strictly on the General Linear Model and the Generalized Linear Model are not appropriate for group-randomized trials, as they do not allow multiple random effects. If used, they can yield Type I error rates that are well above the nominal level. At the same time, analyses based on the General Linear Model and the Generalized Linear Model can be used in the context of two-stage analyses, discussed below. They can also be used in conjunction with methods that will correct for variance inflation either during the analysis or *post hoc,* also discussed below.

Group-randomized trials that involve endpoints that have Gaussian error distributions may be analyzed using methods based on the General Linear Mixed Model. Trials that involve endpoints that have non-Gaussian error distributions may be analyzed using methods based on the Generalized Linear Mixed Model. If properly implemented, such analyses will yield Type I error rates at the nominal level.

There is another line of reasoning and some empirical evidence to support the use of the General Linear Mixed Model for the analysis of data from a group-randomized trial even if the observation-level data have non-Gaussian errors. Consider that whenever there is a moderate number of members in each group, the errors associated with an analysis of group means are expected to be distributed approximately Gaussian by the Central Limit Theorem, even if the observation-level errors are decidedly non-Gaussian. Because a mixed-model analysis assesses the variation of the condition means against the variation of the group means, one would expect that the Central Limit Theorem might allow use of methods based on the General Linear Mixed Model, even when the observation-level errors were non-Gaussian.

Hannan and Murray (1996) recently tested this approach using Monte Carlo simulation methods. They compared analyses based on the Generalized Linear Mixed Model and the General Linear Mixed Model when applied to the data simulated from a very simple group-randomized trial. They varied the magnitude of the intraclass correlation, the prevalence rate of the dichotomous endpoint, and the number of groups per condition; the number of members per group was fixed at 30. Across all their combinations, the analyses based on the General Linear Mixed Model gave Type I and II error rates that were equivalent to those obtained using the Generalized Linear Mixed Model. Hannan and Murray (1996) concluded that as long as there is a moderate number of observations per group and groups per condition, the General Linear Mixed Model provides an appropriate analysis for data from a group-randomized trial, even if the observation-level errors are not Gaussian. Donner and Klar (1996) came to the same conclusion in a separate study.

At this point, it is not known whether this pattern will hold for other non-Gaussian distributions, such as Poisson, though the Central Limit Theorem suggests that it would. Additional studies are needed to further define the boundaries for proper application of the General Linear Mixed Model to data from group-randomized trials involving non-Gaussian errors.

Technical Issues Related to Statistical Models

Estimation of Model Parameters

Whatever the statistical model, exact values for parameters of interest are rarely available. They can be computed only when data are available for the entire population of interest, but most studies are based on samples. Under these conditions, the analyst must estimate the parameters in the model from the sampled data.

A good estimate is both unbiased and precise. An estimate is considered unbiased if the expected value of its sampling distribution is equal to the parameter of interest, and it is considered precise if it has a small standard error. The goal of the analyst is to identify a method that sufficiently limits bias while providing enough precision. Related characteristics are consistency and efficiency. An estimate is consistent if it approaches zero bias with increasing sample size. An estimate is efficient if its standard error is not much larger than that of the most precise estimate. Often these characteristics are achieved asymptotically—that is, when the sample size is large—but may not be achieved in smaller samples.

There are many methods to estimate parameters of interest, and no method is better under all conditions than the other methods. This section will provide a brief review of many of the methods now in use.

Least Squares

Ordinary least squares (OLS). Ordinary least-squares estimation minimizes the sum of squared deviations between the observed data and some function of the parameters estimated from the data. In the common multiple-regression application, OLS minimizes the sum of the squared deviations of the observed data from the predicted values. If the residual errors are independent and identically distributed Gaussian, the OLS estimate is both unbiased and has minimum variance.

Weighted least squares (WLS). OLS assumes that the variance is constant across observations. Weighted least squares is often used when that assumption is not appropriate, such as when the sample sizes vary from cell to cell in the design. The best weight in terms of precision is the inverse of the variance. With the assumption that the variance is constant apart from variations in cell sample size, each cell can be weighted by the inverse of the sample size. WLS then minimizes the weighted sum of the squared deviations between the observed data and the predicted values.

Iterative reweighted least squares (IRLS). In some situations, the variance is related to the parameter being estimated, and so cannot be assumed constant apart from cell sample size. Here not only must a weighted approach be used, but the weights must be recalculated each time the parameters are estimated until the estimates converge to stable values. This method is often called iterative reweighted least squares.

Generalized least squares (GLS). When there is more than one random effect in the model, OLS and its weighted variations are no longer appropriate. OLS estimates of the random effects will be good approximations if the extra variation attributable to the additional random effects is quite small relative to the residual error, but they will become increasingly biased toward zero as that extra variation increases. GLS accommodates multiple random-effects; unfortunately, the simple GLS requires that the random effect parameters be known. When such information is not available, the investigator must estimate those random effects as well as any fixed effects in the model.

Iterative generalized least squares (IGLS). IGLS is one approach available when the investigator must estimate multiple random effects in addition to any fixed effects. Initially, the fixed effects are estimated using OLS or WLS. Then the random effects are estimated from the residuals computed between the observed data and the predicted values computed from the first iteration. The estimates of the random effects are then used in the second iteration to obtain a second set of estimates of the fixed effects, which in turn provide a second set of residuals from which to estimate the random effects. This process continues until the estimates of the fixed and random effects converge to within some predetermined criterion. The estimates of IGLS are consistent and equivalent to maximum-likelihood estimates if the residuals have a Gaussian distribution (Goldstein, 1987).

Maximum Likelihood

Maximum-likelihood estimation seeks estimates that maximize the probability that the values predicted by the estimates agree with the data observed in the study. Quite often, least-squares and maximum-likelihood estimation converge to the same result in a large sample with a Gaussian error distribution. Indeed, under the Gaussian assumption, least-squares estimates are maximum-likelihood estimates, even in finite samples.

Maximum likelihood (ML). In maximum-likelihood estimation, a likelihood function is required to specify the probability distribution of the data as a function of a set of parameters. For balanced data, the values of those parameters are often available directly. For unbalanced data, the values for those parameters are usually obtained by iterative numerical analysis such that the parameter set maximizes the agreement between the observed and predicted values. ML estimates are both consistent and asymptotically efficient. In addition, as the sample size grows large, the sampling distributions of ML estimates become approximately Gaussian.

When ML methods are used to estimate both fixed and random effects, the fixed effects are explicitly involved in the estimation of the random effects. If the fixed effects are not well described by the model, not only will they be poorly estimated, but as a result the random effects also will be poorly estimated. The usual approach to solving this problem is to overspecify the fixed effects in the model, so as to get consistent estimators of the random effects. Unfortunately, this may mean that there are many parameters to be estimated. If the number of parameters is large relative to the number of observations, the random effects will be biased toward zero and the standard errors for the fixed effects will be too small. This can lead to deflated p-values and overstatement of the significance of the findings.

Restricted maximum likelihood (REML). Restricted maximum-likelihood estimation separates the estimation of the fixed and random effects. As a result, REML avoids the problem described above for the ML methods. REML estimates are unbiased and more accurate than ML estimates, as the number of fixed effects is large relative to the number of observations. At the same time, REML often yields a larger mean-square error and so is often less efficient. For balanced data, REML and least-squares estimation yield identical results.

Quasi-Likelihood

There will be occasions where it is not possible to specify the probability distribution of the data as a function of a set of parameters, as is required with ML and REML methods. This will occur, for example, when there are multiple random effects and the data are non-Gaussian, or when the data are not from a member of the exponential family. In these cases, methods based on quasi-likelihood have proven useful.

There is a growing set of estimation methods that fall into this category. Indeed, the set is growing so rapidly that the set presented here cannot be viewed as exhaustive. Instead, this set is intended to convey the flavor of the estimation methods now developing under the rubric of quasi-likelihood.

Quasi-likelihood (QL). As Wedderburn (1974) noted, if one is willing to specify the mean as a function of a set of predictors via a link function, and the variance as a function of the mean via a variance function, then one can estimate the parameters using the score equations from the Generalized Linear Model even without specifying the entire distribution. This approach is termed quasi-likelihood, as the solutions are not stated in terms of a true likelihood function. The QL approach will give the same results as ML if the data are actually from a member of the exponential family and the variance link is correctly specified (McCullagh and Nelder, 1989).

Penalized quasi-likelihood (PQL). In penalized quasi-likelihood (Breslow and Clayton, 1993), the quasi-likelihood is increased by a penalty term based on the assumed structure of the covariance matrix. The PQL approach then seeks a set of parameter estimates that will both maximize the agreement between the observed and predicted values and minimize the penalty term. Minimizing the penalty term serves to shrink the individual deviations from the parameter estimates toward zero and produces what are sometimes called "shrinkage" estimates of the random effects.

Penalized quasi-likelihood with extra-dispersion (PQL+). PQL, as presented by Breslow and Clayton (1993), assumes that the variance observed in the data is equal to the theoretical variance given by the variance function. In practice, the observed variance is often larger or smaller than the theoretical variance. The departure from the theoretical variance is often termed extra-dispersion, though it can be negative as well as positive. Wolfinger and O'Connell (1993) describe an estimation procedure that is equivalent to PQL but allows the extra-dispersion in the data to be estimated and incorporated into the analysis. They originally labeled their estimation method as Restricted Pseudo-Likelihood (REPL), but it also may be labeled as PQL with extra-dispersion, or PQL +.

Marginal quasi-likelihood (MQL). Marginal quasi-likelihood is focused on the marginal relationships between the fixed effects and the endpoint. The link function is specified for the marginal mean and the variance function is also specified based on the marginal mean. Unless the link function is the identity link, the regression coefficients from the MQL will differ from those based on PQL. Under MQL, the regression coefficient will express the change in the population average per unit change in the predictor variable, scaled according to the link function.

Marginal quasi-likelihood with extra-dispersion (MQL+). MQL, as presented by Breslow and Clayton (1993), also assumes that the variance observed in the data is equal to the theoretical variance given by the variance function. As noted above, the observed variance is often larger or smaller than the theoretical variance. MQL + allows the extra-dispersion to be estimated and incorporated into the analysis that otherwise employs MQL.

Estimation of Standard Errors

Any model-based analysis involving two conditions will compare an estimate of the intervention effect to an estimate of the standard error for that intervention effect, with reference to a distribution deemed appropriate for that test statistic. The model for the analysis will vary from study to study depending on the design, the endpoints, and the orientation of the analyst. Regardless of the model, the analyst will need an estimate of the standard error for the intervention effect.

Just as there is no one way to design a group-randomized trial and no one way to analyze its data, there are many alternative methods available for estimation of standard errors. The methods can be divided into two general categories: nonparametric methods and parametric methods. Parametric methods make some assumption about the distribution of the random effects, while nonparametric methods do not. Many of the nonparametric methods are based on variance estimation procedures developed for survey data. Others are based on approximations that are asymptotically consistent. Parametric methods are based on inclusion of design characteristics such as strata or clusters in the model itself.

The nonparametric methods may offer benefits in terms of being robust to violations of the assumptions required for the parametric methods, but they may become unstable if they are based on only a few degrees of freedom, as is often the case in group-randomized trials (Skinner et al., 1989). The parametric methods may not be as robust to violations of their underlying assumptions, but often will be more stable.

Nonparametric Methods

Survey methods. A number of nonparametric methods to estimate standard errors were developed for the analysis of data based on complex sampling designs. Such designs may include multilevel stratification and/or cluster sampling, often in combination with simple random sampling within strata or clusters. The sampling may be done with or without replacement, with equal or unequal selection probabilities, from different sampling frames, etc. Survey samplers recognized long ago that standard-error estimation methods based strictly on simple random sampling were inappropriate under more complex sampling schemes, and sought instead to have the estimation methods reflect the complexity of their survey designs (Kish, 1965). The nonparametric methods evolved as survey samplers struggled as well with the often limited number of strata, clusters, or sampling units available in a given survey, since those design limits often meant few degrees of freedom were available for estimation of standard errors. The parallels between their situation and the usual circumstances extant in a group-randomized trial should be obvious.

The primary nonparametric methods developed for survey data include simple replication (sometimes called the method of random groups), balanced repeat replication (sometimes called the method of balanced half samples), jackknife, bootstrap, and Taylor-series linearization. Of necessity, these methods will be reviewed in general terms here, and the reader is referred to more technical references for additional detail (Wolter, 1985; Efron, 1982; Skinner et al., 1989).

The first four methods are all based on the idea of resampling the data and assessing variation between the samples and the original data set. The four methods differ in the way in which the resampling is done (e.g., with or without replacement, full-size samples or subsamples, etc.) and in the way the variation of the sample estimates relative to the estimate from the original data set is computed. They are generally employed when the parameter of interest is a nonlinear statistic, such as a ratio or regression coefficient, since they offer no computational advantage for linear statistics such as means or differences among means.

The fifth method is the Taylor-series linearization method; it, too, is used for nonlinear statistics. This method differs from the first four in that it does not rely on resampling the data. Instead, a Taylor-series expansion is used to approximate the nonlinear statistic by a linear statistic. In a second step, the standard error of that linear approximation is estimated, usually with standard methods for linear statistics.

Regardless of the method used, once the standard error estimate is available, it is used to assess the significance of the parameter of interest, usually with reference to the standard normal distribution.

Substantial research has been conducted over the last 30 years to assess the utility of these survey methods for estimation of standard errors, and there is wide agreement on several points. In general, these methods will converge to the same result with large numbers of subsamples each based on a large number of clusters. However, as the number of clusters per subsample and the number of subsamples declines, the magnitude of the estimated standard error increases, often well beyond the true value. For example, Skinner et al. (1989, p. 52) note that the estimated standard error may be many times too large when there are only a few clusters per subsample. At the same time, the standard normal approximation will no longer be appropriate when the number of clusters is small, since this corresponds to few degrees of freedom; the t-distribution may often be used in this situation, with df based on the number of clusters (Skinner et al., 1989, p. 57). Finally, the variability of the nonparametric standard errors increases as the number of clusters decreases. The implication for group-randomized trials is not good, given that the cluster in the survey is equivalent to the group in the trial. Many group-randomized trials have only a few groups per condition, and these nonparametric methods for standard error estimation may provide little relief in those cases. Given enough groups per condition, these methods can be expected to give unbiased and reasonably precise estimates of the standard errors.

At this point, it is not possible to define a number of groups per condition below which these survey methods perform poorly and above which they perform well. Indeed, it is not likely that such a clear line of demarcation will ever be possible. Simulation studies would help to clarify the conditions under which these methods may be applied appropriately to data from group-randomized trials.

Empirical-sandwich estimation. Zeger and Liang (1986) introduced a formula that provides robust standard-error estimates based on "sandwiching" an approximate correlation matrix inside two outer layers of matrix algebra that otherwise define the variance of a WLS estimator. Liang and Zeger (1986) incorporated this "sandwich" estimation of standard errors as a central component in their generalized estimating equations (GEE) approach to analysis of correlated data, described later in this chapter. In their original papers, they referred to this method as "robust-sandwich" estimation. More recently, they recognized that the method is robust only asymptotically, and have adopted the label "empirical-sandwich" estimation.

Diggle et al. (1994) provide a good description of this method. Normally, a saturated model can be fit via IRLS for the fixed effects. In that case, WLS is used to estimate an approximate or "working" correlation matrix. If the design includes time-varying covariates, or if the values of time vary among conditions, a saturated model via IRLS for the fixed effects may not be possible. In that case, the fixed effects are modeled in as complex a fashion as is deemed appropriate, and REML is used to estimate the working correlation matrix. Either way, the working correlation matrix is used as the center in the empirical-sandwich formula to estimate the standard errors for the fixed effects. The empirical-sandwich formula is asymptotically consistent against misspecification of the correlation matrix, which is why the method was initially labeled as robust. The chief advantages of the method are that it is asymptotically robust and that the WLS estimation that is the default for the working correlation matrix is quite simple.

Two recent reports suggest that the empirical-sandwich estimator is not appropriate in the context of most group-randomized trials. A paper by Thornquist and Anderson (1992) on the small sample properties of GEEs in group-randomized trials reported that confidence intervals based on the empirical sandwich standard errors and the Gaussian distribution were too narrow. Remediation required use of the *t*-distribution with degrees of freedom based on the number of groups allocated to each condition. More recently, Murray et al. (in press) reported that empirical-sandwich estimation resulted in a very unreliable Type I error rate across a range of conditions common to group-randomized trials when the number of groups per condition was 10 or fewer. As the number of groups per condition increased, the performance of the empirical-sandwich estimator improved, so that when there were 20 or more groups per condition, the Type I error rate was at the nominal level.

Parametric Methods

Parametric methods of standard error estimation derive from the parametric methods for analysis of data, including most regression methods. As a result, the method for estimating the standard error will depend on the method underlying the analysis. The suitability of standard errors based on these parametric methods will of course depend on the suitability of the model fit to the data, which is generally considered in terms of the degree to which the assumptions underlying that model are met in the data at hand. Relative to the nonparametric methods, parametric methods will be more efficient if the model is correctly specified (Diggle et al., 1994). At the same time, they may be more biased if the model is misspecified. Parametric methods for estimation of standard errors are illustrated in Chapters 5 through 8.

Sampling Distributions and Degrees of Freedom

Model-based analyses require that the analyst compare the observed value of a test statistic against the sampling distribution for that test statistic in order to determine how likely it would be for a value of that magnitude to occur by chance. This section will focus on methods for choosing an appropriate sampling distribution and the closely related issue of choosing the appropriate degrees of freedom.

Methods That Do Not Explicitly Involve df

The analyst may be willing to assume that the sampling distribution of the test statistic has a particular form and move directly to compare the observed value against the critical value in the assumed distribution. The critical value is selected such that values that large or larger would be observed only as often as allowed by the specified Type I error rate, usually 5%. With this approach, degrees of freedom are not an issue.

The asymptotic Gaussian approximation. The simplest variation of this approach is to assume that the test statistic is asymptotically Gaussian and reference it to the standard Gaussian or standard normal distribution. If the absolute value of the test statistic exceeds 1.96, the result is declared significant at the 5% level (two-tailed).

This approach is the default method in many computer programs, including many that implement analyses based on multilevel analyses, GEEs, and mixed-model regression. For example, if the method yields a regression coefficient and asymptotic standard error, the p-value may be computed by assessing the ratio of the estimate to its standard error against a Gaussian distribution.

Application of these methods to a group-randomized trial presumes that what is true asymptotically is true in the group-randomized trial at hand. Unfortunately, that presumption is often inappropriate, especially when the design involves a limited number of groups allocated to each study condition. Warnings to this effect are included in texts on multilevel analysis (e.g., Bryk and Raudenbush, 1992, pp. 220–224) and in texts on analysis of complex survey samples (e.g., Skinner et al., 1989, pp. 55–57). Those warnings apply equally to the analysis of group-randomized trials.

The core problem is quite simple. Whenever the standard error is estimated, that estimate will include some error. As a result, the sampling distribution of the test statistic will be wider than the standard Gaussian distribution. Large values of the test statistic are more likely under an estimated sampling distribution than they would be under the standard Gaussian distribution. As a result, it is more likely that the null hypothesis will be rejected when the test statistic is assessed against the standard Gaussian distribution than if it were assessed against a sampling distribution that reflects the error of the estimate.

The magnitude of the problem depends largely on the number of independent units that are used to estimate the standard error. In a group-randomized trial, the only units that are independent are the groups. As the number of groups approaches infinity, the sampling distribution of the test statistic will approach a Gaussian distribution, regardless of the original form. As a result, when the number of groups is quite large, the Gaussian approximation will yield results that are approximately correct. However, when that number is small, the Gaussian approximation will often yield p-values that are too small and confidence intervals that are too narrow.

Thornquist and Anderson's (1992) paper on the small-sample properties of GEEs in group-randomized designs provides a good illustration of this point. They reported that confidence intervals computed with the asymptotic standard errors and the Gaussian distribution were too narrow. Remediation required use of the t-distribution with degrees of freedom based on the number of groups allocated to each condition.

Building the sampling distribution. Rather than assume that the sampling distribution of the test statistic is Gaussian, another approach is to build the sampling distribution of that statistic. This is essentially what is done in the survey-sampling methods of computing standard errors. The various replication and linearization methods actually generate an estimate of the sampling distribution for the test statistic of interest, then assess the probability that a test statistic as large as observed would occur under that estimated sampling distribution. The advantage of this method is that it can be used regardless of the shape of the true sampling distribution. To the extent that the sampling distribution is well estimated, the resulting probabilities and confidence intervals will be unbiased.

Despite the intuitive simplicity of this approach, investigators must remember that it is still based on an estimate of the sampling distribution of the standard error. That estimate is also subject to error at a rate that is inversely related to the number of independent observations. Indeed, Skinner et al. (1989) reported that some survey-sampling methods gave extraordinarily conservative results when the number of independent units was quite small. However, given a sufficient number of groups per condition, it will be possible to build a sampling distribution for the test statistic that will provide an accurate estimate of the probability of the observed result. Additional simulation studies may clarify the conditions under which this approach may be applied appropriately to group-randomization studies.

Methods That Explicitly Involve df

Known distribution with df appropriate to the model. Another approach to identifying the correct sampling distribution is to work with a known distribution, such as a t-, F- or chi-square distribution, with degrees of freedom chosen appropriate to the model. Here degrees of freedom reflect the uncertainty or imprecision of the standard error, with greater uncertainty associated with fewer degrees of freedom. In general, the degrees of freedom will be the number of groups minus the number of parameters estimated in the model, though covariates measured at the member level usually will not affect df computed at the group level. If the sampling distribution follows a t-, F-, or chi-square distribution with the chosen degrees of freedom, then the Type I error rate will be at the nominal level when the test statistic is assessed against that distribution.

The choice of the appropriate distribution depends on the test statistic. A ratio of a sample mean or regression coefficient to its standard error will have a sampling distribution that is t, with degrees of freedom equal to the number of groups minus the number of group-level parameters estimated in the model. A ratio of mean squares will have a sampling distribution that is F, with numerator degrees of freedom equal to one less than the number of levels of the term of interest and denominator degrees of freedom equal to the number of groups minus the number of parameters estimated in the model.

Methods appropriate for *post hoc* corrections. Skinner et al. (1989) provide a detailed discussion of the use of *post hoc* corrections for analyses that otherwise ignore the unit of assignment. These methods generally require the investigator to estimate the *VIF,* defined in Chapter 1. The *VIF* is then used to correct the inflation in the test statistic generated in the member-level analysis. Test statistics such as *F-* and chi-square tests are corrected by dividing the test by *VIF.* Test statistics such as a *t-* or *z*-test are corrected by dividing the test by the square root of the *VIF.* The resulting test statistic is approximately correct if the estimate of the *VIF* is valid for the data at hand, but that test statistic must still be assessed against an appropriate distribution with appropriate degrees of freedom.

The *VIF* may be computed based on either an internal or an external estimate of the *ICC.* Since external estimates are rarely available, it is more common to estimate the *ICC* from the data at hand. The precision of such an internal estimate is determined by the number of groups included in the study. As a result, Skinner et al. (1989) recommended that the degrees of freedom for internally adjusted tests be computed based on the number of groups, not the number of members. Skinner's suggestion leads to degrees of freedom that are equivalent to those that would be obtained as described in the previous section.

Some years earlier, an alternative was suggested by Kish (1965). He suggested computing what he termed effective degrees of freedom by dividing the observation-level degrees of freedom by *VIF.* The test statistic would then be assessed against the effective degrees of freedom. Kish's suggestion has intuitive appeal, as it would scale the degrees of freedom in the same way that the test statistic is scaled. It would often provide a substantial advantage, since the effective degrees of freedom are likely to be greater than the group-level degrees of freedom. Unfortunately, a recent simulation study suggests that for a typical group-randomized trial, effective degrees of freedom yield Type I error rates that are as inflated as those based on observation-level degrees of freedom (Murray et al., 1996). Given that finding, effective degrees of freedom cannot be recommended.

Where an external estimate of the intraclass correlation is available, the *VIF* may be computed with that estimate. If the external estimate can be accepted as a population value, the degrees of freedom can be computed based on the number of observation units (Blair and Higgins, 1986). However, this approach rests on a very strong assumption—that the external estimate is the population value. Investigators should be able to defend that assumption based on considerable experience and data, and be quite cautious in making such a strong assumption in the absence of such experience or data.

Where the investigator has an external estimate of the intraclass correlation but is unwilling to assume that it is a population value, Hannan et al. (1994) suggested that the degrees of freedom be computed based on the precision of the external estimate, with a lower bound determined by the number of groups and the upper bound determined by the number of members. They labeled the estimated degrees of freedom as df^*. This strategy also presumes that the external estimate is valid for the population and circumstances of the study at hand, but does not assume that the external estimate is a population parameter.

The Unit of Analysis in Statistical Models

The phrase *unit of analysis* is the source of much confusion in the context of group-randomized trials.[7] This section will consider both the origin and the meaning of the phrase. It also will review the debate that continues over what the unit of analysis should be in a group-randomized trial. Finally, it will suggest that the attention now given to the unit of analysis is misplaced, and that attention should be focused instead on proper specification of the model for the analysis.

The Confusion

Part of the confusion arises from the fact that there are often so many units from which to choose that investigators and analysts alike may easily and unknowingly choose badly. There are different units of assignment and units of observation. Often there also are units of intervention that differ from both the units of observation and assignment. In some cases, there may be easily defined subunits within the units of assignment, intervention, or observation.

School-based studies provide a good example. Here, schools are allocated to study conditions, making them the unit of assignment. Interventions may be delivered in health classes, making those classes the unit of intervention. Students are usually the primary source of data, making the student the primary unit of observation. At the same time, some data may also be collected at the level of the classroom, the teacher, the school, or the community, so that those sources may also be units of observation. So which unit or subunit is the unit of analysis?

Another source of confusion is that there are many different ways to conduct the analysis. Consider the school-based trial. If the analysis is limited entirely to data from students, does that make the student the unit of analysis? If classroom means are computed first, so that the main analysis is conducted on those means, does that make the classroom the unit of analysis? If data from individual students, classrooms, teachers, and schools are all included in a single analysis, which of those units is the unit of analysis?

Another source of confusion is the intent of the investigators. Most would say that they want to draw inferences about the effect of the intervention program on students like those included in the study. Does that make the student the unit of analysis? Some might want to draw inferences about the effect of the intervention program in other schools like those included in the study. Does that make the school the unit of analysis?

In truth, the proper unit of analysis is determined entirely by the design of the study, including the selection and allocation schemes for groups and members. But the unit of analysis is operationalized in terms of the model specified for the analysis. A unit is the unit of analysis for an effect if and only if that effect is assessed against the variation among those units. It will not matter whether the unit in question is the unit of observation, assignment, or intervention. It will not matter if there are other units represented in the analysis, at either higher or lower levels of aggregation, except as they contribute to the variation of the unit of analysis. And it will not matter what the investigators' intentions are, except as they guide the research design and the specification of the model for the analysis. The only thing that will matter in the determination of the unit of analysis for a particular effect in a particular analysis is the model for that analysis. That model will determine the construction of both the effect and its standard error, and in so doing, the unit of analysis.

The Debate

The debate has focused on what should be the proper unit of analysis for a group-randomized trial. Analysts have argued that the unit of assignment must be the unit of analysis in order to have a valid analysis. As a result, much pressure has come from analysts, including the author, who have urged their colleagues to employ the unit of assignment as the unit of analysis (e.g., Murray, McKinlay et al., 1994).

The basis for this position is that the units of assignment are the only units to be randomized to the study conditions. Because randomization assures independence of errors, that assumption is appropriate only for the units of assignment. According to this position, an analysis conducted at the level of the unit of assignment will carry the nominal Type I error rate, whereas analyses conducted at lower levels in the study hierarchy will carry an inflated Type I error rate. Several simulation studies have reported results consistent with that pattern, providing additional support for this position (Zucker, 1990; Murray et al., 1996; Murray and Wolfinger, 1994).

On the other side of the debate are those who do not want to employ models that specify the unit of assignment as the unit of analysis. Some have resisted because they fear substantial loss of statistical power. As noted in Chapter 1, power almost always will be lower when the unit of assignment, rather than the unit of observation, is the unit of analysis. Some investigators will argue that it doesn't make sense to conduct an analysis that is certain to have low power. Others will argue that it doesn't make sense to do an analysis that is likely to have a high Type I error rate. Both groups are right in their arguments.

Others have resisted because they want to take advantage of the information that is available on the different kinds of units represented in the data. For example, they might argue against an analysis of school means because they want to make adjustment for factors measured at the level of the student. Or they might argue against an analysis of school means because they are interested in sex-specific analyses and want to stratify on the sex of the student. Either way, they would be right in their arguments.

Others have resisted because they didn't work through the issues fully at the time they designed their study and don't want to abandon their project at the analysis stage. They might argue that their study was not designed to support an analysis at the level of the unit of assignment. And they would be right in their argument.

The issue is not whether those who have resisted are right in their arguments, but instead whether they are right in their proposed solutions. Investigators are wrong if they go forward with an analysis known to have a Type I error rate measurably greater than the nominal level. To do so is to risk overstating the significance of the result and misleading the scientists and policy makers who attend to that result. To knowingly conduct and report such an analysis is a clear violation of common standards for scientific conduct and must be discouraged in the strongest possible terms. Investigators do themselves, the research community, and particularly policy makers a substantial disservice when they use inappropriate methods, draw erroneous conclusions, and cause others to waste resources in pursuit of false leads.

Investigators are wrong if they go forward with a study that cannot have adequate power for a proper analysis. To do so is to waste both time and resources, both for themselves and for their sponsors and colleagues. That, too, must be strongly discouraged.

Finally, investigators are wrong if they ignore valuable information at any level in their data in the belief that it cannot be put to good use. Modern methods allow use of data at all levels of a group-randomized trial, while still protecting the validity of the analysis.

A Different Focus

> The question of the proper . . . unit of analysis . . . is answered directly, correctly and implicitly when the proper statistical model is employed.
>
> Hopkins (1982), p. 17

Unfortunately, the focus on the use of the unit of assignment as the unit of analysis has missed entirely the point that this is a necessary but not a sufficient condition for a proper analysis in a group-randomized trial. For many trials, there are several different analytic models that define the unit of assignment as the unit of analysis. However, not all of those models are well matched to the underlying structure of the data. It is important to account for the multiple sources of random variation expected in the data, but also to properly model the structure of the covariance matrix that is defined by those sources.

The focus should be on the selection and proper implementation of a model that is well matched to the underlying structure of the data. Under those conditions, the assumptions underlying the model are satisfied and the analysis will have the nominal Type I error rate. If the study is large enough, it will have adequate power to detect the intervention effect postulated for the trial. If the design and analysis are efficient, the cost of the study will be minimized. If the significance of the research question warrants that cost and the sponsors are satisfied that the trial as proposed can answer the question, the trial should go forward.[8]

For any single trial, there may be several different strategies that can be used to obtain a model that is well matched to the underlying structure of the data. Analysts can choose among those strategies based on familiarity, availability of resources, personal preference, and the like. Of course, the analyst must ensure that the strategy is properly implemented so that the resulting model will in fact be well matched to the data.

General Strategies for Model-Based Inference

Poor Strategies

There are several strategies for the analysis of group-randomized trials that are almost certain to be poorly matched to the underlying structure of the data. As such, they threaten the validity of the analysis through misspecification of the analytic model, either because the analyst has ignored a measurable source of random variation, misrepresented a measurable source of random variation, or misrepresented the pattern of over-time correlation in the data.

These strategies usually carry an inflated Type I error rate; the level of inflation can be substantial. While it is possible for these methods to yield a Type I error rate close to the nominal level, simulation studies have shown that this will not occur under conditions common to most group-randomized trials (Zucker, 1990; Murray et al., 1996; Murray and Wolfinger, 1994).

Analyses That Ignore the Group

This strategy does not include the group in the analysis in any form. As a result, the analysis is based on the General Linear Model and the variation among the conditions is assessed against the average variation within conditions. This strategy maximizes the degrees of freedom for the standard error of the estimate of the intervention effect, since there usually will be many more members than groups. In turn, this often serves to improve power. While that feature may make this strategy appear attractive, it is simply wrong. It leads inevitably to a Type I error rate that is higher than the nominal level, with the magnitude of that inflation directly related both to the magnitude of the intraclass correlation and the number of members per group. Because this strategy cannot yield a valid analysis under conditions commonly found in group-randomized trials, it should not be used.

Analyses That Include the Group as a Nested Fixed Effect

Sometimes the group is included in the analysis as a nested fixed effect in the belief that this will "account" for variation due to the groups. When the group is treated as a fixed effect, the analysis is again based on the General Linear Model and the variation among the conditions is assessed against the average variation within conditions. At first glance, this strategy would appear to have much to offer. The groups are reflected in the analysis, so that variation associated with them appears to be removed from the conditions and from residual error, much as variation associated with a blocking factor is removed when the blocking factor is included in the analysis of data from a randomized-blocks design. The analyst may understand that the treatment of the group as a fixed effect precludes generalization to other groups like those used in the study, but may be willing to limit generalization and speak only about effects observed in the study at hand. Indeed, Hopkins (1983) advocated exactly this strategy as a preliminary step to determine whether the intervention was effective, at least in the sample of groups employed in the study.

   This is a remarkably seductive trap, but a trap nonetheless. Zucker (1990) showed that whenever different groups are nested in each study condition, variation associated with those groups will contribute to the variation of the condition means. Even if that variation is slight, it is multiplied by the number of members per group in the calculation of the variance of the condition means, so that even modest variation associated with the groups can have a substantial effect. If the groups are included as a fixed effect, Zucker (1990) showed that the Type I error rate of the resulting analysis would be inflated, often badly. The only way that the Type I error rate could be maintained at the nominal level was to include the group as a nested random effect. That finding was replicated in full by Murray et al. (1996).

Analyses That Employ a Subgroup as the Unit of Analysis

This strategy would analyze the data at a lower level of aggregation than the group, but at a higher level of aggregation than the member. It requires application of the General or Generalized Linear Mixed Model, specifies the intermediate level as a random effect, but ignores the group. Two recent studies that employed variations on this strategy provide illustrations.

Perry et al. (1992) allocated a single community to each of two conditions, then intervened in all the schools in the intervention community, delivering the intervention to students in those schools. Data were obtained from the individual students. In this case, many schools were nested within each community, and many more students were nested within each school. There was no variation among communities allocated to each condition, since there were no replications, and so the analysis could not be conducted at the level of the community. Instead, Perry et al. (1992) assessed the variation between the two conditions against the average variation among the schools nested within each condition, with the expectation that schools would capture most of the variation that would otherwise be seen among communities in the absence of an intervention effect.[9]

Carleton et al. (1995) also allocated a single community to each of two conditions, then intervened in one of those communities with a variety of programs aimed at the entire population. They conducted several independent surveys each year in each of the two cities, referring to each independent survey as a batch. Carleton et al. (1995) assessed the variation between the two conditions against the average variation among the batches nested within each condition. That analysis was based on the expectation that the batches would capture most of the variation that would otherwise be seen among communities in the absence of an intervention effect (Feldman et al., 1996).[10]

The problem with this strategy is that its validity rests on a strong assumption that cannot be tested in the data. This strategy assumes that the intermediate level accounts for all of the variation that would otherwise be seen among the groups in the absence of an intervention effect. Yet when there is only one group, as in the Perry et al. (1992) and Carleton et al. (1995) studies, the variation due to the group cannot be estimated apart from variation due to condition and so the assumption cannot be tested.

A recent simulation study has shown that there is considerable risk if that strong and untestable assumption is not met. Murray et al. (1996) examined the Type I error rates for analyses in which the variation of the conditions was assessed against the average variation among subgroups nested within the conditions. The magnitude of the intraclass correlation was known, as was the fraction of that correlation explained by the subgroup. Murray et al. (1996) reported that the performance of the test based on the subgroup was, in fact, fairly good when the subgroup accounted for a large fraction of the intraclass correlation. However, the Type I error rate was always higher than for the analysis that assessed the variation of the conditions against the variation of the groups, and the inflation in the Type I error rate was often substantial. As a result, analyses based on subgroups are not recommended.

Analyses That Misspecify the Structure of the Covariance Matrix

Many investigators might argue that correctly identifying all the sources of random variation in their data is challenge enough, and that it is terribly unfair to ask them as well to properly specify the structure of the covariance matrix defined by those sources. Unfortunately, misspecification of the covariance matrix can invalidate what otherwise would appear to be a strong analysis of data from a group-randomized trial. For that reason, careful consideration must be given to the structure of the covariance matrix.

To illustrate, consider a trial that has five annual surveys in each unit of assignment. Because there are more than two time intervals, it is possible to estimate the heterogeneity in the group-specific slopes. An analysis that improperly assumes that those group-specific slopes are homogeneous will carry an inflated Type I error rate, with the magnitude of the inflation directly related to the magnitude of the heterogeneity (Murray et al., in press). In contrast, an analysis that allows that heterogeneity to be estimated will carry a Type I error rate at the nominal level. Both analyses would require application of the General or Generalized Linear Mixed Model. In addition, the variation of the intervention effect would be assessed against the variation among the groups, so that both models might appear valid at first glance. However, they differ substantially in the way that the covariance matrix is structured, and the model that more closely reflects the underlying structure of the data will be valid while the other may not. Murray et al. (in press) reported Type I error rates above 20% for models that improperly specified the structure of the covariance matrix under conditions commonly found in group-randomized trials.

Good Strategies for One or Two Time Intervals

There are a number of strategies that will generally provide a valid analysis of data from a Posttest-Only Control Group Design or a Pretest-Posttest Control Group Design. The four strategies described in this section represent four different ways to implement what is often labeled a mixed-model analysis of variance (ANOVA) or covariance (ANCOVA) (Feldman and McKinlay, 1994; Koepsell et al., 1991; Murray and Hannan, 1990; Murray and Wolfinger, 1994). The first two strategies implement that mixed-model analysis of variance or covariance in two stages, relying on the familiar General or Generalized Linear Model. The last two strategies implement the mixed-model analysis of variance or covariance in a single stage, relying on the General or Generalized Linear Mixed Model. Though these four strategies may seem quite different, all converge asymptotically to the same solution in the absence of measurable confounding or measurable improvement in precision due to adjustment for extraneous variables.

All four mixed-model strategies identify the groups and members as sources of random variation. Given only one or two time intervals, there is no opportunity to misrepresent the pattern of over-time correlation in the data. The major risk for the use of mixed-model analysis of variance or covariance in the context a group-randomized trial is the possibility that the components of variance may be heterogeneous across the study conditions. However, as the number of groups randomly assigned to each condition increases, that risk becomes negligible.

Mixed-Model ANOVA in Two Stages

This strategy was offered in the 1950s as the original solution to the "unit of analysis" problem and is often called a "means analysis." It is a perfectly acceptable though conservative solution to avoid the inflated Type I error rate inherent in the strategies described above as not valid. It is accomplished by computing group means in a first stage, ignoring all the information available on members and/or subgroups. In a second stage, those means are analyzed to assess the intervention effect. In that second stage, the error term is computed at the level of the group, making the group the unit of analysis for that stage.

The means analysis has several advantages. The two stages can be conducted using separate applications of software based on the General Linear Model, as there is only a single source of random variation considered in each stage. This analysis is therefore simple to do and simple to explain. Absent confounding, it will give an unbiased estimate of the intervention effect and its standard error. If a sufficient number of groups are randomized to each condition, it will be a very strong strategy.

Unfortunately, this simple means analysis fails to take into account any member- or intermediate-level factors that might be unevenly distributed among the intervention conditions. In the same way, the investigator will not be able to improve the precision of the intervention-effect estimates by removing extraneous variance attributable to nuisance factors. For these reasons, the means analysis is not a preferred strategy.

Mixed-Model ANCOVA in Two Stages

A simple extension of the means analysis is to employ the General Linear Model in the first stage, with regression adjustment for covariates measured at the member level to compute adjusted group means. In the second stage, those adjusted means would be analyzed using the General Linear Model for a second time to assess intervention effects, with or without additional adjustment for covariates measured at the group level. In that second stage, the error term is still computed at the level of the group, and so the group is still the unit of analysis in the second stage.

This adjusted-means analysis allows for regression adjustment for confounders and other covariates, and so is often preferred over the unadjusted means analysis. At the same time, the analyst must be careful to ensure that the assumptions underlying the adjustments are met. For the typical linear regression application, the major assumptions are that the relationship between each covariate and the endpoint is linear and homogeneous across intervention conditions and that the covariates are not on the causal pathway between the intervention and the endpoint.

This strategy has been used in the analysis of several recent and important group-randomized trials. The paper by Zucker et al. (1995) describes the use of this strategy in the primary analysis of data from the Child and Adolescent Trial for Cardiovascular Health (CATCH). The paper by Murray, Hannan et al. (1994) describes the use of this strategy in the primary analysis of data from the Minnesota Heart Health Program (MHHP).

Mixed-Model ANOVA in One Stage

This analysis requires application of the General Linear Mixed Model, with both the groups and members identified as nested random effects. Variations on this strategy were offered by Hopkins (1982) as a simple alternative to the "means analysis." He pointed out that in a balanced design with no covariates, the test of the intervention effect from this analysis would be identical to that obtained from the means analysis. In the unbalanced case, identical results will be obtained if the means are weighted inverse to their sample size. This is because the designation of the group as a nested random effect identifies the group as the unit of analysis for the intervention effect in the context of the analysis of variance, based on the expected mean squares for that analysis. Unfortunately, without additional modifications, this strategy offers no particular advantage over the means analysis.

Mixed-Model ANCOVA in One Stage

To improve on the previous strategy, the analyst can include regression adjustment for covariates measured at various levels in the design. This analysis also requires application of the General Linear Mixed Model, with both the groups and members identified as nested random effects. However, the regression adjustment for covariates can remove confounding due to unevenly distributed covariates and can also improve the precision of the intervention-effect estimates by removing predictable variation due to extraneous factors. As a result, methods based on this strategy generally are preferred for the analysis of data from group-randomized trials (Feldman and McKinlay, 1994; Koepsell et al., 1991; Murray and Hannan, 1990; Murray and Wolfinger, 1994).

During the last 10 years, software has become available to conduct such single-stage analyses. Here the member-level data are entered into the analysis along with information on the groups. The group is designated as a nested random effect, as is the member. There are a number of methods available based on this strategy, each with its advantages and disadvantages. The three major types of software available under this strategy apply mixed-model regression, multilevel methods, and generalized estimating equations. All three are discussed in detail later in this chapter.

Good Strategies for Two or More Time Intervals

As noted earlier, mixed-model analysis of variance and covariance are generally valid for analysis of data from a group-randomized trial having only one or two time intervals in the design. However, as the number of time intervals increases beyond two, or with continuous surveillance, the mixed-model ANOVA and ANCOVA may no longer be valid. Murray et al. (in press) have shown that the mixed-model ANOVA will become increasingly inappropriate for designs involving more than two time intervals as the heterogeneity of the group-specific time trends increases. Under conditions commonly found in group-randomized trials, the mixed-model ANOVA applied to data having that structure often carried a Type I error rate of 20% or higher. This occurs because the mixed-model ANOVA and ANCOVA assumes that the group-specific slopes are homogeneous, so that there is no component of variance for group slopes. Where that component of variance exists in the data, the standard errors from the mixed-model ANOVA and ANCOVA will be too small, the test statistics too large, the p-values too small, and the significance of the findings overstated. The situation is parallel to what happens when the unit of analysis is ignored altogether in the analysis of data from the Posttest-Only Control Group Design.

Murray et al. (in press) also demonstrated that an alternative approach, commonly labeled a *random-coefficients analysis,* avoids this problem. The random-coefficients analysis provides for a component of variance for group slopes. If variation among those slopes exists in the data, the random-coefficients analysis will apply it correctly in the estimation of the standard error. If no variation among those slopes exists in the data, the random-coefficients analysis will reflect that as well. Murray et al. (in press) reported that the random-coefficients analysis carried the nominal Type I error rate regardless of the degree of heterogeneity across a wide range of conditions common to group-randomized trials.

Strategies With Limited Application

Post Hoc Correction for the Extra Variation

As noted above, Skinner et al. (1989) provide a detailed discussion of the use of *post hoc* corrections for analyses that otherwise ignore the group. These methods generally require the investigator to estimate the *VIF,* defined in Chapter 1. The *VIF* is then used to correct the inflation in the test statistic generated in the observation-level analysis. Test statistics such as *F-* and chi-square tests are corrected by dividing the test by *VIF.* Test statistics such as a *t-* or *z*-test are corrected by dividing the test by the square root of the *VIF.* The resulting test statistic is approximately correct if the estimate of the *ICC* is valid for the data at hand and the test statistic is assessed against an appropriate distribution with appropriate degrees of freedom. This strategy has not been employed to date in a published group-randomized trial, but deserves further investigation.

Mixed-Model ANOVA/ANCOVA for Designs Having More Than Two Time Intervals

As noted above, the mixed-model ANOVA/ANCOVA may not be valid for data from designs having more than two time intervals. At the same time, if the group-specific slopes are homogeneous, it will be valid. Further, it may offer an improvement in power over the random-coefficients analysis, because the degrees of freedom for the standard error of the intervention effect will be greater. Given the risks, the analyst will want to take care to test whether the group-specific slopes are, in fact, homogeneous before reporting results based on this strategy.

Randomization or Permutation Tests

Most of the research on the analysis of data from group-randomized trials has focused on model-based inference. As a result, most of the material presented in this chapter and in the balance of this book is focused on methods that employ model-based inference.

An alternative approach to the analysis of data from a group-randomized trial involves the use of randomization tests, also called permutation tests (e.g., Gail et al., 1996). With this approach, the analyst computes the intervention-effect estimate in the usual way. This can be done in any design, whether cohort or cross-sectional, matched or unmatched, stratified or unstratified, etc. What separates the randomization test from the methods discussed thus far is that it does not assess the observed intervention effect against a model-based or other estimate of the standard error of that intervention effect. Instead, the analyst constructs the distribution of all possible intervention effects under the null hypothesis using the unadjusted or adjusted group-specific means, slopes, or some other group-level statistic, conditional only on the observed data. The observed intervention effect is treated as but one of the possible intervention effects, and the probability of getting a more extreme result under the null hypothesis given the observed data is the proportion of possible intervention effects that are greater in magnitude than the observed effect. For example, if only 3.5% of the possible intervention effects are larger than the observed effect, then the one-tailed p-value attached to the observed effect would be $p = 0.035$. Similarly, if only 3.5% of the possible intervention effects are larger in absolute value than the observed effect, then the two-tailed p-value attached to the observed effect would be $p = 0.035$. Instead of referencing an observed test statistic to an assumed distribution, the observed intervention effect is referenced to the distribution of intervention effects that are possible under the null hypothesis given the observed data.

Randomization tests do not rely on a statistical model for their validity. Instead, they rely on a proper randomization. When the groups are randomized to conditions, each group has the same probability of being assigned to a given condition. Under the null hypothesis of no intervention effect, the observed intervention effect is due not to the intervention but to the chance allocation of groups to conditions. Where the entire distribution of possible intervention effects can be specified, the probability that an effect as large as or larger than that observed is easily obtained, conditional only on the observed values for the groups.

In spite of their conceptual simplicity, randomization tests have been applied in only one community trial. Gail and colleagues at the National Cancer Institute employed this method in the evaluation of the COMMIT trial (COMMIT Research Group, 1995a, b; Gail et al., 1992; Green et al., 1995). Subsequently,

Gail et al. (1996) published an excellent review of the way in which randomization tests can be employed in the evaluation of group-randomized trials.

Of particular interest in the Gail et al. (1996) paper are the results from simulation studies to evaluate the Type I error rate for the randomization test as applied to a variety of designs employed in group-randomized trials. For an unmatched design, they reported that the Type I error rate was nominal when the number of groups per condition was the same in both conditions, even with heterogeneous variances in the two study conditions. However, if the number of groups was not the same in both conditions and the variances were heterogeneous, the Type I error rate was inflated to as much as twice the nominal level. In the matched design, which is balanced by definition, the Type I error rate was nominal unless the number of observations per condition was substantially uneven and the distribution of the intervention effect was substantially asymmetric. Because the investigator can usually ensure that the number of groups per condition is equal and that the number of observations per condition is similar, these constraints will not be a problem in most group-randomized trials.

Gail et al. (1996) also report on simulation studies to examine the impact of regression adjustment for covariates on both power and the Type I error rate for the randomization test. By adding regression adjustments in a preliminary step, Gail et al. (1996) move the randomization test substantially closer to the methods that depend entirely on statistical models for their validity. Indeed, the example provided in Gail et al. (1996) employed the Generalized Linear Mixed Model to generate a residual value for each unit of observation, computed as the difference between the observed value and the value predicted under their model. By taking care to choose covariates that were unrelated to the intervention, the regression model served to adjust the residuals for any imbalance in the distribution of the covariates among the groups, without removing whatever intervention effect might be present. The randomization test was then applied to the residuals rather than to the unadjusted data; it could also have been applied to the adjusted group-level statistics. Gail et al. (1996) report that the adjustment had no effect on the Type I error rate, even when there was substantial confounding with unbalanced data in terms of the number of members per condition. They also report that regression adjustment for covariates appreciably improved power when the covariates were strongly related to the outcome and especially when they were unevenly distributed among the groups, as has been reported for other analysis methods that accommodate regression adjustment for covariates, such as mixed-model regression (Murray and Short, 1995, 1996, 1997).

The finding that the Type I error rate was at the nominal level in most cases is not surprising. Not only is the theoretical basis for the randomization test sound, but the mechanics of the test also suggest that it will do well. At the heart of the test is the requirement that the analyst prepare a single statistic for each unit of assignment in the study, such as a posttest mean, a change score, or a slope. The difference, on average, between the values estimated for the groups in the intervention condition and the values estimated for the groups in the control condition is the estimate of the intervention effect, and its probability is assessed against the distribution of all possible intervention effects given the values observed in the study. Each group statistic reflects not only variation associated with the members of the group, but also variation due to the groups themselves. Because the data are reduced to a single statistic in each group, it is not possible to misrepresent the structure of the covariance matrix.

The sample-size requirements under the randomization test will be the same as for model-based inference procedures, such as mixed-model or multilevel regression. For example, Gail et al. (1996) suggest the sample size methods appropriate to the t-test as a good approximation for estimating sample size for the randomization test. As will be seen in Chapter 9, that is also the basis for sample-size estimation for the model-based methods. As a result, the methods presented in Chapter 9 will be applicable for estimation of sample size for a randomization test as well as for methods based on a specific model.

The findings reported by Gail et al. (1996) suggest that randomization tests can play a useful role in the evaluation of group-randomized trials. Additional research comparing this approach with model-based methods will help to identify the conditions under which either of these methods will be preferred over the other.

Computer Software

These models, methods, and strategies become concrete in the form of the computer software used to analyze the data. The variety of programs now available is quite remarkable and grows almost daily. Many of these programs can be used to analyze data from a group-randomized trial so that the investigator and analyst have considerable flexibility in choosing their software. This section provides general guidance to help investigators and analysts know when and when not to employ different kinds of software for the analysis of data from a group-randomized trial. The focus is on general regression software, as might be used to implement the models described earlier in this chapter. Such software can be used to implement most of the strategies discussed in this chapter, though not all. For example, none of the programs described below will generate the distributions required for the randomization test. Similarly, none will perform *post hoc* corrections. Even so, many of the programs described below can be used in conjunction with manual methods or general-purpose programming languages to implement these methods.

Fixed-Effects Regression

The most common analyses, such as linear regression and ANOVA/ANCOVA, are usually based on the General or Generalized Linear Model and so are appropriate for data with only a single source of random variation. Software to implement those methods is often described as appropriate for fixed-effects models only. These methods can be used to analyze data from a group-randomized trial, but only in the context of the two-stage ANOVA/ANCOVA strategies. These methods cannot be used to conduct a one-stage mixed-model regression analysis, a one-stage random-coefficients analysis, or any other one-stage analysis based on the General or Generalized Linear Mixed Model.

It is impossible to describe all the software that is available for fixed-effects analyses. However, it is possible to provide general guidelines to help identify them. Most programs will be clear that they presume a fixed-effects model and include a statement to that effect in the documentation. If the documentation does not specifically indicate that the software allows multiple random effects, the analyst should presume that it does not. If the documentation indicates that the estimation method is ordinary least squares, the analyst can be certain that the software is designed for fixed-effects analyses only.

Complex Survey Analysis

Methods developed for analysis of complex survey samples apply standard regression methods to generate fixed-effect parameter estimates and nonstandard methods to generate standard errors for those estimates. The available evidence suggests that these methods will be valid when the number of groups per condition is large—for example, 20 or more groups per condition. However, as the number of groups per condition declines, the magnitude of the estimated variances may increase well beyond their true value. At the same time, the standard normal approximation, often used with these methods, will no longer be appropriate when the number of groups is small; the *t*-distribution may be used in this situation, with *df* based on the number of groups. The implication for group-randomized trials is not good, as many group-randomized trials have only a few groups per condition. As a result, software for complex survey analysis may have only limited application in the analysis of data from group-randomized trials.

Wolter (1985) described 14 software programs for regression analysis of complex survey data. He noted that three were "state-of-the-art, well-supported, portable programs," while the remainder were either ill-supported, still in development, or not portable. According to Wolter, the stronger programs in 1985 were Osiris IV (Survey Research Center, University of Michigan), SUDAAN (Research Triangle Institute), and SUPERCARP (Department of Statistics, Iowa State University). Cohen et al. (1988) reviewed the RE-PERR routine in OSIRIS IV, the SURREGR routine in SUDAAN, SU-PERCARP, and NASSREG, a newer program from Westat, Inc. Cohen et al. (1988) reported that all four gave quite similar results across a variety of data sets and analyses. Cohen et al. (1988) favored SUDAAN as the simplest of the programs to use and the most efficient.

As of this writing, four of these programs are still available, though only two remain in active development. SUDAAN Version 6.4 and WESREG Version 1.3, which replaced NASSREG, are available and remain in active development. OSIRIS IV, SUPERCARP, and its personal-computer version, PC CARP, are still available but are no longer in active development.

SUDAAN Version 6.4

SUDAAN is available for IBM-compatible personal computers, DEC VAX mainframes and workstations, SUN Spark Stations, and IBM mainframes (Shah et al., 1995). SUDAAN Version 6.4 uses Zeger and Liang's (1986) generalized estimation equations for parameter estimation. Variance estimation is based in part on the Taylor-series linearization method and yields the empirical-sandwich estimator of Zeger and Liang (1986). Parameters are estimated via maximum likelihood for nonlinear models and via least squares for linear models. Weighted versions are available. Version 6.4 provides linear, logistic, and proportional hazards regression, and log-linear analysis, all with multiple fixed and random effects.

SUDAAN's use of the empirical sandwich estimator for standard errors warrants a special note. As noted earlier, that estimator is asymptotically valid but may perform poorly in the context of group-randomized trials. As a result, SUDAAN may have only limited application in the analysis of data from group-randomized trials.

WESREG Version 1.3

WESREG is a user-written SAS procedure (SAS, Inc., Cary, North Carolina) that can be called in SAS Version 6.08 and subsequent versions. It employs weighted least squares to estimate parameters of multiple-regression models from data based on a complex survey-sampling design. The standard errors for the regression coefficients are estimated using either balanced repeated replications or jackknife replication to reflect the complex sampling design. Test statistics are also computed. Degrees of freedom are computed as the number of replicates used in the calculation of the variance estimates, and so may be quite different from the number of assignment units. The documentation notes that the t- and F-test statistics are "approximately valid only if the number of replicates is approximately equal to the actual degrees of freedom." (WESREG, 1994). As a result, this method may have only limited application in group-randomized trials, again because the number of groups per condition is usually limited.

Mixed-Model Regression

Mixed-model regression methods are based on the General Linear Mixed Model for Gaussian data or on the Generalized Linear Mixed Model for non-Gaussian data (Breslow and Clayton, 1993; Donner, 1984a, 1985; Laird and Ware, 1982; Laird et al., 1987; Stiratelli et al., 1984; Ware, 1985; Wolfinger and O'Connell, 1993). Software based on mixed-model regression estimates both fixed and random effects, usually in an iterative process. Programs based on least-squares estimation often employ IRLS. Here, estimates of fixed effects are obtained, and then random effects are estimated from the residuals; this sequence continues until convergence. Programs based on maximum-likelihood estimation often employ numeric analysis algorithms to obtain REML estimates for the random effects, then solve for the fixed effects using mixed-model regression equations.

Mixed-model regression methods may be used quite effectively to analyze data from group-randomized trials, as long as the analyst takes care to confirm that the assumptions underlying the model fit to the data are appropriate for the underlying structure of the data. Reviews have recently appeared on several of the mixed-model regression programs now available. Kreft et al. (1994) and Hedeker et al. (1994) reviewed BMDP-5V. Murray and Wolfinger (1994) reviewed SAS PROC MIXED.

BMDP-3V

BMDP-3V (Dixon, 1992) is a general mixed-model regression program. It uses ML or REML estimation, can accommodate balanced or unbalanced designs, and is based on the General Linear Mixed Model. It can accommodate several fixed and random effects but assumes that all random effects are normally and identically distributed with constant variance across observations. It does not allow the user to specify a structure for the covariance matrix. *F*-statistics for fixed effects are provided under REML estimation, and LR chi-square statistics for fixed effects are provided under ML estimation.

BMDP-5V

BMDP-5V (Dixon, 1992) is a mixed-model regression program designed especially for analysis of repeated-measures data. It uses ML or REML estimation, can accommodate balanced or unbalanced designs, and is based on the General Linear Mixed Model. It allows the user to specify a structure for the within-subject covariance matrix as compound symmetry, first-order autoregressive, banded or general autoregressive, or unstructured. In addition, the user can specify some other covariance structure, though it must be called as a subroutine. Akaike's Information Criterion (AIC) is given to allow the user to select the best-fitting covariance structure. For all fixed effects, Wald chi-square tests are provided, based on asymptotic standard errors. Asymptotic standard errors and *z*-tests are provided for all random effects. BMDP-5V can accommodate missing data as well as fixed or time-varying covariates. It can accommodate a wide variety of mixed-model designs, particularly with repeated measures.

SAS PROC MIXED

The SAS PROC MIXED (SAS Institute Inc., 1992, 1996; Wolfinger, 1992; Littell et al., 1996) procedure was designed as a general mixed-model regression program. It uses ML, REML, or MIVQUE estimation, can accommodate balanced or unbalanced designs, and is based on the General Linear Mixed Model. It allows the user to specify a structure for the within-subject covariance matrix, but also allows the user to specify a separate structure for the between-subject covariance matrix. Either may be specified as simple, compound symmetry, heterogeneous compound symmetry, unstructured, banded, autoregressive, heterogeneous first-order autoregressive, first-order autoregressive moving average, Toeplitz, banded Toeplitz, several factor analytic structures, Huynh-Feldt, power of the mean, or spatial (spherical, power, exponential, Gaussian, linear, linear log). Both Akaike's Information Criterion (AIC) and Schwarz's Bayesian Information Criterion (BIC) are provided to guide selection of covariance structures. For all fixed effects *F*-tests are provided, and asymptotic standard errors and *z*-tests are provided for all random effects. Several pairwise-difference procedures are available, as are tests of simple main effects for interactions. CONTRAST and ESTIMATE statements allow the user to construct specialized contrasts. MIXED can accommodate missing data as well as fixed or time-varying covariates. It can accommodate a variety of mixed-model designs, including the nested designs common to group-randomized trials.

Murray and Wolfinger (1994) recently evaluated SAS PROC MIXED in the context of group-randomized trials having a Posttest-Only Control Group Design or a Pretest-Posttest Control Group Design. They compared this General Linear Mixed Model program to SAS PROC GLM, a General Linear Model program. They found in simulations that SAS PROC MIXED provided tests for fixed effects that had the nominal Type I error rate, regardless of the degree of confounding attributable to covariates or of the magnitude of the intraclass correlation. In contrast, SAS PROC GLM often yielded a highly inflated Type I error rate. This pattern held across a number of analytic strategies commonly employed in group-randomized trials.

SAS GLIMMIX Macro

The GLIMMIX macro iteratively calls SAS PROC MIXED, and broadly implements the Generalized Linear Mixed Model (Littell et al., 1996; Wolfinger and O'Connell, 1993). It supports a variety of link functions, including the identity, logit, log, reciprocal, and power links. It supports a variety of variance functions, including the binomial, poisson, Gaussian, gamma, and inverse Gaussian. ML estimation is used if there is only one random effect in the model, and REML estimation is used if there are multiple random effects.

Hierarchical or Multilevel Analysis

Hierarchical or multilevel methods may be seen as a special form of mixed-model regression proposed specifically for data that has a hierarchical or multilevel structure (Bryk and Raudenbush, 1992; Cheung et al., 1990; Goldstein, 1987; Hox and Kreft, 1994; Mason et al., 1983; DeLeeuw and Kreft, 1986). In their original form, hierarchical or multilevel methods were based on the General Linear Mixed Model and allowed multiple fixed and random effects; all error distributions were assumed Gaussian. More recently, these methods have been applied to data with non-Gaussian error distributions, and those extensions are based on the Generalized Linear Mixed Model.

The original development of hierarchical or multilevel methods was in educational research, where data are often collected from students nested within classes that are nested within schools that are nested within districts, etc. Those investigators were interested in the relationship between the dependent variable and variables measured at various levels in the hierarchy, and in the interactions among the predictors both within and across levels. They also wanted to allow for sources of random variation at each level.

The typical hierarchical or multilevel analysis is conducted in stages, parallel to the layers in the hierarchy (or to the levels). In the first stage, the endpoint is regressed on observation-level predictors. The coefficients obtained in the first stage are then treated as raw data in a second stage, where predictors at that level are entered into the regression. In theory, this could continue for many levels, though most of the programs now available accommodate only two or three levels. With good attention to model specification and degrees of freedom, hierarchical or multilevel analysis will have broad application in the analysis of data from group-randomized trials.

A number of programs are available for multilevel analyses. Kreft et al. (1994) reviewed GENMOD, HLM, ML3, and VARCL. Hedeker et al. (1994) commented on ML3, HLM, VARCL, and offer their own program for multilevel analysis via macros in SPSS. Raudenbush (1997) discusses the use of hierarchical models for analysis of data from group-randomized trials.

GENMOD

GENMOD fits two-level hierarchical models and uses REML as the method of estimation. Kreft et al. (1994) reported that GENMOD is available only for MS-DOS and MTS operating systems. They also characterized GENMOD as less user-friendly than the other programs they reviewed.

HLM

HLM can fit two- or three-level hierarchical models. HLM uses ML or REML estimation and can accommodate balanced or unbalanced designs. It was originally based on the General Linear Mixed Model, since it could accommodate several fixed and random effects but assumed that all random effects were normally and identically distributed with constant variance across observations. The most recent release extends to Generalized Linear Mixed Models, allowing hierarchical linear models for data with binomial or Poisson error distributions.

ML3

ML3 fits two- or three-level hierarchical linear models. Estimation is via IGLS or RIGLS, which are equivalent to ML and REML estimates, respectively, when the data are Gaussian. Simple hierarchical logistic regression analyses and log-linear modeling analyses are possible. However, a recent report by Rodriguez and Goldman (1995) was critical in its evaluation of ML3 as applied to binary data.

VARCL

VARCL can fit up to nine-level hierarchical models. It can accommodate unbalanced designs but not missing data. Kreft et al. (1994) report that interactions across levels are possible, though not as easily as in other multilevel
programs. Estimation is via Fisher scoring. Unlike most other multilevel programs, VARCL can employ quasi-likelihood methods. It allows the user to
choose among a variety of link and variance functions, permitting multilevel
analyses under the Generalized Linear Mixed Model. However, the recent report by Rodriguez and Goldman (1995) gave a poor review to VARCL.

Generalized Estimating Equations

In their initial paper, Liang and Zeger (1986) noted that one of the barriers to
development of methods for analysis of non-Gaussian data with multiple
sources of random variation was the paucity of information on joint distributions other than the multivariate normal. This was exactly the situation that
led to quasi-likelihood and its variations. Liang and Zeger (1986) simply took
another approach to this problem. They proposed a method based on the marginal distribution of the dependent variable, thereby avoiding the need to specify the form of the joint distribution altogether.

The GEE approach defines the marginal expectation of the dependent variable as a function of the predictor variables, and also assumes that the variance
is a known function of the mean. This part of GEE is a marginal analogue to
the usual Generalized Linear Model and is quite similar to what Breslow and
Clayton (1993) have termed *marginal quasi-likelihood*. The GEE approach
then specifies what is termed a working correlation matrix for the observations,
thereby allowing for multiple random effects. It is this working correlation
matrix that extends GEE to be an analogue of the Generalized Linear Mixed
Model. Standard errors are computed using empirical-sandwich estimation.
The GEE approach gives consistent estimators under relatively weak assumptions about the form of the correlation matrix and can be implemented using
IRLS.

The marginal approach embodied in GEE is sometimes called the
population-averaged approach (Zeger et al., 1988). It contrasts with the more
traditional *subject-specific approach* that is reflected in the mixed-model
regression and multilevel modeling methods described above. In the subject-
specific approach, the random effects are modeled explicitly. In the population-
averaged approach, they are not. Several reports have addressed the appropriate uses for the two approaches (e.g., Breslow and Clayton, 1993; Diggle

et al., 1994) and reached similar conclusions. They have suggested that the subject-specific approach is appropriate when the analyst wants prediction for the individual, but note that the subject-specific approach requires sufficient data per individual to be able to model the individual adequately, and provides consistent estimators only when the correlation matrix is correctly specified. The population-averaged approach requires less data per individual, but cannot provide prediction for individuals. It is most appropriate when the prediction of interest involves populations or subgroups, as is often the case in public health, and provides consistent estimators even when the correlation matrix is misspecified, though only asymptotically.

Current sources of GEE software may be obtained from Zeger or Liang at Johns Hopkins University. At the time of this writing, Zeger listed sources for GEE macros in SAS and SPSS, and a version of GEE in S–Plus (Statistical Sciences, Inc., 1993). All the software identified by Zeger was available at no cost. As noted earlier, SUDAAN Version 6.4 is based on the generalized estimating equations, and the standard errors are based on the empirical-sandwich estimators used by Zeger and Liang (1986). As such, it can be used to conduct analyses quite similar to GEE. In addition, Version 6.11 of SAS PROC MIXED offers the empirical-sandwich estimator as an option, so that it too can be used to conduct analyses quite similar to GEE.

Thornquist and Anderson (1992) presented a paper on the small-sample properties of GEEs in group-randomized designs with data with a Gaussian error distribution. They reported that the GEE estimators of regression coefficient standard errors, residual error, and the *ICC* were negatively biased when the *ICC* was positive, and that the bias increased as the number of groups decreased; the bias was unaffected by the number of members per group. Thus, the bias would be worst in the typical group-randomized trial having a limited number of groups allocated to each condition. The bias in the estimation of the *ICC* could be corrected by replacing the usual moment estimator in GEE with a minimum-variance quadratic unbiased estimator (MIVQUE). The bias in the standard errors of the regression coefficients was corrected by inflating the standard error to reflect the uncertainty in estimation of the fixed effects.[11] Remediation of the confidence intervals required use of the corrected standard error in conjunction with the *t*-distribution rather than the Gaussian distribution.

More recently, Murray et al. (in press) reported that the empirical-sandwich estimation method as implemented in SAS PROC MIXED resulted in very unreliable Type I error rates across a range of conditions common to group-randomized trials. They reported that the Type I error rate was sometimes much too high, sometimes too low, and never at the nominal level in simulations when the number of groups per condition was 10 or fewer. As the number of groups per condition increased, the performance of the empirical-sandwich estimator improved, so that when there were 20 or more groups per condition, the Type I error rate was close to the nominal level.

Because that estimator is such a central feature in GEE methods, these findings suggest that GEEs may have only limited application in the context of group-randomized trials. The available evidence suggests that they be limited to trials having 20 or more groups allocated to each study condition.

Implementation Issues

Investigators and analysts who take care to plan a proper analysis and to select appropriate software will not want to have their good plans spoiled by subtle problems in the implementation of their analysis. Unfortunately, most of the software described in the previous section is complex and the documentation is not always clear. As a result, it can be hard for the user to determine whether the analysis will be properly implemented.

This section reviews two of the common problems that can occur during the implementation of an analysis of data from a group-randomized trial.

The Non-Negativity Constraint

Most software based on maximum likelihood or quasi-maximum likelihood estimation imposes a non-negativity constraint such that variance component estimates are not allowed to drop below zero (Swallow and Monahan, 1984). This constraint often allows the likelihood algorithm to converge more rapidly. In addition, a large negative variance estimate can make it impossible for the software to calculate the likelihood. In this case, the non-negativity constraint can keep the analysis from failing altogether.

On the surface, this constraint makes sense. A negative variance component is a statistical non sequitur, though it has meaning in the context of a negative *ICC*. However, not only are true negative *ICC*s uncommon, it becomes increasingly likely that the estimate will be negative by chance alone as the true value approaches zero.

At the same time, preventing negative variance components might inflate the average variance component, reduce the average test statistic, inflate the average *p*-value, and so deflate the Type I error rate, especially given a small variance component and a test statistic based on limited degrees of freedom. Murray et al. (1996) reported exactly that pattern in a simulation study designed in part to assess the impact of the non-negativity constraint in the context of group-randomized trials. They found that preventing negative variance components drove the Type I error rate toward zero. They also found that the Type I error rate was maintained at the nominal level only when negative estimates were permitted. In other words, to prevent negative *ICCs* is to make the nominal Type I error rate more stringent, even given a proper analysis. While this has the positive effect of reducing the Type I error rate, it will simultaneously have the negative effect of reducing power. Indeed, the power will drop off very sharply as the Type I error rate becomes more stringent. These findings suggest that investigators should avoid the non-negativity constraint in the context of analyses of group-randomized trials. Murray et al. (in press) drew a similar conclusion in a study of random-coefficient models.

Several popular programs, including SAS PROC MIXED and HLM, routinely prevent negative variance estimates. As shown by Murray et al. (1996), this can result in a dramatic reduction in the Type I error rate and an equally dramatic and far more deleterious reduction in the power of the trial. Power is enough of a problem in group-randomized trials, and no investigator will want the hurdle raised substantially higher, especially without any warning, simply as a result of a subtle default in the analysis software.

Software That Only Appears to Support Mixed Models

Some widely used programs are often misinterpreted as appropriate for group-randomized trials when in fact they are not. An excellent example is SAS PROC GLM (SAS, 1992). The documentation for this program states clearly that it presumes a fixed-effects model. However, the program allows the user to designate some terms as random effects. It also allows the analyst to construct *F*-tests based on an analysis of expected mean squares that reflect those random-effect designations. As a result, many investigators believe that they are conducting a mixed-model analysis when they employ those features. Unfortunately, this is not the case, and the results can be wildly inaccurate (Murray and Wolfinger, 1994). When the user properly constructs *F*-tests using the random statement with the test option, the fixed-effects *F*-tests generated by SAS PROC GLM will have a Type I error rate that approaches the nominal level, even when the data involve multiple random effects, but only if the data are balanced and there is no measurable confounding due to covariates included in the analysis. When the data are unbalanced or when there is measurable confounding, the fixed-effects *F*-tests generated by SAS PROC GLM will have a Type I error rate that may be much too large or much too small. The only certainty is that it will not be at the nominal level.

SAS PROC GLM is not the only fixed-effects program that allows the user to designate effects as random, potentially lulling the analyst into thinking that it will perform a proper one-stage mixed-model analysis. Investigators and analysts should take care to ensure that the documentation specifically includes support for multiple random effects in the analysis, not just in the labeling.

Summary

Given a good design, care should be taken to ensure that the analytic method is appropriate for the design. For model-based inference, that will require that the model be well matched to the underlying structure of the data. Analyses based on the General Linear Mixed Model are appropriate for group-randomized trials in which the endpoints have errors distributed Gaussian, while analyses based on the Generalized Linear Mixed Model are appropriate generally when the errors are non-Gaussian. Analyses based on the General Linear Mixed Model may also be appropriate for group-randomized trials in which the errors are non-Gaussian, so long as there is at least a moderate number of observations per group and groups per condition.

Given one or two time intervals, mixed-model ANOVA/ANCOVA is well supported for use in the analysis of data from group-randomized trials. Given more than two time intervals and measurable heterogeneity among assignment-unit slopes, those methods will have an inflated Type I error rate and random-coefficients models are recommended instead.

Methods such as those designed for analysis of complex survey data, those that employ the empirical sandwich formula for estimation of error variances, and those that assume a standard normal distribution, will generally not be appropriate for group-randomized trials unless those trials involve an unusually large number of groups per condition (e.g., ≥ 20). Other methods, such as analyses that ignore variation due to groups, analyses that delete nonsignificant components of variance, analyses based on *post hoc* corrections of fixed-effects analyses, analyses based on batches or subunits, and analyses that employ effective degrees of freedom, require strong assumptions that often cannot be well tested. Investigators who wish to employ those methods must provide evidence that the assumptions are appropriate.

Randomization tests provide an alternative to model-based inference. Though not yet studied extensively in the context of group-randomized trials, the available literature suggests that this approach can give quite satisfactory results. Additional research is required to compare model-based methods and randomization tests to identify the conditions under which one approach is favored over the other.

There is at present a wide variety of software available to implement these methods. No one program can be recommended as better than the alternatives. Investigators should consider their own level of knowledge, as well as that of their colleagues and staff, as they select software products. Whatever the software, analysts should take care that the method is implemented as intended.

Endnotes

1. The random-effects covariance matrix is the matrix that summarizes the nature of and relationships among the random effects. The simplest analytic model, based on the General Linear Model, has a single variance component, σ_e^2, presumed constant for all observations. More complex analytic models may include other sources of random variation. Those sources may be reflected in differences in variances observed in different subsets of the data, or in correlations among observations taken from the same groups or members. Even more complex designs may include variations in those correlations either over time or in different subsets of the data. The patterns can get quite complex. Wolfinger and O'Connell (1993) provide a good overview of many of the patterns that are found and of methods that can be used to choose among them. Further information is provided in Chapter 8.

2. Methods to assess goodness of fit are not as well developed for complex mixed models as they are for simpler models based on the General Linear Model. Interested readers are referred to a discussion on these issues in McCullagh and Nelder (1989) and to recent articles by Wolfinger (1993), Kass and Wasserman (1995), Kass and Raftery (1995), and Berger and Pericchi (1996).

3. Models that have no fixed effects are called random-effects models. They have not been used in the analysis of data from group-randomized trials.

4. Arithmetic operations will not be commutative across all transformations. Depending on the nature of the operations applied to the data after the initial transformation, reverse transformation may not yield a result that effectively represents the same result in the original scale. This issue is illustrated in Chapter 7.

5. Note that $^{-1}$ denotes the inverse, not the reciprocal, so that $g^{-1}(\cdot) \times g(\cdot) = 1$. As a result, the form of the inverse link function will depend upon the link function. For example, if the link function is the logit and P is the probability of the outcome of interest, $\ln\left(\frac{P}{1-P}\right)$, then the inverse link function is:

$$\frac{\exp\left(\ln\left(\frac{P}{1-P}\right)\right)}{1+\exp\left(\ln\left(\frac{P}{1-P}\right)\right)}$$

6. If the observations were means, the weighting factor for a given mean would be the number of observations contributing to that mean. If the observations were the raw data, then $\omega_i = 1$.

7. The phrase "the level of the analysis" is often used interchangeably with "unit of analysis"; both are widely misunderstood.

8. The phrase "can answer the question" is important. It is rarely the case that the research team can know the answer in advance of the trial. If they did, it would be a waste of time and resources to do the study. Indeed, one of the issues raised in Chapter 2's discussion of planning a trial was the need to document that the question had not yet been answered. Having said that, it is important that all concerned, both the investigators and the sponsors, be willing to accept the answer whatever it is. It may be that the intervention

proves effective. It may be that it does not. The investigators and the sponsors must be prepared to accept either answer and move forward on that basis. Null findings can be just as important as positive findings, even if they are less exciting initially.

9. It is important to note that the author was a coauthor on the Perry et al. (1992) paper. At the time the analysis for that paper was conducted, the dangers associated with an analysis at the level of the subunit were not well understood.

10. Similarly, it is important to note that at the time the batch analysis was employed for the Carleton et al. (1995) paper, the dangers associated with that analysis were not well understood. The Feldman et al. (1996) paper documents those dangers.

11. This problem exists in ML estimation and is corrected in REML; Thornquist and Anderson's finding of the same problem in their work may be due to the fact that GEE uses IRLS, which converges to ML.

5

Analyses for Nested Cross-Sectional Designs

Organization of the Chapter

The Analyses

This chapter presents analyses appropriate for data from nested cross-sectional designs. One chapter cannot cover all the designs and analyses possible within this class of designs, but it can represent the major variations. Following the recommendations in Chapter 4, these analyses are based on the General Linear Mixed Model or the Generalized Linear Mixed Model.

Notation

There is no standard notation in textbooks of statistics and research design. Even so, there are some conventions that are widely followed. Consistent with those conventions, Greek symbols are used in this book when their meaning is well established, such as the mean (μ), intervention effect (Δ), variance (σ^2), and residual error (ε), and for certain algebraic functions such as summation (Σ). The expression σ_e^2 is used to refer to the residual-error variance, regardless of the design. Similarly, the expression σ_Δ^2 is used to refer to the variance of the intervention effect, regardless of the structure of Δ.

Unfortunately, there are no conventions for symbols, subscripts, and indexes used to represent the terms of interest. Indeed, one of the most common features in notational systems is that the characters bear no relationship to the terms they identify. Because such systems are difficult to learn, the notation employed here avoids that pattern. Instead, fixed and random effects are represented by the uppercase of the first letter of the variable name as a reminder of the effect to which the character refers. Similarly, the number of levels of each effect are represented by the lowercase of the first letter of the variable name.

Member, M_i ($i = 1 \ldots m$), identifies the unit of observation. Group,

G_k ($k=1\ldots g$), identifies the unit of assignment. Time, T_j ($j=1\ldots t$), identifies the intervals during which measurements are taken on the groups and members. Condition, C_l ($l=1\ldots c$), identifies the study conditions. Strata, S_p ($p=1\ldots s$), identifies one stratification factor. Block, B_q ($q=1\ldots b$), identifies a second stratification factor when necessary.

All random effects are in bold type, while fixed effects are in plain type. Because fixed and random effects are distinguished in this manner, all expected mean squares are presented in terms of variance components. For example, the variation among the levels of condition is defined as σ_c^2 instead of

$$\sum_{i=1}^{c} C_i^2/(c-1).$$

Degrees of freedom are abbreviated as *df*. Numerator degrees of freedom are abbreviated as *ndf* and denominator degrees of freedom are abbreviated as *ddf*.

Posttest-Only Control Group Design

The strengths and weaknesses of this design were presented in Chapter 3. Absent randomization of a large number of identifiable groups to each condition, this is a particularly weak design and no analysis can make up for its weaknesses. With randomization of a large number of identifiable groups to each condition, this design can be quite strong. Either way, there are two major options available for the analysis. The simpler unadjusted analysis is presented first, followed by the adjusted analysis. Examples are provided in Chapter 7.

Unadjusted Analysis of Posttest Data

The Model

In the unadjusted analysis of posttest data, the model is:

$$Y_{i:k:l} = \mu + C_l + G_{k:l} + \varepsilon_{i:k:l} \tag{5.1}$$

Here the observed value ($Y_{i:k:l}$) for the ith member nested within the kth group nested within the lth condition is expressed as a function of the grand mean (μ), the effect of the lth condition (C_l), and the realized value of the kth group ($G_{k:l}$). Any difference between the predicted and observed values is left to the residual error ($\varepsilon_{i:k:l}$).

In most group-randomized trials, condition is a fixed effect. In order to account for the positive intraclass correlation expected in the data, $G_{k:l}$ must be included in the analysis as a random effect; simulation studies have shown that failure to do so, in the presence of measurable intraclass correlation, will result in a Type I error rate that is inflated, often badly (Zucker et al., 1990; Murray and Wolfinger, 1994; Murray et al., 1996). The two random effects allow for correlation among members within a group ($G_{k:l}$) and for random variation among the members ($\varepsilon_{i:k:l}$).

The Intervention Effect

In the familiar ANOVA, the F-statistic assesses the variation among the condition means against the variation among the group means. The null hypothesis is that the variation due to the conditions is zero. When there are only two conditions, the numerator of the F-statistic is based on a single df and it is more convenient to use the t-statistic. In that case, the intervention effect is the difference between the two condition means and the null hypothesis is that the difference is zero. For the intervention and control conditions, the intervention effect is:

$$\Delta = (\overline{Y}_{..I} - \overline{Y}_{..C}) \tag{5.2}$$

The Expected Mean Squares

The expected mean squares for this analysis are shown in Table 5.1. The MS_c has three components: residual error (σ_e^2), a weighted component of variance due to the groups ($m\sigma_{g:c}^2$), and a weighted component of variance due to condition ($mg\sigma_c^2$). The test of the null hypothesis is $MS_c/MS_{g:c}$.

The Variance of the Intervention Effect

When the intervention effect is defined as the difference between two condition means, the variance of that intervention effect under the null hypothesis is:

Table 5.1. Expected Mean Squares for the Unadjusted Analysis of Data From a Nested Cross-Sectional Posttest-Only Control Group Design

Source	df	E(MS)	MS
Condition	$c-1$	$\sigma_e^2 + m\sigma_{g:c}^2 + mg\sigma_c^2$	MS_c
Group:C	$c(g-1)$	$\sigma_e^2 + m\sigma_{g:c}^2$	$MS_{g:c}$
Member:G:C	$gc(m-1)$	σ_e^2	MS_e

$$\sigma_\Delta^2 = 2\left(\frac{MS_{g:c}}{mg}\right)$$ (5.3)

Here there are m members per group and g groups per condition. The derivation of this variance is presented in Chapter 9.

Assumptions

The model for this analysis provides for two sources of random variation. If there are additional sources in the data, the model is misspecified and the Type I and II error rates are unknown.

Under the General Linear Mixed Model, the two random effects are assumed to be independent and distributed as $G_{k:l} \approx N(\sigma_{g:c}^2)$ and $\varepsilon_{i:k:l} \approx N(\sigma_e^2)$. Under the Generalized Linear Mixed Model, the data are assumed to have a non-Gaussian distribution of a particular form.

Under the Generalized Linear Mixed Model, it is the linear predictor η_i that is assumed to be a linear function of the fixed and random effects, not the expected value μ_i (cf. Chapter 4). As a result, readers should understand that the simple presentation of the model and the material that flows from it (the definition of intervention effect, the expected mean squares, and the variance of the intervention effect) are correct only with a Gaussian distribution and an identity link. Conceptually, the presentation is equally applicable given any variance and link functions, but in the scale defined by the link function and with the distribution appropriate to the variance function.

Even without reliance on the Generalized Linear Mixed Model, this analysis appears to be robust to violation of the normality assumption for the residual-error distribution, given a moderate number of groups and members (Hannan and Murray, 1996). It also provides substantial protection against violations of the independence assumption as the most likely form of dependence is modeled explicitly via $G_{k:l}$.

This analysis specifies only one source of systematic variation among the study conditions, C_l. Any factor other than the intervention that favors one condition over the other serves to bias the estimate of the intervention effect; the bias may be positive or negative, large or small. If hundreds of groups are randomized to each condition, the investigator can assume that all potential sources of bias are evenly distributed among the conditions. Given the usual state of affairs in a group-randomized trial, where fewer than 10 groups are assigned to each condition, that is a strong assumption, one that is untestable and that the investigator should avoid. Without randomization of a large number of groups to each condition, the design is often uninterpretable because the risk for bias is very high. If bias is present, the true Type I and II error rates are unknown.

This analysis also assumes that all groups and members respond to the intervention in the same way. Violations reduce power by reducing the precision of the intervention effect.

Strengths and Weaknesses

The strength of this analysis lies in its simplicity. The major weakness is that it assumes that any difference observed between the intervention and control conditions is due to the intervention. A second weakness is that any variation not attributable to condition is left to the group or to residual error. Such variation serves only to reduce power by reducing the precision of the estimate of the intervention effect. Absent randomization of a large number of groups to each condition, this is a weak design that cannot be remedied in the analysis.

Adjusted Analysis of Posttest Data

In the adjusted analysis, covariates are added to the analysis to reduce confounding, to improve the precision of the estimate of the intervention effect, or both. Covariates can be measured at any level and are written generically as X_o ($o = 1 \ldots x$). Covariates measured at the group level and member level are distinguished as X_g and X_m.

The Model

The model for the adjusted analysis is:

$$Y_{i:k:l} = \mu + C_l + \sum_{o=1}^{x} \beta_o(X_{oi:k:l} - \overline{X}_o \ldots) + G_{k:l} + \varepsilon_{i:k:l} \qquad (5.4)$$

This model differs from the model for the unadjusted analysis presented above only by addition of the covariates. For each covariate, the portion of $Y_{i:k:l}$ that is explained by the difference between the observed value and sample mean on the covariate $(X_{oi:k:l} - \overline{X}_o \ldots)$ is attributed to the covariate. Any difference that remains between the predicted and observed value is left to the residual error $(\varepsilon_{i:k:l})$.

In most group-randomized trials, condition is a fixed effect. The random effects allow for correlation among members within a group $(G_{k:l})$ and for random variation among the members $(\varepsilon_{i:k:l})$.

The Intervention Effect

In the familiar ANCOVA, the F-statistic assesses the variation among the adjusted condition means against the variation among the adjusted group means. The null hypothesis is that the variation due to the conditions is zero. When there are only two conditions, the numerator of the F-statistic is based on a single df and it is more convenient to use the t-statistic. In that case, the intervention effect is the difference between the adjusted condition means and the null hypothesis is that the difference is zero. For the intervention and control conditions, the intervention effect is:

$$\Delta = (\overline{Y}_{..I} - \overline{Y}_{..C}) - \sum_{o=1}^{x} \beta_o (\overline{X}_{o..I} - \overline{X}_{o..C}) \qquad (5.5)$$

The Expected Mean Squares

The expected mean squares for this analysis are shown in Table 5.2. Note that the covariates are not shown in the table except as they affect the df for the other terms. The MS_c has three components: residual error (σ_e^2), a weighted component of variance due to the groups ($m\sigma_{g:c}^2$), and a weighted component of variance due to condition ($mg\sigma_c^2$). The test of the null hypothesis is $MS_c/MS_{g:c}$.

For each covariate measured at the group level (x_g), df associated with that covariate are lost from $MS_{g:c}$. For each covariate measured at the member level (x_m), df associated with that covariate are lost from MS_e. Because df at the group level are generally limited and are critical for power, use of covariates measured at the group level should be restricted to those that either correct confounding or measurably reduce the variance of the intervention effect.

Table 5.2. Expected Mean Squares for the Adjusted Analysis of Data From a Nested Cross-Sectional Posttest-Only Control Group Design

Source	df	E(MS)	MS
Condition	$c-1$	$\sigma_e^2 + m\sigma_{g:c}^2 + mg\sigma_c^2$	MS_c
Group:C	$c(g-1) - x_g$	$\sigma_e^2 + m\sigma_{g:c}^2$	$MS_{g:c}$
Member:G:C	$gc(m-1) - x_m$	σ_e^2	MS_e

The Variance of the Intervention Effect

When the intervention effect is defined as the difference between two adjusted condition means, the variance of that intervention effect under the null hypothesis is:

$$\sigma_\Delta^2 = 2\left(\frac{MS_{g:c}}{mg}\right) \tag{5.6}$$

Here there are m members per group and g groups per condition. The $MS_{g:c}$ reflects the regression adjustment for covariates. A more detailed presentation on the impact of this procedure on the variance components is reserved for Chapter 9.

Selection of Covariates

Selection of covariates is complicated in a group-randomized trial because they can be measured at multiple levels. For example, group as well as member characteristics may be used as covariates, either separately or in combination. In general, the investigator should seek to identify factors likely to be related to the endpoints prior to the collection of data so that they can be measured and considered as possible covariates at the time of the analysis. Those factors vary according to the content of the study, and no list can be suggested that would be appropriate for all studies. In particular, it would be dangerous to assume that adjustment for basic demographic variables such as age and sex would be sufficient for all studies. Instead, covariates must be chosen based on the substantive area of the research.

Once the data are available, the pool of potential covariates can be examined in preliminary analyses to determine if they explain variation among groups or members. The potential covariates that pass this initial screening can be examined during the analysis to determine whether there is evidence of confounding or whether they explain significant variation after adjustment for other factors in the model.

Confounding is assessed by comparing the unadjusted coefficient for condition with the adjusted coefficient. If the adjustment changes the coefficient by a degree that the investigator deems important, then confounding is established and the adjusted analysis should be used. The presence or absence of confounding is determined on the basis of judgment, not on the basis of any statistical test.

Even if there is no evidence of meaningful confounding, the investigator can retain covariates that explain significant variation in the outcome, for they can improve the precision of the analysis even if they do not remove bias.

Three recent papers have focused on the issues of covariate selection and assessment of covariate utility in the context of group-randomized trials, and the reader may find those helpful (Murray and Short, 1995, 1996, 1997).

Assumptions

The assumptions for this analysis include those from the unadjusted analysis for this design, and violations have similar effects. In addition, this analysis allows variation in the endpoint to be attributed to the covariates included in the model. As a result, the investigator must be cognizant of several assumptions attached to the use of the regression adjustment for these covariates.

First, the endpoint is assumed to be linearly related to each covariate. Violations can result in upward or downward bias in the estimate of the intervention effect, so this assumption should be tested. Since nonlinear relationships are rarely more than quadratic, the addition of a quadratic term (X_o^2) often provides a simple method both to estimate the degree of nonlinearity and to test for its significance. Higher-order polynomials may be added as needed. Alternatively, the covariate may be broken into quartiles or quintiles and dummy-coded indicator variables used to represent those levels; more than five levels are rarely needed to reflect the extent of the nonlinear relationship (Kish, 1987).

Second, the regression slopes for each covariate are assumed homogeneous across the conditions. Here, violations reduce the power of the analysis. This assumption is also easily tested, by inclusion of terms reflecting a possible interaction between condition and the covariate in question (CX_g or CX_m). For fixed-effect covariates, the interaction is a fixed effect and is tested against $MS_{g:c}$. The null hypothesis for any such interaction is that the regression slopes are homogeneous across the conditions. The test for that hypothesis has lower power than for the main effect of condition, so care should be taken when interpreting the results of such a test, with attention given to the magnitude of the interaction as well as the p-value of the test. In addition, since extra df are lost at the group level for each interaction between condition and a covariate measured at that level, analysts should be very selective in their use of such interactions.

Third, the regression slopes for each covariate are assumed to be homogeneous across groups within each condition. While this is generally a plausible assumption, violations reduce the power of the analysis. This assumption is also easily tested, by inclusion of terms reflecting a possible interaction between the groups and the covariate in question (GX_g or GX_m). The interaction would be a random effect and tested against residual error. The null hypothesis for the interaction term is that the regression slopes are homogeneous. The test for that hypothesis has lower power than for the main effect of the covariate, so care should be taken when interpreting the results of such a test, with attention given to the magnitude of the interaction as well as the p-value of the test.

Fourth, it is assumed that the intervention has no effect on the covariates. This is the same as assuming that the covariates are not on the causal pathway between the intervention and the endpoint. Violations reduce the power for the test for the intervention by reducing the intervention-effect estimate; as a result, violations should be avoided. This is a particularly difficult issue for the Posttest-Only Control Group Design, because it is not possible to select covariates that were measured prior to the intervention. Under these circumstances, the investigator must be especially careful to select covariates that cannot be influenced by the intervention; demographic and other immutable characteristics are candidates, but only if they are related to the endpoint.

This analysis also assumes that all groups and members respond to the intervention in the same way. Violations reduce power by reducing the precision of the intervention effect.

Strengths and Weaknesses

This analysis is stronger than the unadjusted analysis for the same design. To the extent that the covariates capture biases that otherwise would be confounded with condition, the regression adjustment may reduce bias. In addition, the adjusted analysis is usually more powerful than the unadjusted analysis because the variance components in $MS_{g:c}$ are often reduced. However, that does not always happen. It is quite possible for the adjusted $MS_{g:c}$ to be larger than the unadjusted $MS_{g:c}$. In that case, power is reduced.

If no group-level covariates are used, the ddf are the same in the adjusted and unadjusted analyses, so any improvement in power accrues only from the regression adjustment for covariates. If group-level covariates are used, any improvement in power is offset by the reduction in power from the reduction in the ddf available for the test of the intervention effect.

Regression adjustment for covariates is subject to a variety of weaknesses and misuses. Chief among them for this design is that the investigator cannot know whether all differences among the conditions that are not associated with the intervention have been removed by the regression adjustment. To the extent that any remain, they are confounded with condition and bias the estimate of the intervention effect; that bias can be negative or positive, large or small. The only effective solution to this problem is to randomize a large number of groups to each condition, so that randomization has an opportunity to evenly distribute confounding influences among the conditions. Because this strategy is rarely possible in the context of group-randomized trials, the Posttest-Only Control Group Design is not generally recommended.

Quite apart from that problem, random measurement error in the covariates can both reduce power and bias the estimates of the regression slopes. Where there is only a single covariate, the effect is an underadjustment. With multiple covariates, the multiple measurement errors can result in a net over- or under-adjustment. This can result in spurious intervention effects, either positive or negative, large or small. The best way to avoid such problems is to choose covariates that are well measured.

Inclusion of a laundry list of covariates in an effort to correct for sources of bias uses *df*, often inflates the variance of the estimate of the intervention effect, and creates a greater opportunity for violations of assumptions and measurement error. Unless the covariates are well chosen, they may not serve to reduce bias or improve precision.

As noted in Chapter 3, the Posttest-Only Control Group Design is a weak design in the absence of randomization of a large number of groups to each condition. While the adjusted analysis is better than the unadjusted analysis, it cannot make up for an inherently weak design.

Pretest-Posttest Control Group Design

In the nested cross-sectional version of this design, data are collected in each condition before and after the intervention has been delivered in the intervention condition. As discussed in Chapter 3, this is much stronger design than the Posttest-Only Control Group Design. It is also the most common of the nested cross-sectional designs.

A number of options exist for analysis of data from this design. For example, the pretest data could be ignored; because that option results in the analyses discussed earlier in this chapter, no further attention is given to it here. As another option, time can be included as a factor in the analysis, crossed with condition. This option has as its two major variations an unadjusted analysis and an analysis that includes regression adjustments for covariates. Examples are provided in Chapter 7.

Unadjusted Time × Condition Analysis

The Model

In the unadjusted time × condition analysis, the model is:

$$Y_{i:jk:l} = \mu + C_l + T_j + TC_{jl} + G_{k:l} + TG_{jk:l} + \varepsilon_{i:jk:l} \qquad (5.7)$$

Here the observed value ($Y_{i:jk:l}$) for the ith member nested within the kth group and l^{th} condition and observed at the jth time is expressed as a function of the grand mean (μ), the effect of the lth condition (C_l), the effect of the jth time (T_j), the joint effect of the lth condition and the jth time (TC_{jl}), the realized value of the kth group ($G_{k:l}$), and the realized value of the combination of the kth group and j^{th} time ($TG_{jk:l}$). Any difference between this predicted value and the observed value is allocated to the residual error ($\varepsilon_{i:jk:l}$).

In most group-randomized trials, condition, time, and their interaction are fixed effects. In order to account for the positive intraclass correlation expected in the data, $G_{k:l}$ and $TG_{jk:l}$ must be included in the analysis as random effects; simulation studies have shown that failure to do so, in the presence of measurable intraclass correlation, will result in a Type I error rate that is inflated, often badly (Zucker et al., 1990; Murray and Wolfinger, 1994; Murray et al., 1996). The three random effects allow for correlation among members within a group ($G_{k:l}$), for correlation among members within a time $\times$ group survey ($TG_{jk:l}$), and for random variation among the members ($\varepsilon_{i:jk:l}$).

The Intervention Effect

In the familiar ANOVA, the F-statistic assesses the variation among the time $\times$ condition means against the variation among the time $\times$ group means. The null hypothesis is that the variation due to conditions over time is zero. When there are only two conditions and two time intervals, the numerator of the F-statistic is based on a single df and it is more convenient to use the t-statistic. In that case, the intervention effect is the net difference and the null hypothesis is that the net difference is zero. For the intervention and control conditions, the intervention effect is:

$$\Delta = (\overline{Y}_{..2I} - \overline{Y}_{..1I}) - (\overline{Y}_{..2C} - \overline{Y}_{..1C}) \qquad (5.8)$$

The Expected Mean Squares

The expected mean squares are shown in Table 5.3. The MS_{tc} has three components: residual error (σ_e^2), a weighted component of variance due to the interaction of time with group ($m\sigma_{tg:c}^2$), and a weighted component of variance due to the intervention ($mg\sigma_{tc}^2$). The test of the null hypothesis is $MS_{tc}/MS_{tg:c}$.

The Variance of the Intervention Effect

When the intervention effect is defined as the net difference over two time intervals between two conditions, the variance of that intervention effect under the null hypothesis is:

Table 5.3. Expected Mean Squares for the Unadjusted Analysis of Data From a Nested Cross-Sectional Pretest-Posttest Control Group Design

Source	df	E(MS)	MS
Condition	$c-1$	$\sigma_e^2 + mt\sigma_{g:c}^2 + mtg\sigma_c^2$	MS_c
Group:C	$c(g-1)$	$\sigma_e^2 + mt\sigma_{g:c}^2$	$MS_{g:c}$
Time	$t-1$	$\sigma_e^2 + m\sigma_{tg:c}^2 + mgc\sigma_t^2$	MS_t
TC	$(t-1)(c-1)$	$\sigma_e^2 + m\sigma_{tg:c}^2 + mg\sigma_{tc}^2$	MS_{tc}
TG:C	$(t-1)c(g-1)$	$\sigma_e^2 + m\sigma_{tg:c}^2$	$MS_{tg:c}$
Member:TG:C	$tgc(m-1)$	σ_e^2	MS_e

$$\sigma_\Delta^2 = 2*2\left(\frac{MS_{tg:c}}{mg}\right) \tag{5.9}$$

Here there are m members in each time $\times$ group survey and g groups per condition. The $MS_{tg:c}$ reflects the repeat observations on the same groups. A more detailed presentation on the impact of this procedure on the variance components is reserved for Chapter 9.

Assumptions

This analysis provides for three sources of random variation. If there are additional sources in the data, the model is misspecified and the true Type I and II error rates are unknown.

Under the General Linear Mixed Model, the random effects are assumed to be independent and distributed as $G_{k:l} \approx N(0,\sigma_{g:c}^2)$, $TG_{jk:l} \approx N(0,\sigma_{tg:c}^2)$, and $\varepsilon_{i:jk:l} \approx N(0,\sigma_e^2)$. With the important caveats noted earlier in this chapter, the analysis can be extended to non-Gaussian data by assuming a different distribution for $\varepsilon_{i:jk:l}$ and a different link function. The analysis would then represent an application of the Generalized Linear Mixed Model.

Even without reliance on the Generalized Linear Mixed Model, this analysis appears to be robust to violation of the normality assumption for the residual error distribution, given a moderate number of groups and members (Hannan and Murray, 1996). It also provides substantial protection against violations of the independence assumption as the most likely forms of dependence are modeled explicitly via $G_{k:l}$ and $TG_{jk:l}$.

This analysis assumes that any net difference observed between the intervention and control conditions is due to the intervention. Any source of bias that would serve to favor one condition over the other serves to bias the estimate of the intervention effect. That bias may be positive or negative, large or small. In the presence of such bias, the true Type I and II error rates are unknown.

This analysis also assumes that all groups and members respond to the intervention in the same way. Violations reduce power by reducing the precision of the intervention effect.

Strengths and Weaknesses

A major advantage of this analysis over those presented for the Posttest-Only Control Group Design is the availability of pretest data in both conditions and the inclusion of those data in the analysis. This allows for an adjustment for baseline levels, as the intervention effect is assessed as a net difference in the intervention condition relative to the control condition. Because it is more difficult to suggest plausible alternative explanations for net differences than for simple differences, this feature provides a better defense against sources of bias than was available in the Posttest-Only Control Group Design.

Even so, there is no guarantee that the study conditions are similar in all respects at baseline. To the extent that there are different trends operating among the conditions, they remain as a threat to the validity of the unadjusted analysis in the form of differential maturation or secular trends.

This analysis often has less power than either analysis discussed for the Posttest-Only Control Group Design. The *ddf* for condition are the same, but the intervention effect in this analysis involves a net difference rather than a simple difference. Power is always less for a more complicated effect such as a net difference relative to a less complicated effect such as a simple difference, all other factors constant. Thus, a larger study may be required to achieve the same power. This issue is discussed further in Chapter 9.

Adjusted Time × Condition Analysis

Regression adjustment for covariates can be used to remove variability due to covariates from the time × condition analysis. Because different members are seen at each time in a nested cross-sectional design, the covariates must be measured concurrent with measurement of the endpoint. As a result, this regression adjustment is not the same as an adjustment for baseline values that might be used in a nested cohort design. Even so, regression adjustment for covariates can be helpful, such as adjusting for height, weight, room temperature, or arm circumference for blood pressure readings. To the extent that such factors are unevenly distributed among conditions, they would induce confounding if ignored. To the extent that they explain variation among groups or members, they would reduce power if ignored. As in the Posttest-Only Control Group Design, covariates can be measured at any level.

The Model

The model for the adjusted analysis is:

$$Y_{i:jk:l} = \mu + C_l + T_j + TC_{jl} + \sum_{o=1}^{x} \beta_o(X_{oi:jk:l} - \overline{X}_{o \cdot \ldots}) + G_{k:l} + TG_{jk:l} + \varepsilon_{i:jk:l}$$

(5.10)

This model differs from the model for the unadjusted analysis only by addition of the covariates. For each covariate, the portion of $Y_{i:jk:l}$ that is explained by the difference between the observed value and sample mean on the covariate, $(X_{oi:jk:l} - \overline{X}_{o \cdot \ldots})$, is attributed to the covariate.

In most community trials, condition, time, and their interaction are fixed effects. The random effects allow for variation and correlation as described for the unadjusted analysis.

The Intervention Effect

In the familiar ANCOVA, the F-statistic assesses the variation among the adjusted time $\times$ condition means against the variation among the adjusted time $\times$ group means. The null hypothesis is that the variation due to conditions over time is zero. When there are only two conditions and two time intervals, the numerator of the F-statistic is based on a single df and it is more convenient to use the t-statistic. In that case, the intervention effect is the adjusted net difference and the null hypothesis is that the adjusted net difference is zero. For the intervention and control conditions, the intervention effect is:

$$\Delta = (\overline{Y}_{\cdot \cdot 2I} - \overline{Y}_{\cdot \cdot 1I}) - (\overline{Y}_{\cdot \cdot 2C} - \overline{Y}_{\cdot \cdot 1C}) - \sum_{o=1}^{x} \beta_o((\overline{X}_{o \cdot \cdot 2I} - \overline{X}_{o \cdot \cdot 1I}) - (\overline{X}_{o \cdot \cdot 2C} - \overline{X}_{o \cdot \cdot 1C}))$$

(5.11)

The Expected Mean Squares

The expected mean squares for this analysis are shown in Table 5.4. Note that the covariates are not shown in the table except as they affect the df for the other terms. The MS_{tc} has three components: residual error (σ_e^2), a weighted

Table 5.4. Expected Mean Squares for the Adjusted Analysis of Data From a Nested Cross-Sectional Pretest-Posttest Control Group Design

Source	df	E(MS)	MS
Condition	$c-1$	$\sigma_e^2 + mt\sigma_{g:c}^2 + mtg\sigma_c^2$	MS_c
Group:C	$c(g-1)-x_g$	$\sigma_e^2 + mt\sigma_{g:c}^2$	$MS_{g:c}$
Time	$t-1$	$\sigma_e^2 + m\sigma_{tg:c}^2 + mgc\sigma_t^2$	MS_t
TC	$(t-1)(c-1)$	$\sigma_e^2 + m\sigma_{tg:c}^2 + mg\sigma_{tc}^2$	MS_{tc}
$TG:C$	$(t-1)c(g-1)-x_g$	$\sigma_e^2 + m\sigma_{tg:c}^2$	$MS_{tg:c}$
Member:TG:C	$tgc(m-1)-x_m$	σ_e^2	MS_e

component of variance due to the interaction of time with group ($m\sigma_{tg:c}^2$), and a weighted component of variance due to the intervention ($mg\sigma_{tc}^2$). The test of the null hypothesis is $MS_{tc}/MS_{tg:c}$.

For each covariate measured at the group level (x_g), *df* associated with that covariate are lost from $MS_{g:c}$ and from $MS_{tg:c}$. For each covariate measured at the member level (x_m), *df* are lost from MS_e.

The Variance of the Intervention Effect

When the intervention effect is defined as the adjusted net difference over two time intervals between two conditions, the variance of that intervention effect under the null hypothesis is:

$$\sigma_\Delta^2 = 2 * 2\left(\frac{MS_{tg:c}}{mg}\right) \qquad (5.12)$$

Here there are *m* members per time × group survey and *g* groups per condition. The $MS_{tg:c}$ reflects the repeat observations on the same groups, as well as the regression adjustment for covariates. A more detailed presentation of the impact on those procedures on the variance components is reserved for Chapter 9.

Assumptions

The assumptions for this analysis include those from the unadjusted analysis for this design and those related to the regression adjustment for covariates for the Posttest-Only Control Group Design. Violations have effects as described in those sections.

Strengths and Weaknesses

Relative to the adjusted analysis of the Posttest-Only Control Group Design, a larger study is required for the adjusted analysis in the Pretest-Posttest Control Group Design to achieve the same power because the intervention effect is an adjusted net difference instead of an adjusted simple difference. However, relative to the unadjusted analysis of the Pretest-Posttest Control Group design, a smaller study is required to the extent that the regression adjustment for covariates reduces the variance of the intervention effect.

On balance, this analysis is the strongest of the four presented thus far. By virtue of having and using baseline data, it provides a better defense against the problems that threaten the validity of the analysis of data from a Posttest-Only Control Group Design. By virtue of including regression adjustment for covariates, it is often more powerful and less affected by potential sources of bias than the unadjusted analysis presented in the previous section. Given random assignment of a modest number of groups to each condition, this can be a strong design and a good analysis, provided the assumptions underlying the analysis are met.

Stratification or Matching in the Analysis

As discussed in Chapter 3, there are three quite different reasons to employ *a priori* stratification or matching in the design. First, an *a priori* stratified or matched design is preferred whenever the investigators want to ensure balance across conditions on an important potential source of bias. Second, an *a priori* stratified design is preferred whenever the investigators have an *a priori* interest in testing whether the intervention effect is different across strata defined by characteristics of the groups. Third, an *a priori* matched design can improve the precision of the analysis of the main effect for condition to the extent that the matching factors are well correlated with the primary endpoints. Similarly, an *a priori* stratified design can improve the precision of the analysis of the main effect of condition, but only if the stratum-specific effects are homogeneous.

It is certainly possible to employ *a priori* stratification or matching in order to control the influence of an important confounding variable without reflecting that design feature in the analysis. If the investigator has no interest in stratum-specific effects and expects only limited improvement in precision, then an unstratified or unmatched analysis is preferred. However, if the investigator expects different intervention effects among the strata, a stratified analysis should be used. And if the investigator expects that there can be a measurable improvement in power, a stratified or matched analysis is preferred.

Stratification also can be employed in the analysis even if it was not part of the design. This is often called *post hoc* stratification. It is applied after the data are collected, as part of the analysis, and involves stratification on one or more member characteristics rather than on one or more group characteristics.

The null hypothesis in any stratified analysis in which stratum is a fixed effect is that the stratum-specific intervention effects are homogeneous. As a result, the focus of the sections on stratified analyses in which stratum is a fixed effect is on the test of that null hypothesis. If that null hypothesis is rejected, the investigator should report the stratum-specific results, along with the test of the null hypothesis from the stratified analysis. If that null hypothesis is not rejected, the investigator should report that result and then collapse across strata. At that point, the analysis reverts to an unstratified analysis as presented in earlier sections of this chapter. The stratification factor should be retained as a covariate if there is evidence that it reduces confounding or improves precision.

It should be noted that the power for alternatives to the null hypothesis in the stratified analysis is much less than for alternatives in the unstratified analysis, all other factors constant. This is because the null hypothesis in the stratified analysis involves a more complex intervention effect than in the unstratified analysis. Power is always less for more complex effects than for simpler effects. Because of the substantial difference in sample-size requirements, the investigator must determine in advance whether the stratified null hypothesis is critical, and if it is, plan a large enough study to have sufficient power to assess it.

In contrast, the null hypothesis in any stratified analysis in which stratum is a random effect, as well as in any matched analysis, is simply that there is no intervention effect. There is no interest in whether the intervention effect is homogeneous across strata or matched sets. Instead, interest is in whether the intervention effect is significant given the variation associated with the strata or the matched sets.

This section shows how to include stratification and matching in the analysis. *A priori* and *post hoc* stratification are presented separately, as they require different analyses. Matching is considered as a special case of *a priori* stratification. The adjusted analysis from the Pretest-Posttest Control Group Design is used to illustrate these analyses, though stratification and matching can be used with any of the designs in this chapter.

A Priori Stratification With Stratum as a Fixed Effect

When the investigator is interested only in the levels of the stratification factor that are included in the design, stratum is a fixed effect. As an example, consider a multicenter group-randomized trial in which the investigators are interested only in the centers included in the trial. Such studies may develop because a single research center cannot operate a study large enough to address the research question of interest. Or it may be that a single research center does not have access to all the populations or subgroups of interest. Under these conditions, investigators from multiple centers may join together to organize a multicenter group-randomized trial. Such trials have common intervention and evaluation protocols, common training and quality control, and frequent meetings of the investigators from each of the centers. Often a coordinating center manages the collection and analysis of the data and provides expertise on design and analysis for the study.

If the investigators really are interested only in *narrow inferences* about the specific centers included in the study, center is included in the analysis as a fixed effect and the analysis presented in the this section is appropriate. However, if the investigators really want to make *broad inferences* about other centers "like those employed in the study," center must be included as a random effect and the analysis presented in the section that follows this one is appropriate.

The Model

The model for the Pretest-Posttest Control Group Design that includes *a priori* stratification with regression adjustment for covariates is:

$$Y_{i:jk:lp} = \mu + C_l + S_p + CS_{lp} + T_j + TC_{jl} + TS_{jp} + TCS_{jlp}$$
$$+ \sum_{o=1}^{x} \beta_o(X_{oi:jk:lp} - \bar{X}_{o.\ ....}) + G_{k:lp} + TG_{jk:lp} + \varepsilon_{i:jk:lp}$$

$$(5.13)$$

The S_p ($p = 1 \ldots s$) are the strata. Stratum is added both as a main effect and as a series of interactions with the other fixed effects. This adds four fixed effects to the unstratified model for the Pretest-Posttest Control Group Design. Note that the notation $G_{k:lp}$ reflects the nesting of the groups within the cells defined by the condition × stratum interaction.

In most group-randomized trials, condition, time, and their interaction are fixed effects. In this design, stratum is also a fixed effect; as are all its interactions involving condition and time. In order to account for the positive intraclass correlation expected in the data, $G_{k:lp}$ and $TG_{jk:lp}$ must be included in the analysis as random effects; simulation studies have shown that failure to do so, in the presence of measurable intraclass correlation, will result in a Type I error rate that is inflated, often badly (Zucker et al., 1990; Murray and

Wolfinger, 1994; Murray et al., 1996). The three random effects allow for correlation among the members within a group $(G_{k:lp})$, for correlation among the members within a time $\times$ group survey $(TG_{jk:lp})$, and for random variation among the members $(\varepsilon_{i:jk:lp})$.

The Intervention Effect

In the familiar ANCOVA, the F-statistic assesses the variation among the adjusted time $\times$ condition $\times$ stratum means against the variation among the adjusted time $\times$ group means. The null hypothesis is that the variation due to conditions over time and across strata is zero. When there are only two conditions, two time intervals, and two strata, the numerator of the F-statistic is based on a single df and it is more convenient to use the t-statistic. In that case, the intervention effect is defined as the difference between the two strata in their adjusted net differences. The null hypothesis is that the difference between the two strata is zero.

The Expected Mean Squares

The expected mean squares for this analysis are shown in Table 5.5. Note that the covariates are not shown in the table except as they affect the df for the other terms. The MS_{tcs} has three components: residual error (σ^2_e), a weighted component of variance due to the interaction of time with group $(m\sigma^2_{tg:cs})$, and a weighted component of variance due to the intervention $(mg\sigma^2_{tcs})$. The test of the null hypothesis is $MS_{tcs}/MS_{tg:cs}$.

Table 5.5. Expected Mean Squares for the Adjusted Analysis of Data From a Nested Cross-Sectional Pretest-Posttest Control Group Design With *A Priori* Stratification and Stratum as a Fixed Effect

Source	df	E(MS)	MS
Condition	$c-1$	$\sigma^2_e + mt\sigma^2_{g:cs} + mtgs\sigma^2_c$	MS_c
Strata	$s-1$	$\sigma^2_e + mt\sigma^2_{g:cs} + mtgc\sigma^2_s$	MS_s
CS	$(c-1)(s-1)$	$\sigma^2_e + mt\sigma^2_{g:cs} + mtg\sigma^2_{cs}$	MS_{cs}
Group:CS	$cs(g-1)-x_g$	$\sigma^2_e + mt\sigma^2_{g:cs}$	$MS_{g:cs}$
Time	$t-1$	$\sigma^2_e + m\sigma^2_{tg:cs} + mgcs\sigma^2_t$	MS_t
TC	$(t-1)(c-1)$	$\sigma^2_e + m\sigma^2_{tg:cs} + mgs\sigma^2_{tc}$	MS_{tc}
TS	$(t-1)(s-1)$	$\sigma^2_e + m\sigma^2_{tg:cs} + mgc\sigma^2_{ts}$	MS_{ts}
TCS	$(t-1)(c-1)(s-1)$	$\sigma^2_e + m\sigma^2_{tg:cs} + mg\sigma^2_{tcs}$	MS_{tcs}
TG:CS	$(t-1)cs(g-1)-x_g$	$\sigma^2_e + m\sigma^2_{tg:cs}$	$MS_{tg:cs}$
M:TG:CS	$tgcs(m-1)-x_m$	σ^2_e	MS_e

For each covariate measured at the group level (x_g), a degree of freedom is lost from $MS_{g:cs}$ and from $MS_{tg:cs}$. For each covariate measured at the member level (x_m), a degree of freedom is lost from MS_e.

The Variance of the Intervention Effect

When the intervention effect is defined as the contrast between two strata in their net difference over two time intervals between two conditions, the variance of that intervention effect under the null hypothesis is:

$$\sigma_\Delta^2 = 2 * 2 * 2 \left(\frac{MS_{tg:cs}}{mg} \right) \tag{5.14}$$

Here m is the number of observations in each time $\times$ group survey and g is the number of groups in each condition $\times$ stratum cell. The $MS_{tg:cs}$ reflects the stratification, the repeat observations on the same groups, and the regression adjustment for covariates. A more detailed presentation on the impact of those procedures on the variance components is reserved for Chapter 9.

Assumptions

This analysis provides for three sources of random variation. If there are additional sources in the data, the model is misspecified and the true Type I and II error rates are unknown.

Under the General Linear Mixed Model, the random effects are assumed to be independent and distributed as $G_{k:lp} \approx N(0, \sigma_{g:cs}^2)$, $TG_{jk:lp} \approx N(0, \sigma_{tg:cs}^2)$, and $\varepsilon_{i:jk:lp} \approx N(0, \sigma_e^2)$. With the important caveats noted earlier in this chapter, the analysis can be extended to non-Gaussian data by assuming a different distribution for $\varepsilon_{i:jk:lp}$ and a different link function. The analysis would then represent an application of the Generalized Linear Mixed Model.

Even without reliance on the Generalized Linear Mixed Model, this analysis appears to be robust to violation of the normality assumption for the residual-error distribution, given a moderate number of groups and members (Hannan and Murray, 1996). It also provides substantial protection against violations of the independence assumption as the most likely forms of dependence are modeled via $G_{k:lp}$ and $TG_{jk:lp}$.

The assumptions for this analysis include those related to the regression adjustment for covariates; violations have effects as described earlier. The stratified analysis carries the additional assumption that the relationship between each covariate and the endpoint is constant across the strata. Violations reduce power by reducing the precision of the intervention effect. This assumption may be tested via interaction terms involving the strata and the covariates.

Strengths and Weaknesses

The primary advantage and rationale of reflecting the *a priori* stratification in the analysis is that it provides a test of the null hypothesis that the intervention effect is homogeneous across the strata. That is simply assumed in an unstratified analysis. The stratified analysis is the only approach that provides a test of this null hypothesis.

The primary weakness of reflecting the *a priori* stratification in the analysis is that the power for the test of the null hypothesis is more limited than for the test of the main effect for condition, all other factors constant. This is because the null hypothesis in the stratified analysis involves a more complex intervention effect than in the unstratified analysis. Because of the substantial difference in sample size requirements, the investigator must determine in advance whether the stratified null hypothesis is critical, and if it is, plan a large enough study to have sufficient power to assess it.

A Priori Stratification With Stratum as a Random Effect

In the analysis presented in the previous section, the levels of the stratification factor included in the design were the only levels of interest. As a result, stratum was a fixed effect and inferences were limited to those levels. There are other circumstances in which the levels of the stratification factor represent some larger population of levels to which the investigator wishes to generalize any findings. Under these circumstances, stratum is included as a random effect.

A good example is the multicenter group-randomized trial in which the investigators want to generalize to other centers like those used in the study. When the investigators are interested in such *broad inferences,* center must be included in the analysis as a random effect. It is that action and its proper implementation that provides the statistical basis for any such broad inference, as opposed to the more *narrow inference* available when center is included as a fixed effect.[1]

The Model

Consider a multicenter group-randomized trial with a pretest and a posttest, two conditions, several centers, and groups nested within the cells of the condition × center interaction. The model for this analysis is:

$$Y_{i:jk:lp} = \mu + C_l + T_j + TC_{jl} + \sum_{o=1}^{x} \beta_o(X_{oi:jk:lp} - \overline{X}_{o\cdots\cdots}) + S_p$$
$$+ CS_{lp} + G_{k:lp} + TS_{jp} + TCS_{jlp} + TG_{jk:lp} + \varepsilon_{i:jk:lp} \qquad (5.15)$$

All four effects involving stratum are now shown as random effects.

In most group-randomized trials, condition, time, and their interaction are fixed effects. Because the investigator wants the analysis to provide a statistical basis for generalization to other strata like those employed in the study, stratum and its interactions are random effects. In order to account for the positive intraclass correlation expected in the data, $G_{k:lp}$ and $TG_{jk:lp}$ must be included in the analysis as random effects; simulation studies have shown that failure to do so, in the presence of measurable intraclass correlation, will result in a Type I error rate that is inflated, often badly (Zucker et al., 1990; Murray and Wolfinger, 1994; Murray et al., 1996). The seven random effects allow for correlation among members within a stratum (S_p), within a condition $\times$ stratum cell (CS_{lp}), within a group ($G_{k:lp}$), within a time $\times$ stratum survey (TS_{jp}), within a time $\times$ condition $\times$ stratum survey (TCS_{jlp}), within a time $\times$ group survey ($TG_{jk:lp}$), and for random variation among the members ($\varepsilon_{i:jk:lp}$). Note that S_p, CS_{lp} and TCS_{jlp} are no longer fixed effects of interest, but are instead sources of random variation.

The Intervention Effect

When stratum is a random effect, the intervention is represented by the time $\times$ condition interaction. When stratum is a random effect, the strata themselves are of no particular interest and instead the interest is in whether the intervention effect is significant given the variation associated with the strata. In other words, the interest is in generalizing to the larger population of strata that they represent; the strata play no role in the definition of the intervention effect, though they do play an important role in the variance of that effect.

In the familiar ANCOVA, the F-statistic assesses the variation among the adjusted time $\times$ condition means against the variation among the adjusted time $\times$ group means. The null hypothesis is that the variation due to conditions over time is zero. When there are only two conditions and two time intervals, the numerator of the F-statistic is based on a single df and it is more convenient to use the t-statistic. In that case, the intervention effect is the adjusted net difference and the null hypothesis is that the adjusted net difference is zero. For the intervention and control conditions, the intervention effect is:

$$\Delta = (\overline{Y}_{\cdot\cdot2I} - \overline{Y}_{\cdot\cdot1I}) - (\overline{Y}_{\cdot\cdot2C} - \overline{Y}_{\cdot\cdot1C}) - \sum_{o=1}^{x} \beta_o((\overline{X}_{o\cdot\cdot2I} - \overline{X}_{\cdot\cdot1I}) - (\overline{X}_{o\cdot\cdot2C} - \overline{X}_{o\cdot\cdot1C}))$$
$$(5.16)$$

Table 5.6. Expected Mean Squares for the Adjusted Analysis of Data From a Nested Cross-Sectional Pretest-Posttest Control Group Design with *A Priori* Stratification and Stratum as a Random Effect

Source	df	E(MS)	MS
Condition	$c-1$	$\sigma_e^2 + mt\sigma_{g:cs}^2 + mgt\sigma_{cs}^2 + mgts\sigma_c^2$	MS_c
Strata	$s-1$	$\sigma_e^2 + mt\sigma_{g:cs}^2 + mgtc\sigma_s^2$	MS_s
CS	$(c-1)(s-1)$	$\sigma_e^2 + mt\sigma_{g:cs}^2 + mgt\sigma_{cs}^2$	MS_{cs}
Group:CS	$cs(g-1) - x_g$	$\sigma_e^2 + mt\sigma_{g:cs}^2$	$MS_{g:cs}$
Time	$t-1$	$\sigma_e^2 + m\sigma_{tg:cs}^2 + mgc\sigma_{ts}^2 + mgcs\sigma_t^2$	MS_t
TC	$(t-1)(c-1)$	$\sigma_e^2 + m\sigma_{tg:cs}^2 + mg\sigma_{tcs}^2 + mgs\sigma_{tc}^2$	MS_{tc}
TS	$(t-1)(s-1)$	$\sigma_e^2 + m\sigma_{tg:cs}^2 + mgc\sigma_{ts}^2$	MS_{ts}
TCS	$(t-1)(c-1)(s-1)$	$\sigma_e^2 + m\sigma_{tg:cs}^2 + mg\sigma_{tcs}^2$	MS_{tcs}
TG:CS	$(t-1)cs(g-1) - x_g$	$\sigma_e^2 + m\sigma_{tg:cs}^2$	$MS_{tg:cs}$
M:TG:CS	$tgcs(m-1) - x_m$	σ_e^2	MS_e

The Expected Mean Squares

The expected mean squares for this analysis are shown in Table 5.6. Note that the covariates are not shown in the table except as they affect the *df* for the other terms. The MS_{tc} has four components: residual error (σ_e^2), a weighted component of variance due to the interaction of time with group ($m\sigma_{tg:cs}^2$), a weighted component of variance due to the interaction of time with group and stratum ($mg\sigma_{tcs}^2$), and a weighted component of variance due to the intervention ($mgs\sigma_{tc}^2$). The test of the null hypothesis is MS_{tc}/MS_{tcs}.

For each covariate measured at the group level (x_g), *df* associated with that covariate are lost from $MS_{g:cs}$ and from $MS_{tg:cs}$. For each covariate measured at the member level (x_m), *df* are lost from MS_e.

The Variance of the Intervention Effect

When the intervention effect is defined as the net difference over two time intervals between two conditions, the variance of that intervention effect under the null hypothesis is:

$$\sigma_\Delta^2 = 2*2\left(\frac{MS_{tcs}}{mgs}\right) \tag{5.17}$$

Here *m* is the number of observations in each time × group survey, *g* is the number of groups in each condition × stratum cell, and *s* is the number of strata. The MS_{tcs} reflects the stratification on center, the repeat observations on the same groups, and the regression adjustment for covariates. A more detailed presentation on the impact of those procedures on the variance components is reserved for Chapter 9.

Assumptions

This analysis provides for seven sources of random variation. If there are additional sources in the data, the model is misspecified and the true Type I and II error rates are unknown.

Under the General Linear Mixed Model, the random effects are assumed to be independent and distributed as $S_p \approx N(0, \sigma_s^2)$ $CS_{lp} \approx N(0, \sigma_{cs}^2)$ $G_{k:lp} \approx N(0, \sigma_{g:cs}^2)$, $TS_{jp} \approx N(0, \sigma_{ts}^2)$, $TCS_{jlp} \approx N(0, \sigma_{tcs}^2)$, $TG_{jk:lp} \approx N(0, \sigma_{tg:cs}^2)$, and $\varepsilon_{k:jk:lp} \approx N(0, \sigma_e^2)$. With the important caveats noted earlier in this chapter, the analysis can be extended to non-Gaussian data by assuming a different distribution for $\varepsilon_{i:jk:lp}$ and a different link function. The analysis would then represent an application of the Generalized Linear Mixed Model.

Even without reliance on the Generalized Linear Mixed Model, this analysis appears to be robust to violation of the normality assumption for the residual error distribution, given a moderate number of groups and members (Hannan and Murray, 1996). It also provides substantial protection against violations of the independence assumption as the most likely forms of dependence are modeled via $G_{k:lp}$ and $TG_{jk:lp}$ and the random effects involving stratum.

The remaining assumptions made for the stratified analysis presented in the previous section also apply to this analysis. Violations have a similar effect.

Strengths and Weaknesses

The strengths and weaknesses described in the previous section apply equally here. The major additional advantage that accompanies modeling stratum as a random effect is that the investigator has the statistical basis for generalizing any findings to other strata like those used in the study.

Matching in the Analysis

The matched analysis is a simplified version of the analysis presented in the preceding section. That is because the matched-pairs design is an example of *a priori* stratification in which stratum is a random effect. What separates the matched analysis from the usual *a priori* stratified analysis is that there is only one group per cell instead of several. To avoid introducing new terminology, the term *stratum* is used here to refer to the matched sets.

The Model

The model for the Pretest-Posttest Control Group Design that includes matching and regression adjustment for covariates is:

$$Y_{i:jlp} = \mu + C_l + T_j + TC_{jl} + \sum_{o=1}^{x} \beta_o(X_{oi:jlp} - \overline{X}_{o \cdots}) + S_p + CS_{lp} + TS_{jp}$$
$$+ TCS_{jlp} + \varepsilon_{i:jlp}$$

$$(5.18)$$

In most group-randomized trials, condition, time, and their interaction are
fixed effects. In the matched analysis, the investigator has no interest in the
matched sets per se, and is simply using matching in an effort to control
confounding due to the matching variable or to improve the precision of the
analysis. To provide a statistical basis for generalization to other strata like
those employed in the study, stratum and its interaction with time are random
effects. In order to account for the positive intraclass correlation expected in
the data, CS_{lp} and TCS_{jlp} must be included in the analysis as random effects.
The five random effects allow for correlation among members within the
matched sets (S_p), correlation among the members within the condition $\times$
stratum cells (CS_{lp}), correlation among the members within the time $\times$ stratum surveys (TS_{jp}), correlation among the members within the time $\times$ condition $\times$ stratum surveys (TCS_{jlp}), and for random variation among the members
$(\varepsilon_{i:jlp})$.

Note that there are no $G_{k:lp}$ and $TG_{jk:lp}$ terms in the model. This is because
they cannot be estimated in the matched design apart from CS_{lp} and TCS_{jlp}
because there is only one group in each time $\times$ condition $\times$ stratum cell.

The Intervention Effect

As in the previous section, the intervention effect is represented by the time
$\times$ condition interaction. In the familiar ANCOVA, the F-statistic assesses the
variation among the adjusted time $\times$ condition means against the variation
among the adjusted time $\times$ condition $\times$ stratum means. The null hypothesis
is that the variation due to conditions over time is zero. When there are only
two conditions and two time intervals, the numerator of the F-statistic is based
on a single df and it is more convenient to use the t-statistic. In that case, the
intervention effect is the adjusted net difference and the null hypothesis is that
the adjusted net difference is zero. For the intervention and control conditions,
the intervention effect is:

$$\Delta=(\bar{Y}_{\cdot\cdot2I}-\bar{Y}_{\cdot\cdot1I})-(\bar{Y}_{\cdot\cdot2C}-\bar{Y}_{\cdot\cdot1C})-\sum_{o=1}^{x}\beta_o((\bar{X}_{o\cdot\cdot2I}-\bar{X}_{o\cdot\cdot1I})-\bar{X}_{o\cdot\cdot2C}-\bar{X}_{o\cdot\cdot1C}))$$

(5.19)

The Expected Mean Squares

The expected mean squares for this analysis are shown in Table 5.7. Note that the covariates are not shown in the table except as they affect the df for the other terms. The MS_{tc} has three components: residual error (σ_e^2), a weighted component of variance due to the interaction of time with condition and stratum ($m\sigma_{tcs}^2$), and a weighted component of variance due to the intervention ($ms\sigma_{tc}^2$). The test of the null hypothesis is MS_{tc}/MS_{tcs}.

For each covariate measured at the group level (x_g), degrees of freedom associated with that covariate are lost from MS_{cs} and from MS_{tcs}. For each covariate measured at the member level (x_m), degrees of freedom associated with that covariate are lost from MS_e.

The Variance of the Intervention Effect

When the intervention effect is defined as the adjusted net difference over two time intervals between two conditions, the variance of that intervention effect under the null hypothesis is:

$$\sigma_\Delta^2 = 2*2\left(\frac{MS_{tcs}}{ms}\right)$$

(5.20)

Table 5.7. Expected Mean Squares for the Adjusted Analysis of Data from a Nested Cross-Sectional Pretest-Posttest Control Group Design with *A Priori* Matching

Source	df	E(MS)	MS
Condition	$c-1$	$\sigma_e^2+mt\sigma_{cs}^2+mts\sigma_c^2$	MS_c
Strata	$s-1$	$\sigma_e^2+mtc\sigma_s^2$	MS_s
CS	$(c-1)(s-1)-x_g$	$\sigma_e^2+mt\sigma_{cs}^2$	MS_{cs}
Time	$t-1$	$\sigma_e^2+mc\sigma_{ts}^2+mcs\sigma_t^2$	MS_t
TC	$(t-1)(c-1)$	$\sigma_e^2+m\sigma_{tcs}^2+ms\sigma_{tc}^2$	MS_{tc}
TS	$(t-1)(s-1)$	$\sigma_e^2+mc\sigma_{ts}^2$	MS_{ts}
TCS	$(t-1)(c-1)(s-1)-x_g$	$\sigma_e^2+m\sigma_{tcs}^2$	MS_{tcs}
M:TCS	$tcs(m-1)-x_m$	σ_e^2	MS_e

Here m is the number of observations at each time $\times$ condition $\times$ stratum survey and s is the number of strata. The MS_{tcs} reflects the matching, the repeat observations on the same groups, and the regression adjustment for covariates. A more detailed presentation on the impact of those procedures on the variance components is reserved for Chapter 9.

Assumptions

This analysis provides for five sources of random variation. If there are additional sources in the data, the model is misspecified and the true Type I and II error rates are unknown.

Under the General Linear Mixed Model, the random effects are assumed to be independent and distributed as $S_p \approx N(0,\sigma_s^2)$, $CS_{lp} \approx N(0,\sigma_{cs}^2)$, $TS_{jp} \approx N(0,\sigma_{ts}^2)$, $TCS_{jlp} \approx N(0,\sigma_{tcs}^2)$, and $\varepsilon_{i:jlp} \approx N(0,\sigma_e^2)$. With the important caveats noted earlier in this chapter, the analysis can be extended to non-Gaussian data by assuming a different distribution for $\varepsilon_{i:jlp}$ and a different link function. The analysis would then represent an application of the Generalized Linear Mixed Model.

Even without reliance on the Generalized Linear Mixed Model, this analysis appears to be robust to violation of the normality assumption for the residual-error distribution, given a moderate number of groups and members (Hannan and Murray, 1996). It also provides substantial protection against violations of the independence assumption as the most likely forms of dependence are modeled via CS_{lp}, TCS_{jlp} and the other random effects involving stratum.

The assumptions for this analysis include those related to regression adjustment for covariates and violations have the same effect.

The matched analysis does not provide a test of whether the intervention effect is homogeneous across the matched sets. That is simply assumed and is usually untestable in the matched analysis.[2] Violations reduce power by reducing the precision of the estimate of the intervention effect.

The matched analysis also assumes that the relationship among each covariate and the endpoint is constant across the matched sets. Violations reduce power by reducing the precision of the estimate of the intervention effect. Of course, this assumption may be tested by inclusion of interaction terms involving the strata and the covariates of concern in the analysis.

Strengths and Weaknesses

If effective, matching has two advantages. First, it controls for the potential confounding influence of the matching factor. Second, it improves the precision of the estimate of the intervention effect.

The degree to which matching controls the potential confounding influence of the matching factor depends on the quality of the matching. If groups are well matched, control is good. If groups are poorly matched, residual confounding may still bias the estimate of the intervention effect.

The degree to which the precision of the estimate of the intervention effect is improved depends on the magnitude of the matching correlation. As the matching correlation increases, the cells become more homogeneous, improving power. To the extent that matching also accounts for some of the variation among the groups, the *VIF* for this design is also reduced, further improving power. However, as was the case for the *a priori* stratified analysis, the matching correlation is a correlation at the group level, and so is usually much smaller than if it were at the member level. As a result, the improvement in power from matching is usually much smaller in a group-randomized trial than in a clinical trial. Making matters worse, the *ddf* for the intervention effect in a matched analysis are reduced by half compared to the unmatched analysis, for they are based on the number of matched sets, not the number of groups. If the gain in power from the matching correlation is less than the loss in power from the reduced *ddf*, the matched analysis is actually less powerful than the unmatched analysis (Martin et al., 1993). The reader is referred to the discussion of these issues in Chapter 3.

Post Hoc Stratification

With *post hoc* stratification, the investigator is interested only in the levels of the stratification factor that are included in the analysis. As a result, stratum is a fixed effect.

The Model

The model for the Pretest-Posttest Control Group Design that includes *post hoc* stratification on a member characteristic with regression adjustment for covariates is:

$$Y_{i:jkp:l} = \mu + C_l + S_p + CS_{lp} + T_j + TC_{jl} + TS_{jp} + TCS_{jlp} + \sum_{o=1}^{x} \beta_o(X_{oi:jkp:l} - \bar{X}_{o\cdot\ldots}) $$
$$+ G_{k:l} + TG_{jk:l} + GS_{kp:l} + TGS_{jkp:l} + \varepsilon_{i:jkp:l}$$

$$(5.21)$$

Stratum is added both as a main effect and as a series of interactions with the other fixed effects. In addition, stratum interacts with group and time × group.

This adds four fixed effects and two random effects to the adjusted analysis for the unstratified version of this design.

In most group-randomized trials, condition, time, and their interaction are fixed effects. With *post hoc* stratification, the investigator is interested only in the levels of the stratification factor that are included in the analysis, so that stratum is a fixed effect, as are its interactions with the other fixed effects. In order to account for the positive intraclass correlation expected in the data, $G_{k:l}$, $GS_{kp:l}$, $TG_{jk:l}$, and $TGS_{jkp:l}$ must be included in the analysis as random effects. The five random effects allow for correlation among members within a group ($G_{k:l}$), for correlation among members within a group × stratum cell ($GS_{kp:l}$), for correlation among members within a time × group survey ($TG_{jk:l}$), for correlation among members within a time × group × stratum survey ($TGS_{jkp:l}$), and for random variation among the members ($\varepsilon_{i:jkp:l}$).

The Intervention Effect

With *post hoc* stratification, the intervention effect is represented by the time × condition × stratum interaction. In the familiar ANCOVA, the *F*-statistic assesses the variation among the adjusted time × condition × stratum means against the variation among the adjusted time × group × stratum means. The null hypothesis is that the variation due to conditions over time and across strata is zero. When there are only two conditions, two time intervals, and two strata, the numerator of the *F*-statistic is based on a single *df* and it is more convenient to use the *t*-statistic. In that case, the intervention effect is defined as the difference between the two strata in their adjusted net differences. The null hypothesis is that the difference between the two strata is zero.

The Expected Mean Squares

The expected mean squares for this analysis are shown in Table 5.8. Note that the covariates are not shown in the table except as they affect the *df* for the other terms. The MS_{tcs} has three components: residual error (σ_e^2), a weighted component of variance due to the interaction of time with group and stratum ($m\sigma_{tgs:c}^2$), and a weighted component of variance due to the intervention ($mg\sigma_{tcs}^2$). The test of the null hypothesis is $MS_{tcs}/MS_{tgs:c}$.

For each covariate measured at the group level (x_g), a degree of freedom is lost from $MS_{g:c}$, $MS_{gs:c}$, $MS_{tg:c}$, and from $MS_{tgs:c}$. For each covariate measured at the member level (x_m), a degree of freedom is lost from MS_e.

Table 5.8. Expected Mean Squares for the Adjusted Analysis of Data from a Nested Cross-Sectional Pretest-Posttest Control Group Design with *Post Hoc* Stratification

Source	df	E(MS)	MS
Condition	$c-1$	$\sigma_e^2 + mts\sigma_{g:c}^2 + mtgs\sigma_c^2$	MS_c
Group:C	$c(g-1)-x_g$	$\sigma_e^2 + mts\sigma_{g:c}^2$	$MS_{g:c}$
Strata	$s-1$	$\sigma_e^2 + mt\sigma_{gs:c}^2 + mtgc\sigma_s^2$	MS_s
CS	$(c-1)(s-1)$	$\sigma_e^2 + mt\sigma_{gs:c}^2 + mtg\sigma_{cs}^2$	MS_{cs}
GS:C	$c(g-1)(s-1)-x_g$	$\sigma_e^2 + mt\sigma_{gs:c}^2$	$MS_{gs:c}$
Time	$t-1$	$\sigma_e^2 + ms\sigma_{tg:c}^2 + mgsc\sigma_t^2$	MS_t
TC	$(t-1)(c-1)$	$\sigma_e^2 + ms\sigma_{tg:c}^2 + mgs\sigma_{tc}^2$	MS_{tc}
TG:C	$(t-1)c(g-1)-x_g$	$\sigma_e^2 + ms\sigma_{tg:c}^2$	$MS_{tg:c}$
TS	$(t-1)(s-1)$	$\sigma_e^2 + m\sigma_{tgs:c}^2 + mgc\sigma_{ts}^2$	MS_{ts}
TCS	$(t-1)(c-1)(s-1)$	$\sigma_e^2 + m\sigma_{tgs:c}^2 + mg\sigma_{tcs}^2$	MS_{tcs}
TGS:C	$(t-1)c(g-1)(s-1)-x_g$	$\sigma_e^2 + m\sigma_{tgs:c}^2$	$MS_{tgs:c}$
M:TGS:C	$tgsc(m-1)-x_m$	σ_e^2	MS_e

The Variance of the Intervention Effect

When the intervention effect is defined as the contrast between two strata in their adjusted net difference over two time intervals between two conditions, the variance of that intervention effect under the null hypothesis is:

$$\sigma_\Delta^2 = 2*2*2\left(\frac{MS_{tgs:c}}{mg}\right) \tag{5.22}$$

Here m is the number of members in each time $\times$ group $\times$ stratum survey and g is the number of groups in each condition. The $MS_{tgs:c}$ reflects the stratification, the repeat observations on the same groups, and the regression adjustment for covariates. A more detailed discussion of the impact of those procedures on the variance components is reserved for Chapter 9.

Assumptions

The analysis provides for five sources of random variation. If there are additional sources in the data, the model is misspecified and the true Type I and II error rates are unknown.

Under the General Linear Mixed Model, the random effects are assumed to be independent and distributed as $G_{k:l} \approx N(0,\sigma_{g:c}^2)$, $GS_{kp:l} \approx N(0,\sigma_{gs:c}^2)$, $TG_{jk:l} \approx N(0,\sigma_{tg:c}^2)$, $TGS_{jkp:l} \approx N(0,\sigma_{tgs:c}^2)$, and $\varepsilon_{i:jkp:l} \approx N(0,\sigma_e^2)$. With the important caveats noted earlier in this chapter, the analysis can be extended to non-Gaussian data by assuming a different distribution for $\varepsilon_{i:jkp:l}$ and a different link function. The analysis would then represent an application of the Generalized Linear Mixed Model.

Even without reliance on the Generalized Linear Mixed Model, this analysis appears to be robust to violation of the normality assumption for the residual error distribution, given a moderate number of groups and members (Hannan and Murray, 1996). It also provides substantial protection against violations of the independence assumption as the most likely forms of dependence are modeled explicitly via $G_{k:l}$, $GS_{kp:l}$, $TG_{jk:l}$, and $TGS_{jkp:l}$.

In other respects, the assumptions for the *post hoc* stratified analysis are the same as for the *a priori* stratified analysis. Violations have the same effect.

Strengths and Weaknesses

As was the case for *a priori* stratification, the primary advantage of the *post hoc* stratified analysis is that it provides a test of whether the intervention effect is homogeneous across the subgroups defined by the strata.

Also like *a priori* stratification, the power for the test of the null hypothesis is less than for the test of the main effect for condition, all other factors constant. This is because the intervention effect in the stratified analysis is more complex than in the unstratified analysis.

Additional Baseline or Follow-up Intervals

Additional baseline and/or follow-up intervals can be included in the design, extending the simple Pretest-Posttest Control Group Design. Chapters 2 and 3 review the general benefits of such an extension for the validity of the design. This section presents analysis methods for these *Extended Designs.*

In each of the previous examples in this chapter, time was modeled as a categorical variable, both as a main effect and in any interactions. This is appropriate when the data are collected during one or two discrete time intervals, such as during time-limited baseline and follow-up surveys. When additional discrete intervals are added to the design, or when data collection is continuous, the investigator can continue to model time categorically but can also consider analyses in which time is modeled as a continuous variable. This section considers the analysis of data from an Extended Design in which time is modeled as a categorical variable and as a continuous variable. Extensions of the now familiar mixed-model ANOVA/ANCOVA are presented first, followed by a presentation of a random-coefficients model.

The Traditional Mixed-Model ANOVA/ANCOVA

It is quite straightforward to extend the analyses presented for the Pretest-Posttest Control Group Design to incorporate additional levels of time. Indeed, the only changes involve the definition and interpretation of the intervention effect.

The Model

The model for the Extended Design is the same as for the Pretest-Posttest Control Group Design (cf. Equations 5.7 and 5.10). The addition of more intervals increases the value of t in the T_j ($j=1 \ldots t$) notation, but has no other effect on the model.

The Intervention Effect

In the familiar ANOVA, the F-statistic assesses the variation among the time $\times$ condition means against the variation among the time $\times$ group means. The null hypothesis is that the variation due to conditions over time is zero. With more than two time intervals, the intervention effect can no longer be reduced to a net difference over time even if there are only two conditions.

The Expected Mean Squares and Variance of the Intervention Effect

The expected mean squares and the variance of the intervention effect are unchanged from those presented for the Pretest-Posttest Control Group Design (Tables 5.3 and 5.4 and Equations 5.9 and 5.12). However, the null hypothesis is now that $TC_{jl} = 0$ for all j and l.

ddf for Fixed Effects

In any group-randomized trial, the df of greatest interest are the ddf for the test of the intervention effect. That figure is a function of the number of groups per condition, and the number of times, conditions, and *post hoc* strata, if any.[3] The tables of expected mean squares presented in earlier sections provide formulae for the ddf for each of the analyses considered thus far. In each case, the number of observations taken at each time in each group played no role in computing the ddf for the intervention effect, though the formulae assumed that there were multiple observations in each cell in the design.

Those formulae must be adapted for more complex situations. For example, they don't address explicitly the issue of empty cells in the design or of different numbers of time intervals among the groups. To accurately determine the *ddf* for a complex design, the investigator should create the multidimensional matrix defined by the number of groups per condition, and the number of times, conditions, and *post hoc* strata, if any. The investigator can then determine the number of cells in that matrix that have more than one observation. That figure represents the total *df* available at the group level. The investigator can then partition those *df* among the terms in the model. In the traditional mixed-model ANOVA/ANCOVA, the *df* not allocated to other sources is available as the *ddf* for the test of the intervention effect.[4]

Assumptions

Because the model for this analysis is the same as for the Pretest-Posttest Control Group Design, the assumptions also are the same. The reader is referred to the presentation earlier in this chapter for a review of the assumptions and the effect of their violation.

Careful examination of the way in which the time $\times$ group component of variance is estimated reveals a subtle but important feature of those assumptions that emerges only when there are three or more time intervals included in the design. The time $\times$ group component of variance is estimated as the variance of the deviations of the time $\times$ group means from their time $\times$ condition mean. Implicit in this estimation method is the assumption that each group in a given condition shares a common time trend or slope that is unique to that condition. So long as there is no measurable deviation of the group-specific slopes from that common slope, the mixed-model ANOVA/ANCOVA has a nominal Type I error rate for the test of the intervention effect, regardless of the number of time intervals included in the design and in the analysis (Murray et al., in press). However, whenever there is any measurable deviation among the group-specific slopes relative to the common slope, the variance of the intervention effect in the mixed-model ANOVA/ANCOVA is too small and the Type I error rate is inflated. Murray et al. (in press) demonstrated that the inflation in the Type I error rate increases as the component of variance for the group slopes represents a larger and larger fraction of the total variation in the data.

Importantly, the mixed-model ANOVA/ANCOVA has a nominal Type I error rate even in the presence of measurable heterogeneity of the group-specific patterns so long as there are only two time intervals included in the design. That is because there is no estimable variation among the deviations of the time $\times$ group means from their time $\times$ condition mean apart from their deviation from the presumed common slope. However, as is clear from the results reported by Murray et al. (in press), as soon as $t > 2$ and the group-specific slopes are heterogeneous, the mixed-model ANOVA/ANCOVA has an inflated Type I error rate.

Other assumptions may apply to this analysis as well. For example, if regression adjustment for covariates is included, then the assumptions associated with that procedure apply. Similarly, if stratification or matching is included in the analysis, the assumptions associated with those procedures apply. Violations have effects as described earlier.

Strengths and Weaknesses

This analysis makes no assumption about the pattern of the intervention effect over time. A significant TC interaction means that some of the TC means are different from others, but the analysis isn't structured to find a particular pattern. Absent information suggesting a specific pattern, the investigator may want to cast such a broad net.

Another strength of the traditional mixed-model ANOVA/ANCOVA is that the ddf are greater than in the random-coefficients analysis. In general, power for an omnibus F-test improves as the number of means increases, because the ndf and ddf increase. In this example, the ndf for TC are computed as $(c-1)(t-1)$ and increase from 1 when there are only two surveys to 4 when there are five surveys or 9 when there are 10 surveys. Similarly, the ddf for TC are computed as $(t-1)c(g-1)$ and increase from $2(g-1)$ when there are two surveys to $8(g-1)$ when there are five surveys and $18(g-1)$ when there are 10 surveys. In contrast, the ndf and ddf for the random coefficients analysis remain fixed at $(c-1)$ and $c(g-1)$, respectively. When the assumptions underlying the traditional mixed-model ANOVA/ANCOVA are met, that analysis has better power than the random-coefficients analysis.

The major weakness of the traditional mixed-model ANOVA/ANCOVA is that it has an inflated Type I error rate in the presence of measurable heterogeneity among the group-specific slopes when there are more than two time intervals included in the design. Under those conditions, it is simply not a valid analysis. The ANOVA/ANCOVA approach continues to be useful when there are only one or two time intervals in the design, or when preliminary testing indicates that the group-specific slopes are homogeneous. However, caution is required for such preliminary tests, as the asymptotic standard error for a variance component is not well estimated when the variance component is near zero. In addition, the degrees of freedom for the preliminary test may be quite limited, thereby limiting its power. For these reasons, the prudent course is to forgo the extra power that may come with the traditional mixed-model ANOVA/ANCOVA and employ an analysis method that has a nominal Type I error rate even in the presence of measurable heterogeneity among the group-specific slopes. That method is the random-coefficients analysis, described later in this chapter.

The fact that the traditional mixed-model ANOVA/ANCOVA makes no assumption about the pattern of the intervention effect over time both a strength and a weakness. It was listed above as a strength because it puts no constraints on the pattern to be detected. However, this is also a weakness, for the power to detect such a diffuse and general intervention effect is poor if that effect in fact can be predicted. In that case, the more targeted analysis has better power.

The Trend Analysis in the Mixed-Model ANOVA/ANCOVA

The analysis presented in this section is patterned generally after the trend analysis for factorial and repeated-measures designs. Readers may find it helpful to review trend analysis in general experimental design texts (e.g., Kirk, 1982; Winer et al., 1991). It can also be seen as an extension of Koepsell et al.'s (1991) planned contrasts.

Coding Time as a Continuous Variable

To treat time as a continuous variable, it must be scaled in real time, with an appropriate zero point. A logical zero point is the time at which the intervention began, and a natural way to scale T_j is to assign values that represent the time between a given survey and the zero point, using zero or negative values for baseline surveys and positive numbers for surveys conducted after the intervention began.

Specifying an Intervention Pattern

Consider possibilities for the baseline period, illustrated in Figure 5.1. The conditions might share a common baseline trend, with the same slope and the same intercept (A). The conditions might have parallel baseline trends, with a common slope but different intercepts (B). The conditions might have nonparallel baseline trends, with different slopes and different intercepts (C). Given a sufficient number of baseline time intervals, the slopes might have nonlinear as well as linear components (D).

Consider next the intervention period, illustrated in Figure 5.2. The control condition might maintain its baseline trend while the intervention condition changes; that change might be gradual (E) or abrupt (F) and it might be sustained (E or F) or transient (G). The control condition might change as well, in a fashion that is only gradually or immediately different from the intervention

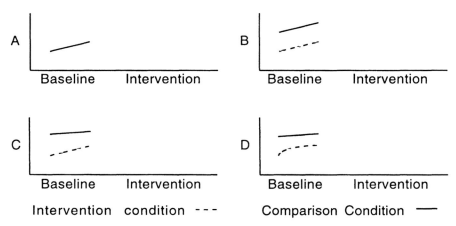

Figure 5.1. Four possible patterns during the baseline period for the extended nested cross-sectional design.

condition (H). There are many patterns, and the investigators must select the pattern that makes the most sense given the endpoints, the intervention, and the results from related studies.

Once the investigator has chosen a pattern, the challenge to the analyst is to create an analysis that provides a test of that pattern. The method must reflect the design and ought to maximize the power available to test the alternative hypothesis defined by the chosen pattern. Koepsell et al. (1991) suggested this approach in their discussion of planned contrasts for group-

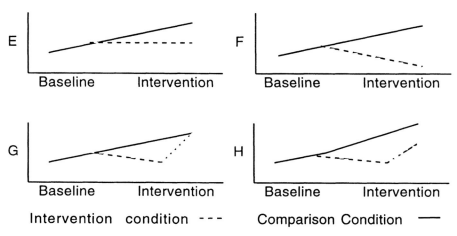

Figure 5.2. Four possible patterns during the intervention period for the extended nested cross-sectional design.

randomized trials. Murray, Hannan et al. (1994) extended that work as part of the development of the analysis methods for the data from the Minnesota Heart Health Program (MHHP).

The approach described by Murray, Hannan et al. (1994) was originally suggested by Peter Hannan and is built around a reallocation of the df at the group level. Hannan recognized that the upper limit for the ddf for the test of the intervention effect is the number of time $\times$ group cells having multiple observations, as that number defines the total df available at the group level if there are no *post hoc* strata. He sought to partition those df so as to optimize the number for the test of the intervention effect.

In the traditional Pretest-Posttest Control Group Design and in the Extended Design in which time is treated as a categorical variable, $(t–1)$ df are allocated for time. Another $(c–1)(t-1)$ df are allocated for the time $\times$ condition interaction, for a total of $c(t-1)$ df. This representation of time puts no constraints on the relationship between time and the endpoint or on the pattern of that relationship across conditions. As such, it allows for higher-order interactions for time (e.g., time $\times$ time) and time $\times$ condition (e.g., condition $\times$ time $\times$ time), limited only by the number of time intervals in the design, t.

Hannan noted that the $c(t-1)$ df could be reduced by treating the main effect for time as a continuous variable and by assuming one or more of those higher-order interactions to be zero. For example, if the time trend for the endpoint in the control condition is modeled as linear and the intervention effect is modeled as linear but with a different slope, the $c(t-1)$ df are reduced to two. Hannan saw that this approach could mean a net savings in df, which would become available for the ddf for the test of the intervention effect, based on the repartition of the total df at the group level.

Pooling the saved df into the ddf for the test of the intervention effect is based on the assumption that the model for the time trend and for the intervention effect adequately fits the data. If the specified model is adequate, the increased ddf improve the power for that test for the intervention effect. In addition, power is improved if the modeled intervention effect captures most of the variation among the time $\times$ group means, which it should if the model fits the data.

The Model

This approach is illustrated using an analysis patterned after that reported for the primary risk factor analyses from the Minnesota Heart Health Program (MHHP) (Luepker et al., 1994; Murray, Hannan et al., 1994). The original analyses modeled time in terms of years from the onset of intervention, but defined years in terms of time as intended in the design. The analyses presented here reflect time as implemented. In addition, the original analysis modeled the intervention effect as a series of year-specific departures from the secular trend estimated from all non-intervention data. The analysis presented here treats time as a continuous variable with linear and quadratic components. The secular trend is constructed using all the non-intervention observations, pooling data from the intervention and comparison communities, as was done in the original analysis. The intervention effect is modeled as a departure from the secular trend, also with linear and quadratic components.

This model is written as:

$$Y_{i:jk:l} = \mu + C_l + T_{(\text{lin})}t_j + T_{(\text{quad})}t_j^2 + T_{(\text{lin})}t_j C_l + T_{(\text{quad})}t_j^2 C_l$$
$$+ \sum_{o=1}^{x} \beta_o(X_{oi:jk:l} - \overline{X}_{o\cdots}) + G_{k:l} + TG_{jk:l} + \varepsilon_{i:jk:l}$$

$$(5.23)$$

In the previous section (The Traditional Mixed-Model ANOVA/ANCOVA) the j levels of time were represented by $j-1$ indicator variables. In this analysis, time is represented by a linear term, $T_{(\text{lin})}$, which is multiplied by the value of time for each observation and by a quadratic term, $T_{(\text{quad})}$, which is multiplied by the squared value of time for each observation. Those terms were defined by the MHHP investigators so that the intervention and comparison data were pooled in the definition of $T_{(\text{lin})}$ and $T_{(\text{quad})}$ prior to the onset of the intervention.

In the previous section (The Traditional Mixed-Model ANOVA/ANCOVA) the tc levels of the time $\times$ condition interaction were represented by $(t-1)$ $(c-1)$ indicator variables. In this model, the interaction is represented by c-1 linear terms, $T_{(\text{lin})}C_l$, and by c-1 quadratic terms, $T_{(\text{quad})}C_l$, with all defined so that they are constrained to zero during the baseline period.

Importantly, time is not treated as a continuous variable in the random effects in this analysis. The term $TG_{jk:l}$ is identical to the same term in the traditional mixed-model ANOVA/ANCOVA. It is the treatment of time as a categorical variable in the random effects that allows the analyst to pool *df* saved from the fixed effects into the *ddf* already available for $TG_{jk:l}$.

The Intervention Effect

In this analysis, the intervention effect is defined as the variation in the regression lines fit to the study conditions after regression adjustment for the covariates. The null hypothesis is that the variation is zero. Given just two conditions, the intervention effect is a difference between two regression lines. The first is the common secular trend fit with linear and quadratic components to the data from both conditions prior to the intervention and to the data from the control condition after the onset of the intervention. The second is the departure from that common secular trend in the intervention condition after the onset of the intervention; it also has linear and quadratic components. The null hypothesis is that the difference between the two regression lines is zero. Note that because of the way that the $T_{(\text{lin})}C_l$ and $T_{(\text{quad})}C_l$ terms are parameterized in this example, the difference between the two regression lines is represented directly by those terms.

The Expected Mean Squares

The expected mean squares for this analysis are shown in Table 5.9. Note that the covariates are not shown in the table except as they affect the *df* for the other terms.

The *E(MS)* and *df* for Condition and Group:*C* are constructed in the usual manner. The *E(MS)* for Time is replaced by the *E(MS)* for the linear and quadratic components of time. The usual *df* for Time, $t-1$, are reduced to 1 each for the two components, with the remainder falling to *TG:C*. The *E(MS)* for *TC* is replaced by the *E(MS)* for the linear and quadratic components of the time × condition interaction. The usual *df* for *TC*, $(t-1)(c-1)$, are reduced to 1 each for the two components, with the remainder falling to *TG:C*. As a result, the *df* for *TG:C* is written as res_{tgc}. It is computed as the total *df* at the group level, *tgc*, minus the *df* used for the terms above it in the table.

The $MS_{t(\text{quad})c}$ has three components: residual error (σ_e^2), a weighted component of variance due to the interaction of time with group ($m\sigma_{tg:c}^2$), and a weighted component of variance due to the intervention ($mg\sigma_{t(\text{quad})c}^2$). The test of the null hypothesis of no quadratic intervention effect is $MS_{t(\text{quad})c}/MS_{tg:c}$. If that null hypothesis is accepted, the $T_{(\text{quad})}C$ term would be removed and

Table 5.9. Expected Mean Squares for an Adjusted Analysis of Data from An Extended Nested Cross-Sectional Design in Which Time is Modeled as a Continuous Variable in the Fixed Effects

Source	df	E(MS)	MS
Condition	$c-1$	$\sigma_e^2 + mt\sigma_{g:c}^2 + mgt\sigma_c^2$	MS_c
Group:C	$c(g-1)-x_g$	$\sigma_e^2 + mt\sigma_{g:c}^2$	$MS_{g:c}$
Time(lin)	1	$\sigma_e^2 + m\sigma_{tg:c}^2 + mgc\sigma_{t(\text{lin})}^2$	$MS_{t(\text{lin})}$
Time(quad)	1	$\sigma_e^2 + m\sigma_{tg:c}^2 + mgc\sigma_{t(\text{quad})}^2$	$MS_{t(\text{quad})}$
$T(\text{lin})C$	$c-1$	$\sigma_e^2 + m\sigma_{tg:c}^2 + mg\sigma_{t(\text{lin})c}^2$	$MS_{t(\text{lin})c}$
$T(\text{quad})C$	$c-1$	$\sigma_e^2 + m\sigma_{tg:c}^2 + mg\sigma_{t(\text{quad})c}^2$	$MS_{t(\text{quad})c}$
TG:C	res_{tgc}	$\sigma_e^2 + m\sigma_{tg:c}^2$	$MS_{tg:c}$
M:TG:C	$tgc(m-1)-x_m$	σ_e^2	MS_e

the analysis rerun. The test of the null hypothesis of no linear intervention effect is then $MS_{t(\text{lin})c}/MS_{tg:c}$.

For each covariate measured at the group level (x_g), df associated with that covariate are lost from $MS_{g:c}$ and from $MS_{tg:c}$. For each covariate measured at the member level (x_m), df are lost from MS_e.

The Variance of the Intervention Effect

Because of the way that the terms are parameterized in this analysis, the $T_{(\text{lin})}C$ and $T_{(\text{quad})}C$ terms directly represent the difference between the two conditions. The variance of that difference under the null hypothesis is:

$$\sigma_\Delta^2 = \frac{MS_{tg:c}}{\sigma_{e(tc)}^2 \, (mtgc - f - 1)} \tag{5.24}$$

Here m is the number of members per group, t is the number of time intervals, g is the number of groups per condition, c is the number of conditions, f is the number of fixed-effect parameters in the model, and $\sigma_{e(tc)}^2$ is the residual variation in time. This variance has a different form that those presented in the previous sections because the intervention effect is defined in terms of regression lines rather than means. The $MS_{tg:c}$ reflects any reduction due to repeat measurements on the same groups and due to the regression adjustment for covariates. It also reflects the modeling of time with linear and quadratic components and of the intervention effect with linear and quadratic components. Further development of this variance is provided in Chapter 9.

The ddf for the Variance of the Intervention Effect

Because the random-effects portion of the model is the same as in the previous section, the *ddf* for the variance of the intervention effect are computed in the same way. Note that in this analysis, the fixed effects require fewer *df* than was the case in the traditional mixed-model ANOVA/ANCOVA, so that additional *df* are available for the *ddf* for the variance of the intervention effect.

Assumptions

Because the random-effects portion of the model is the same as in the analyses presented earlier for the Pretest-Posttest Control Group design, the assumptions are also the same. The reader is referred to those earlier sections for a review of those assumptions and the effect of their violation.

The assumption of homogeneity of the group-specific slopes as discussed in the previous section applies equally to the linear trend analysis in the mixed-model ANOVA/ANCOVA. Notably, the inflation of the Type I error rate associated with violation of that assumption is even greater in the linear trend analysis than in the traditional mixed-model ANOVA/ANCOVA (Murray et al., in press). This is because the variance of the intervention effect in the linear trend analysis is always smaller than the variance of the intervention effect in the traditional mixed-model ANOVA/ANCOVA. Murray et al. (in press) demonstrated that the inflation in the Type I error rate increases as the component of variance for the group slopes represents a larger and larger fraction of the total variation in the data.

Even if the assumption of homogeneity of the group-specific slopes is reasonable, the analyst should be aware of the additional assumptions that accompany the pattern for the two regression lines. In the example above, the model assumed that the slopes for the two conditions were identical during baseline, as the common secular trend was estimated from all non-intervention data. The example also assumed that there were linear and quadratic components to the common secular trend and that those two components adequately described that trend. The example also assumed that the intervention effect was a departure from the secular trend fit to the other data and captured by a linear and quadratic component. Other models may make other assumptions, and the analyst should take care to gauge the appropriateness of those assumptions, through tests if possible and through logic otherwise.

Other assumptions may apply to this analysis as well. For example, if regression adjustment for covariates is included, then the assumptions associated with that procedure apply. Similarly, if stratification or matching is included in the analysis, the assumptions associated with those procedures apply. Violations have effects as described in those earlier sections.

Strengths and Weaknesses

When the assumptions for this analysis are met and the specified pattern for the intervention effect reflects the pattern in the data, this analysis has more power than either the traditional mixed-model ANOVA/ANCOVA or the random-coefficients analysis.

The major weakness of the linear trend analysis in the mixed-model ANOVA/ANCOVA is that it has an inflated Type I error rate in the presence of measurable heterogeneity among the group-specific slopes. In the presence of such heterogeneity, it is simply not a valid analysis. The ANOVA/ANCOVA approach is useful when preliminary testing indicates that the group-specific slopes are homogeneous. However, as noted in the previous section, caution is required for such preliminary tests. The prudent course is to forgo the extra power that may come with the linear trend analysis in the mixed-model ANOVA/ANCOVA and employ an analysis method that has a nominal Type I error rate even in the presence of measurable heterogeneity among the group-specific slopes. That method is the random-coefficients analysis.

The Random-Coefficients Analysis

The mixed-model ANOVA/ANCOVA for the Extended Design included a component of variance for groups nested within conditions. This component allows for correlation among the members within a group. Another way to think of the same component is that it allows for a random intercept for each group. This perspective sets the stage for the random-coefficients analysis, which is also a mixed-model regression analysis, but one that allows both random intercepts and random slopes for each group. Those slopes may be linear, quadratic, etc. In addition, the slopes and intercepts may covary or be independent.

Random-coefficients models have been used widely in education (e.g., Bryk and Raudenbush, 1992) and sociology (e.g., Hox and Kreft, 1994). They have been proposed for use in the analysis of data from longitudinal studies in epidemiology (e.g., Dwyer et al., 1992; Rutter and Elashoff, 1994). Quite recently, they have been recommended for group-randomized trials that have more than two time intervals (Murray et al., in press). Even so, none of the papers published to date from group-randomized trials in public health has used a random-coefficients model in the analysis.

There are at least two reasons for this pattern. First, most group-randomized trials involve only one baseline and a single follow-up survey. Given such a data-collection schedule, the random-coefficients model offers no advantage. Second, most of the methodologically oriented papers published on group-randomized trials in public health have recommended the ANOVA/ANCOVA version of the mixed-model regression analysis (e.g., Feldman and McKinlay, 1994; Koepsell et al., 1991; Murray and Hannan, 1990; Murray and Wolfinger, 1994). Prior to Murray et al. (in press), none had identified the dangers associated with the assumption of homogeneity among the group-specific slopes that is attached to the ANOVA/ANCOVA and none had suggested the random-coefficients approach as an alternative.

That pattern is likely to change over the next few years. The Murray et al. (in press) paper will draw attention to the issue, as will publication of this book. In addition, there is now under way a multicenter group-randomized trial that has specified a random-coefficients model for its primary analysis (Feldman et al., under review).

The Model

Random-coefficients models focus on time trends, in both the fixed- and the random-effects portions of the model. The simplest random-coefficients model focuses on linear time trends and is:

$$Y_{i:jk:l} = \mu + C_l + T_{(\text{lin})}t_j + T_{(\text{lin})}t_jC_l + G_{k:l} + T_{(\text{lin})}t_jG_{k:l} + \varepsilon_{i:jk:l} \quad (5.25)$$

As in the linear trend analysis in the mixed-model ANOVA/ANCOVA, time is represented by a linear term, $T_{(\text{lin})}$, which is multiplied by the value of time for each observation. In the random coefficients model, this applies both to the fixed and to the random effects. The fixed effect $T_{(\text{lin})}$ represents an average slope for the control condition, the interaction $T_{(\text{lin})}C$ represents the average departure from that slope observed in the intervention condition, and $T_{(\text{lin})}G$ represents the random departures from those averages that define the group-specific slopes.

In most group-randomized trials, condition, time, and their interaction are fixed effects. In order to account for the heterogeneity among the group-specific intercepts and slopes expected in the data, $G_{k:l}$ and $T_{(\text{lin})}G_{k:l}$ must be included in the analysis as random effects; a recent simulation study showed that failure to do so, in the presence of measurable heterogeneity, will result in a Type I error rate that is inflated, often badly (Murray et al., in press). The three random effects allow for variation among the group-specific intercepts $(G_{k:l})$, for variation among the group-specific slopes $(T_{(\text{lin})}G_{k:l})$, and for random variation among the members $(\varepsilon_{i:jk:l})$.

The Intervention Effect

In this analysis, the F-statistic assesses the variation among the condition mean slopes against the variation among the group-specific slopes. The null hypothesis is that the variation due to the conditions is zero. When there are only two conditions, the numerator of the F-statistic is based on a single df and it is more convenient to use the t-statistic. In that case, the intervention effect is the difference between the condition mean slopes and the null hypothesis is that the difference is zero.

The Expected Mean Squares

The expected mean squares for the random-coefficients analysis are shown in Table 5.10. The $MS_{t(\text{lin})c}$ has three components: residual error for the group-specific slope $\left(\dfrac{\sigma_{e(y)}^2}{\sigma_{e(t)}^2(mt-f-1)}\right)$, a component of variance due to the heterogeneity among the group-specific slopes $(\sigma_{t(\text{lin})g:c}^2)$ and a weighted component of variance due to the intervention $(g\sigma_{t(\text{lin})c}^2)$. The test of the null hypothesis of no intervention effect is given as $MS_{t(\text{lin})c}/MS_{t(\text{lin})g:c}$.

Though no covariates were included in this analysis, they certainly could be. For each covariate measured at the group level (x_g), df associated with that covariate are lost from $MS_{g:c}$ and from $MS_{t(\text{lin})g:c}$. For each covariate measured at the member level (x_m), df are lost from MS_e.

Table 5.10. Expected Mean Squares for a Random-Coefficients Analysis of Data from an Extended Nested Cross-Sectional Design in Which Time is Modeled as a Linear Term in Both the Fixed and Random Effects

Source	df	E(MS)	MS
Condition	$c-1$	$\sigma^2_{e(y)}\left(\dfrac{mt-1}{mt(mt-f-1)}+\dfrac{\bar{t}^2}{\sigma^2_{e(t)}(mt-f-1)}\right)+\sigma^2_{g:c}+g\sigma^2_c$	MS_c
Group:C	$c(g-1)$	$\sigma^2_{e(y)}\left(\dfrac{mt-1}{mt(mt-f-1)}+\dfrac{\bar{t}^2}{\sigma^2_{e(t)}(mt-f-1)}\right)+\sigma^2_{g:c}$	$MS_{g:c}$
Time(lin)	1	$\dfrac{\sigma^2_{e(y)}}{\sigma^2_{e(t)}(mt-f-1)}+\sigma^2_{t\,(\mathrm{lin})g:c}+gc\sigma^2_{t\,(\mathrm{lin})}$	$MS_{t(\mathrm{lin})}$
T(lin)C	$c-1$	$\dfrac{\sigma^2_{e(y)}}{\sigma^2_{e(t)}(mt-f-1)}+\sigma^2_{t\,(\mathrm{lin})g:c}+g\sigma^2_{t\,(\mathrm{lin})c}$	$MS_{t(\mathrm{lin})c}$
T(lin)G:C	$c(g-1)$	$\dfrac{\sigma^2_{e(y)}}{\sigma^2_{e(t)}(mt-f-1)}+\sigma^2_{t\,(\mathrm{lin})g:c}$	$MS_{t(\mathrm{lin})g:c}$
M:TG:C	$gc(mt-2)$	$\sigma^2_{e(y)}$	MS_e

The Variance of the Intervention Effect

When the intervention effect is defined as the difference between two condition mean slopes, the variance of that intervention effect under the null hypothesis is:

$$\sigma^2_\Delta = 2\left(\frac{MS_{t(\mathrm{lin})g:c}}{g}\right) \tag{5.26}$$

Here g is the number of groups in each condition. The $MS_{t(\mathrm{lin})g:c}$ reflects any reduction due to repeat measurements on the same groups. It also reflects the modeling of the linear time trend in each group. Further development of this variance is provided in Chapter 9.

Assumptions

This analysis provides for three sources of random variation. If there are additional sources in the data, the model is misspecified and the true Type I and II error rates are unknown.

Under the General Linear Mixed Model, the random effects are assumed to be distributed as $G_{k:l} \approx N(0,\sigma^2_{g:c})$, $T_{(\mathrm{lin})}G_{k:l} \approx N(0,\sigma^2_{t(\mathrm{lin})g:c})$, and $\varepsilon_{i:jk:l} \approx N(0,\sigma^2_e)$. Both $G_{k:l}$ and $T_{(\mathrm{lin})}G_{k:l}$ are assumed to be independent of $\varepsilon_{i:jk:l}$; however, $G_{k:l}$ and $T_{(\mathrm{lin})}G_{k:l}$ are allowed to covary. With the important caveats noted earlier in this chapter, the analysis can be extended to non-Gaussian data by assuming a different distribution for $\varepsilon_{i:jk:l}$ and a different link function. The analysis would then represent an application of the Generalized Linear Mixed Model.

It is unclear whether the random-coefficients analysis is robust to violation of the normality assumption for the residual error given a moderate number of groups and members; however, the Central Limit Theorem suggests that it would be. The recent report by Murray et al. (in press) confirms that the random-coefficients analysis provides substantial protection against violations of the independence assumption as the most likely forms of dependence are modeled explicitly via $G_{k:l}$ and $T_{(\text{lin})}G_{k:l}$.

This analysis also assumes that the nonlinear components of time and its interactions in the fixed- and random-effects portions of the model are zero. Their degrees of freedom are pooled with the degrees of freedom for MS_e.

This is but one random-coefficients model that could have been written for an Extended Design. Others might differ both in the structure assumed for the fixed-effects portion of the model as well as the random-effects portion. In general, the analyst should take care that the fixed-effects portion of the model reflects the assumed structure of the condition mean slopes and that the random-effects portion reflects the assumed structure of the group-specific slopes.

Strengths and Weaknesses

The major strength of this analysis is that it accommodates whatever level of heterogeneity among the group-specific slopes exists in the data. As a result, it has the nominal Type I error rate whatever that level of heterogeneity might be, even if it is zero (Murray et al., in press). The random-coefficients analysis is the only analysis of the three considered for Extended Designs that has this feature.

Another strength of the random-coefficients analysis is that it can accommodate nonlinear trends over time as well. The analysis presented above included only linear components for time, but quadratic terms could be added.

Another strength of the random-coefficients analysis is that it provides a test of whether there is measurable heterogeneity among the group-specific slopes. That test is available for the null hypothesis $\sigma^2_{t(\text{lin})g:c}=0$. Many of the programs that provide estimates of the variance components also provide information to assess that null hypothesis.[5]

The major weakness of the random-coefficients analysis is that it is less efficient and therefore less powerful than the mixed-model ANOVA/ANCOVA analyses when the assumptions underlying the ANOVA/ANCOVA are satisfied. However, the loss of efficiency appears to be modest and may well prove a fair price to pay for the protection against inflation in the Type I error rate that occurs with the mixed-model ANOVA/ANCOVA analyses when there is measurable heterogeneity among the group-specific slopes.

Summary

This chapter has reviewed analysis methods for the nested cross-sectional designs that are most likely to be used in group-randomized trials. Most of the analysis methods were based on mixed-model ANOVA/ANCOVA and stand as extensions of the familiar ANOVA/ANCOVA methods used in comparative trials that do not involve group randomization. All reflect the additional components of variance due to the nested designs that characterize group-randomized trials. Several simulation studies have now demonstrated that these analyses have the nominal Type I error rate across a wide range of characteristics common to community trials, as long as only one or two time intervals are included in the design (Zucker, 1990; Murray and Wolfinger, 1994; Murray et al., 1996).

When more than two time intervals are included in the design, analysts must consider the possibility that there is heterogeneity among the time trends operating across the groups within each condition. Where no measurable heterogeneity exists, the mixed-model ANOVA/ANCOVA methods still have the nominal Type I error rate. However, in the presence of measurable heterogeneity among the group-specific slopes, the mixed-model ANOVA/ANCOVA methods have an inflated Type I error rate, and the degree of inflation is directly related to the degree of heterogeneity. Given measurable heterogeneity among the group-specific slopes, the appropriate analysis is based on a random-coefficients model, wherein separate random intercepts and slopes are allowed for each group. Such models accommodate whatever degree of heterogeneity exists among the group-specific slopes.

Endnotes

1. A strict interpretation of the meaning of a random effect would also require that the centers be selected at random from the larger population of centers that they are to represent. However, this is rarely possible in practice, as participating centers are generally chosen on the basis of the merit of their grant applications. However, by including the center as a random effect, one still has the statistical basis to generalize to the larger population of centers that the participating centers fairly represent.

2. It may be possible to stratify the matched sets according to levels on the matching factors. This is easiest when the groups are matched closely on a single variable. For example, if groups are matched on population size, it may be possible to stratify the matched sets into those that are quite large, those that are of medium size, and those that are small.

The new stratification factor would be a fixed effect, while pairs would continue to be a random effect. This would allow the investigator to examine whether the intervention effect is the same in those three strata. However, such stratification may be impossible if the groups are matched on several variables with more flexible requirements for a match.

3. *A priori* strata are not included in this list, because they would be accounted for in the number of groups per condition.

4. This is exactly the same pattern as in studies based on allocation of individuals to conditions, but at a higher level of aggregation. The total *df* in a clinical trial, for example, is the number of individuals included in the study, minus one for the grand mean; after allocation of *df* to the terms in the model, the remainder, or residual-error *df,* is available as the *ddf* for the intervention effect.

5. Significance tests for variance components are illustrated in Chapter 7. That chapter also provides a discussion of alternative methods and problems associated with such tests.

6

Analyses for Nested Cohort Designs

This chapter presents analyses appropriate for data from nested cohort designs. As with nested cross-sectional designs, it is impossible to cover all the designs and analyses within this class of designs in a single chapter, but the major variations can be shown. These analyses are based on the General Linear Mixed Model or the Generalized Linear Mixed Model (see Chapter 4).

Posttest-Only Control Group Design

The primary difference between the cohort and cross-sectional versions of the Posttest-Only Control Group Design is the eligibility criteria used to select members for the posttest survey. In the cross-sectional version, the members need not have been present at the beginning of the study. In the cohort version, only members who were present at the beginning of the study are eligible for the posttest survey. Even with this difference in eligibility criteria, the analysis of the data is identical in the two versions of the design. Those methods are presented in Chapter 5.

The nested cohort version of this design faces the same threats to validity as the nested cross-sectional version. Those threats are reviewed in Chapters 2, 3, and 5. With many groups randomized to each condition, it can be a strong design. Absent that feature, it is a weak design and should be avoided.

Pretest-Posttest Control Group Design

In the nested cohort version of the Pretest-Posttest Control Group Design, data are collected from the same members in each condition both before and after the intervention has been delivered in the intervention condition. This design allows the analyst to remove variation attributable to the members from the variance of the intervention effect. When there is a sufficient number of groups randomized to each condition, it can be a very strong design. As a result, it is the most common of the nested cohort designs employed in group-randomized trials.

A number of options exist for analysis of data from this design. In the first option, the pretest data are ignored and the analysis is conducted using only posttest data. This option duplicates the analyses discussed in Chapter 5 and so it is not discussed here. As a second option, time can be included as a factor in the analysis, crossed with condition. Such an analysis is often called a repeated-measures analysis, because in a nested cohort design, there are repeat observations on both the groups and the members. As a third option, covariates can be added to the repeated-measures analysis, either to reduce confounding or improve efficiency. As a fourth option, the posttest data can be analyzed with regression adjustment for covariates measured at baseline, thereby including time-related information without modeling time explicitly in the analysis. Options 2–4 are presented in the next three sections.

Unadjusted Time × Condition Analysis

The Model

In the unadjusted time × condition analysis, the model is:

$$Y_{ij:k:l} = \mu + C_l + T_j + TC_{jl} + G_{k:l} + M_{i:k:l} + TG_{jk:l} + MT_{ij:k:l} + \varepsilon_{ij:k:l} \quad (6.1)$$

Here the observed value ($Y_{ij:k:l}$) for the ith member at the jth time and nested within the kth group and the lth condition is expressed as a function of the grand mean (μ), the effect of the lth condition (C_l), the effect of the jth time (T_j), the joint effect of the jth time and the lth condition (TC_{jl}), the realized value of the kth group ($G_{k:l}$), the realized value of the ith member ($M_{i:k:l}$), the realized value of the combination of the jth time and the kth group ($TG_{jk:l}$), and the realized value of the combination of the ith member and j^{th} time ($MT_{ij:k:l}$). Any difference between this predicted value and the observed value is allocated to the residual error ($\varepsilon_{ij:k:l}$).

In most group-randomized trials, condition, time, and their interaction are fixed effects. In order to account for the positive intraclass correlation expected in the data, $G_{k:l}$ and $TG_{jk:l}$ must be included in the analysis as random effects. The three random effects carried over from the nested cross-sectional version of this design allow for correlation among members within a group ($G_{k:l}$), for correlation among members within a time × group survey ($TG_{jk:l}$), and for random variation among the members ($\varepsilon_{ij:k:l}$). The $M_{i:k:l}$ term allows for correlation among the repeat observations taken on the same member. The $MT_{ij:k:l}$

allows for correlation among replicate measurements on the same member during a single survey. If such replicates are available, $MT_{ij:k:l}$ is estimable apart from $\varepsilon_{ij:k:l}$. If no replicate measures are taken on the same member during a single survey, those components cannot be estimated separately.

The Intervention Effect

In the ANOVA, the F-statistic assesses the variation among the time $\times$ condition means against the variation among the time $\times$ group means. The null hypothesis is that the variation due to conditions over time is zero. When there are only two conditions and two time intervals, the numerator of the F-statistic is based on a single df and it is more convenient to use the t-statistic. In that case, the intervention effect is the net difference and the null hypothesis is that the net difference is zero. For the intervention and control conditions, the intervention effect is:

$$\Delta = (\overline{Y}_{.2 \cdot I} - \overline{Y}_{.1 \cdot I}) - (\overline{Y}_{.2 \cdot C} - \overline{Y}_{.1 \cdot C}) \tag{6.2}$$

The Expected Mean Squares

The expected mean squares are shown in Table 6.1, presuming no replicate measurements on the same member during a single time $\times$ group survey. The MS_{tc} has four components: residual error (σ_e^2), a component of variance due to the interaction of member with time ($\sigma_{mt:g:c}^2$), a weighted component of variance due to the interaction of time with group ($m\sigma_{tg:c}^2$), and a weighted component of variance due to the intervention ($mg\sigma_{tc}^2$). The test of the null hypothesis is $MS_{tc}/MS_{tg:c}$.

Table 6.1. Expected Mean Squares for the Unadjusted Time $\times$ Condition Analysis of Data From a Nested Cohort Pretest-Posttest Control Group Design

Source	df	E(MS)	MS
Condition	$c-1$	$\sigma_e^2 + t\sigma_{m:g:c}^2 + mt\sigma_{g:c}^2 + mtg\sigma_c^2$	MS_c
Group:C	$c(g-1)$	$\sigma_e^2 + t\sigma_{m:g:c}^2 + mt\sigma_{g:c}^2$	$MS_{g:c}$
Member:G:C	$gc(m-1)$	$\sigma_e^2 + t\sigma_{m:g:c}^2$	MS_m
Time	$t-1$	$\sigma_e^2 + \sigma_{mt:g:c}^2 + m\sigma_{tg:c}^2 + mgc\sigma_t^2$	MS_t
TC	$(t-1)(c-1)$	$\sigma_e^2 + \sigma_{mt:g:c}^2 + m\sigma_{tg:c}^2 + mg\sigma_{tc}^2$	MS_{tc}
TG:C	$(t-1)c(g-1)$	$\sigma_e^2 + \sigma_{mt:g:c}^2 + m\sigma_{tg:c}^2$	$MS_{tg:c}$
MT:G:C	$(t-1)gc(m-1)$	$\sigma_e^2 + \sigma_{mt:g:c}^2$	MS_e

The Variance of the Intervention Effect

When the intervention effect is defined as the net difference over two time intervals between two conditions, the variance of that intervention effect under the null hypothesis is:

$$\sigma_\Delta^2 = 2 * 2\left(\frac{MS_{tg:c}}{mg}\right) \tag{6.3}$$

Here there are m members in each time $\times$ group survey and g groups per condition. The $MS_{tg:c}$ reflects the repeat observations on the same groups and members; details are provided in Chapter 9.

Assumptions

This analysis provides for five sources of random variation. If there are additional sources in the data, the model is misspecified and the true Type I and II error rates are unknown.

Under the General Linear Mixed Model, the random effects are assumed to be independent and distributed as $G_{k:l} \approx N(0, \sigma_{g:c}^2)$, $M_{i:k:l} \approx N(0, \sigma_{m:g:c}^2)$, $TG_{jk:l} \approx N(0, \sigma_{tg:c}^2)$, $MT_{ij:k:l} \approx N(0, \sigma_{mt:g:c}^2)$, and $\varepsilon_{ij:k:l} N(0, \sigma_e^2)$. With the important caveats noted in Chapter 5, the analysis can be extended to non-Gaussian data by assuming a different distribution for $\varepsilon_{ij:k:l}$ and a different link function. The analysis would then represent an application of the Generalized Linear Mixed Model.

Even without reliance on the Generalized Linear Mixed Model, this analysis appears to be robust to violation of the normality assumption for the residual-error distribution, given a moderate number of groups and members (Hannan and Murray, 1996). It also provides substantial protection against violations of the independence assumption as the most likely forms of dependence are modeled via $G_{k:l}$, $TG_{jk:l}$, and $M_{i:k:l}$.

The traditional repeated-measures ANOVA also assumes that the within-member random-effects covariance matrices are both homogeneous and circular (Winer et al., 1991).[1] There are many patterns that meet this assumption, but one of the most familiar is compound symmetry. Here all the main diagonal elements have the same value, equal to the sum of the member and member $\times$ time components of variance, and all the off-diagonal elements have the same value, equal to the member component of variance. The repeated-measures analysis is robust to modest violations of the homogeneity of variance and covariance assumptions. Unfortunately, within-member F-tests, including the test for the intervention effect, are not robust to violations of the circularity assumption.[2] Instead, they become increasingly liberal as the degree of noncircularity increases (Winer et al., 1991; Keselman and Keselman, 1993).

Recent advances have greatly reduced the limitations formerly imposed by these assumptions (cf. Diggle et al., 1994). The alternative error functions available under the Generalized Linear Mixed Model allow the analyst to match the assumed and realized distributions. Several software programs based on the General Linear Mixed Model (e.g., SAS PROC MIXED and BMD P5V) and Generalized Linear Mixed Model (e.g., SAS GLIMMIX macro) allow the analyst to model between- and within-member heterogeneity if it is present in the data, thereby avoiding those homogeneity assumptions altogether (cf. Littell et al., 1996). Finally, some programs based on the General Linear Mixed Model (e.g., BMDP 5V and SAS PROC MIXED) and the Generalized Linear Mixed Model (e.g., SAS GLIMMIX macro) allow the analyst to model a noncircular pattern for the within-member random-effects covariance matrices, thereby avoiding the circularity assumption as well. As a result, the analyst has greater flexibility with regard to these assumptions than in the past.[3]

Regardless of the assumed error structure and pattern of the random-effects covariance matrices, the unadjusted time × condition analysis does carry several other assumptions. This analysis assumes that any net difference observed between the intervention and control conditions is due to the intervention. Any source of bias that would serve to favor one condition over the other is completely confounded with the variation due to condition, and serves to bias the estimate of the intervention effect. That bias may be positive or negative, large or small. In the presence of such bias, the true Type I and II error rates are unknown.

This analysis also assumes that all groups and members respond to the intervention in the same way. Violations reduce power by reducing the precision of the intervention effect.

Strengths and Weaknesses

The primary advantage of this design and analysis over its cross-sectional counterpart is that repeat observations are available on the same members as well as on the same groups. Variation due to member is partitioned from the other components of variance; to the extent that members respond consistently over time, this improves the power of this analysis. In turn, this may translate into a smaller and less expensive study.

Like its cross-sectional counterpart, the intervention effect is assessed as a net difference in the intervention condition relative to the control condition.

Because it is more difficult to suggest plausible alternative explanations for net differences than for simple differences, this feature provides a better defense against bias.

Even so, there is no guarantee that the study conditions are similar in all respects at baseline, especially in the absence of randomization of a sufficient number of groups to each condition. To the extent that such differences may generate different trends over time, they remain as a threat to the validity of the unadjusted analysis.

Adjusted Time × Condition Analysis

Regression adjustment for covariates may be used to remove variability due to covariates from the time × condition analysis. Because the same members are seen at each time in a nested cohort design, the covariates can be measured either at baseline only or at each time interval in the survey schedule. Covariates measured at baseline only are called *fixed covariates*. Covariates that change over time are called *time-varying* or *time-dependent covariates.*

Regression adjustment for covariates can be very helpful in a nested cohort design. To the extent that the covariates are related to the endpoint and unevenly distributed among conditions, they would induce confounding if ignored. To the extent that they explain residual variation, they would reduce power if ignored.

The Model

The model for the adjusted analysis is:

$$Y_{ij:k:l} = \mu + C_l + T_j + TC_{jl} + \sum_{o=1}^{x} \beta_o(X_{oij:k:l} - \overline{X}_{o....})$$
$$+ G_{k:l} + M_{i:k:l} + TG_{jk:l} + MT_{ij:k:l} + \varepsilon_{ij:k:l} \tag{6.4}$$

This model differs from the model for the unadjusted analysis only by addition of the covariates. For each covariate, the portion of $Y_{ij:k:l}$ that is explained by the difference between the observed value and sample mean on the covariate, $(X_{oij:k:l} - \overline{X}_{o....})$, is attributed to the covariate.

In most group-randomized trials, condition, time, and their interaction are fixed effects. The random effects allow for variation and correlation as described for the unadjusted analysis.

The Intervention Effect

In the ANCOVA, the F-statistic assesses the variation among the adjusted time $\times$ condition means against the variation among the adjusted time $\times$ group means. The null hypothesis is that the variation due to conditions over time is zero. When there are only two conditions and two time intervals, the numerator of the F-statistic is based on a single df and it is more convenient to use the t-statistic. In that case, the intervention effect is the adjusted net difference and the null hypothesis is that the adjusted net difference is zero. For the intervention and control conditions, the intervention effect is:

$$\Delta = (\bar{Y}_{.2 \cdot I} - \bar{Y}_{.1 \cdot I}) - (\bar{Y}_{.2 \cdot C} - \bar{Y}_{.1 \cdot C})$$
$$- \sum_{o=1}^{x} \beta_o ((\bar{X}_{o \cdot 2 \cdot I} - \bar{X}_{o \cdot 1 \cdot I}) - (\bar{X}_{o \cdot 2 \cdot C} - \bar{X}_{o \cdot 1 \cdot C})) \qquad (6.5)$$

Close inspection of the regression-adjustment portion of this formula reveals a detail often missed even by otherwise well-informed investigators and analysts. The regression coefficient is multiplied by the over-time difference in covariate values between the two conditions. For covariates that do not change their value over time—that is, covariates measured only at baseline—this difference is zero and so the regression adjustment is zero. In other words, regression adjustment for fixed covariates has no effect on the estimate of the intervention effect or on the test of that effect. For this reason, there is rarely any point to adding fixed covariates to a repeated-measures analysis.[4]

The Expected Mean Squares

The expected mean squares for this analysis are shown in Table 6.2. Note that the covariates are not shown in the table except as they affect the df for the other terms. The MS_{tc} has four components: residual error (σ_e^2), a component of variance due to the interaction of member with time ($\sigma_{mt:g:c}^2$), a weighted component of variance due to the interaction of time with group ($m\sigma_{tg:c}^2$), and a weighted component of variance due to the intervention ($mg\sigma_{tc}^2$). The test of the null hypothesis is $MS_{tc}/MS_{tg:c}$.

For each fixed covariate measured at the group level, df associated with that covariate (x_{gf}) are lost from $MS_{g:c}$. For each fixed covariate measured at the member level, df associated with that covariate (x_{mf}) are lost from $MS_{m:g:c}$. For each time-varying covariate measured at the group level, df associated with that covariate (x_{gv}) are lost from $MS_{g:c}$ and $MS_{tg:c}$. For each time-varying covariate measured at the member level, df associated with that covariate (x_{mv}) are lost from $MS_{m:g:c}$ and $MS_{mt:g:c}$. Because df at the group level are generally limited and are critical for power, use of covariates at that level should be

Table 6.2. Expected Mean Squares for the Adjusted Time $\times$ Condition Analysis of Data From a Nested Cohort Pretest-Posttest Control Group Design

Source	df	E(MS)	MS
Condition	$c-1$	$\sigma_e^2 + t\sigma_{m:g:c}^2 + mt\sigma_{g:c}^2 + mtg\sigma_c^2$	MS_c
Group:C	$c(g-1)-x_{gf}-x_{gv}$	$\sigma_e^2 + t\sigma_{m:g:c}^2 + mt\sigma_{g:c}^2$	$MS_{g:c}$
Member:G:C	$gc(m-1)-x_{mf}-x_{mv}$	$\sigma_e^2 + t\sigma_{m:g:c}^2$	$MS_{m:g:c}$
Time	$t-1$	$\sigma_e^2 + \sigma_{mt:g:c}^2 + m\sigma_{tg:c}^2 + mgc\sigma_t^2$	MS_t
TC	$(t-1)(c-1)$	$\sigma_e^2 + \sigma_{mt:g:c}^2 + m\sigma_{tg:c}^2 + mg\sigma_{tc}^2$	MS_{tc}
TG:C	$(t-1)c(g-1)-x_{gv}$	$\sigma_e^2 + \sigma_{mt:g:c}^2 + m\sigma_{tg:c}^2$	$MS_{tg:c}$
MT:G:C	$(t-1)gc(m-1)-x_{mv}$	$\sigma_e^2 + \sigma_{mt:g:c}^2$	MS_e

restricted to those that either correct confounding or measurably reduce the variance of the intervention effect. Note that while the symbols used to represent the variance components are the same as in the unadjusted analysis, those components reflect any reduction in variation due to the regression adjustment for the covariates.

The Variance of the Intervention Effect

When the intervention effect is defined as the adjusted net difference over two time intervals between two conditions, the variance of that intervention effect under the null hypothesis is:

$$\sigma_\Delta^2 = 2 * 2\left(\frac{MS_{tg:c}}{mg}\right) \tag{6.6}$$

Here there are m members per time $\times$ group survey and g groups per condition. The $MS_{tg:c}$ reflects the repeat observations on the same groups and members and the regression adjustment for covariates; details are provided in Chapter 9.

Assumptions

The assumptions for this analysis include those from the unadjusted analysis for this design and those related to the regression adjustment for covariates presented in Chapter 5. Violations have effects as described in those sections. In addition, this analysis assumes that the regression coefficients for each covariate are the same when estimated within members as between members. That assumption is reasonable so long as the intervention cannot affect the value of the covariate (Winer, 1971, p. 801).

Strengths and Weaknesses

Relative to the unadjusted analysis for this design, the adjusted analysis is more efficient to the extent that the regression adjustment for covariates reduces the variance of the intervention effect. Given random assignment of a modest number of groups to each condition, this can be a strong design and a good analysis, provided the assumptions underlying the analysis are met. In addition, the formulation of the intervention effect as a net change is intuitively attractive to many investigators.

The repeated-measures approach suffers from three weaknesses that reduce its utility in the analysis of data from a group-randomized trial. First, it is not robust to inadequate modeling of the pattern of the within-member covariance matrices across any between-member grouping factors, including condition. If the within-member covariance matrices are not well modeled, the Type I and II error rates are unknown. Second, the only covariates that serve any purpose in terms of regression adjustment are those that can change values over time; this often serves to limit the utility of the adjustment procedure. Third, the intervention effect is defined as a net difference; other factors constant, the variance of that effect is larger than for the major alternative, the simple difference, thereby reducing power compared to that alternative.

Mixed-Model Analysis of Covariance

The major alternative to the repeated-measures approach involves analysis of posttest data with regression adjustment for covariates. As before, covariates are added to the model to reduce confounding, to improve the precision of the estimate of the intervention effect, or both. Covariates are often measured at baseline and may include the baseline measure of the primary endpoint. Regression adjustment for covariates of this kind can be more effective in minimizing the threats to the validity of the design.

The Model

The mixed-model ANCOVA is written as:

$$Y_{i:k:l} = \mu + C_l + \sum_{o=1}^{x} \beta_o (X_{oi:k:l} - \bar{X}_{o \cdot \cdot \cdot}) + G_{k:l} + \varepsilon_{i:k:l} \tag{6.7}$$

This model is identical to the model presented in Chapter 5 for the adjusted analysis of data from a nested cross-sectional study based on a Posttest-Only Control Group Design (cf., Eq. 5.4). The observed value ($Y_{i:k:l}$) for the ith

member nested within the kth group nested within the lth condition is expressed as a function of the grand mean (μ), the effect of the lth condition (C_l), the effect of the covariates (X_o), and the realized value of the kth group $(G_{k:l})$. For each covariate, the portion of $Y_{i:k:l}$ that is explained by the difference between the observed value and sample mean on the covariate $(X_{oi:k:l} - \overline{X}_{o\cdot\cdot})$ is attributed to the covariate. Any difference that remains between the predicted and observed value is left to the residual error $(\varepsilon_{i:k:l})$.

In most group-randomized trials, condition is a fixed effect. In order to account for the positive intraclass correlation expected in the data, $G_{k:l}$ must be included in the analysis as a random effect. Simulation studies have shown that failure to do so, in the presence of measurable intraclass correlation, will result in a Type I error rate that is inflated, often badly (Zucker, 1990; Murray and Wolfinger, 1994; Murray et al., 1996). The two random effects allow for correlation among members within a group $(G_{k:l})$ and for random variation among the members $(\varepsilon_{i:k:l})$.

The Intervention Effect

In the ANCOVA, the F-statistic assesses the variation among the adjusted condition means against the variation among the adjusted group means. The null hypothesis is that the variation due to the conditions is zero. When there are only two conditions, the numerator of the F-statistic is based on a single df and it is more convenient to use the t-statistic. In that case, the intervention effect is the difference between the two adjusted condition means and the null hypothesis is that the difference is zero. For the intervention and control conditions, the intervention effect is:

$$\Delta = (\overline{Y}_{\cdot\cdot I} - \overline{Y}_{\cdot\cdot C}) - \sum_{o=1}^{x} \beta_o(\overline{X}_{o\cdot\cdot I} - \overline{X}_{o\cdot\cdot C}) \qquad (6.8)$$

The Expected Mean Squares

The expected mean squares for this analysis are shown in Table 6.3; they are identical to those shown previously in Table 5.2. Note that the covariates are not shown in the table except as they affect the df for the other terms. The MS_c has three components: residual error (σ_e^2), a weighted component of variance due to the groups $(m\sigma_{g:c}^2)$, and a weighted component of variance due to the intervention $(mg\sigma_c^2)$. The test of the null hypothesis is $MS_c/MS_{g:c}$.

For each covariate measured at the group level (x_g), df associated with that covariate are lost from $MS_{g:c}$. For each covariate measured at the member level (x_m), df associated with that covariate are lost from MS_e.

Table 6.3. Expected Mean Squares for the Analysis of Posttest Data With Regression Adjustment for Baseline Values for Data From a Nested Cohort Pretest-Posttest Control Group Design

Source	df	E(MS)	MS
Condition	$c-1$	$\sigma_e^2 + m\sigma_{g:c}^2 + mg\sigma_c^2$	MS_c
Group:C	$c(g-1) - x_g$	$\sigma_e^2 + m\sigma_{g:c}^2$	$MS_{g:c}$
Member:G:C	$gc(m-1) - x_m$	σ_e^2	MS_e

The Variance of the Intervention Effect

When the intervention effect is defined as the difference between two conditions, the variance of that intervention effect under the null hypothesis is:

$$\sigma_\Delta^2 = 2\left(\frac{MS_{g:c}}{mg}\right) \tag{6.9}$$

Here there are m members per group and g groups per condition. The $MS_{g:c}$ reflects the regression adjustment for covariates included in the model, which may include adjustment for baseline values; details are provided in Chapter 9.

Selection of Covariates

The discussion on the selection of covariates presented in Chapter 5 is equally relevant here. The investigator should seek to identify factors likely to be related to the primary endpoint prior to the collection of data so that they can be measured and considered as possible covariates at the time of the analysis. In most cases, measurement of the primary endpoint at baseline provides the single best covariate for inclusion in the analysis. This is because the baseline score on the primary endpoint is likely to be more highly related to the posttest score on the primary endpoint than any other variable that could be measured at baseline. As such, it often provides the best possible adjustment for any baseline differences in levels for the primary endpoint.

Assumptions

The assumptions presented in Chapter 5 for the adjusted analysis of the Posttest-Only Control Group Design apply equally in this case. The fourth assumption was that the intervention has no effect on the covariates. That assumption is much more plausible in the nested cohort design because it is possible to select as covariates variables that were measured during the base-line survey. Such values cannot possibly be affected by the intervention.

Covariates measured at posttest may be included in the analysis. However, caution must be used to ensure that any covariates measured at posttest were not influenced by the intervention.

Strengths and Weaknesses

This analysis provides three major advantages over the repeated-measures analysis described in the previous section. It provides one major advantage over the comparable analysis for its nested cross-sectional counterpart.

First, this analysis avoids altogether assumptions about the pattern of the within-member covariance matrices. Even with the regression adjustment for covariates measured at baseline, this analysis is a completely between-member analysis. Second, this analysis can adjust the posttest results for baseline val-ues on important covariates, including the primary endpoint. The power and validity of such adjustments are often greater than for adjustment for concur-rent covariates. Third, the intervention effect is modeled as a simple adjusted difference and so is less complex than the net difference in the repeated-measures approach. All other factors constant, the power for a simple differ-ence is greater than for a net difference.

The advantage over the comparable analysis in the nested cross-sectional design has already been discussed. Use of baseline measures as covariates avoids questions about the independence of the covariates and the intervention effect and also is likely to do a better job of adjusting for baseline differences that might otherwise bias the results of the study.

Most of the weaknesses associated with regression adjustment for covariates that were discussed in Chapter 5 apply equally here. This is certainly true in terms of the cautions against including a laundry list of covariates, against measurement error in covariates, and against residual confounding.

Stratification or Matching in the Analysis

This section shows how to include stratification and matching in the analysis of data from a nested cohort design; examples are provided in Chapter 8. *A priori* and *post hoc* stratification are presented separately, as they require dif-ferent analyses. Matching is considered as a special case of *a priori* stratifica-tion. These analyses are illustrated for the adjusted time × condition analysis from the Pretest-Posttest Control Group Design and for the ANCOVA as ap-plied to the same design.

A Priori Stratification in the Adjusted Time × Condition Analysis

In *a priori* stratification, the groups are nested within the cells defined by the condition × stratum interaction. In the nested cohort version of this design, members in each group are followed over time as a cohort to assess the effect of the intervention. When the investigator is interested only in the levels of the stratification factor that are included in the design, stratum is a fixed effect.

The Model

The model for the Pretest-Posttest Control Group Design that includes *a priori* stratification with regression adjustment for covariates is:

$$Y_{ij:k:lp} = \mu + C_l + S_p + CS_{lp} + T_j + TC_{jl} + TS_{jp} + TCS_{jlp}$$
$$+ \sum_{o=1}^{x} \beta_o (X_{oij:k:lp} - \overline{X}_{o\cdots}) \qquad (6.10)$$
$$+ G_{k:lp} + M_{i:k:lp} + TG_{jk:lp} + MT_{ij:k:lp} + \varepsilon_{ij:k:lp}$$

Stratum is added both as a main effect and as a series of interactions with the other fixed effects. This adds four fixed effects to the unstratified model presented earlier in this chapter. Note that the notation $G_{k:lp}$ reflects the nesting of the groups within the cells defined by the condition × stratum interaction.

In most group-randomized trials, condition, time, and their interaction are fixed effects. In this design, stratum is also a fixed effect, as are all its interactions involving condition and time. In order to account for the positive intraclass correlation expected in the data, $G_{k:lp}$ and $TG_{jk:lp}$ must be included in the analysis as random effects. The three random effects carried over from the nested cross-sectional version of this design allow for correlation among members within a group ($G_{k:lp}$), for correlation among members within a time × group survey ($TG_{jk:lp}$), and for random variation among the members ($\varepsilon_{ij:k:lp}$). The $M_{i:k:lp}$ term allows for correlation among the repeat observations taken on the same member. The $MT_{ij:k:lp}$ allows for correlation among replicate measurements on the same member during a single survey. If such replicates are available, $MT_{ij:k:lp}$ is estimable apart from $\varepsilon_{ij:k:lp}$. If no replicate measures are taken on the same member during a single survey, those components cannot be estimated separately.

The Intervention Effect

In the ANCOVA, the *F*-statistic assesses the variation among the adjusted time × condition × stratum means against the variation among the adjusted time

$\times$ group means. The null hypothesis is that the variation due to conditions over time and across strata is zero. When there are only two conditions, two time intervals, and two strata, the numerator of the F-statistic is based on a single df and it is more convenient to use the t-statistic. In that case, the intervention effect is defined as the difference between the two strata in their adjusted net differences. The null hypothesis is that the difference between the two strata is zero.

The Expected Mean Squares

The expected mean squares for this analysis are shown in Table 6.4. Note that the covariates are not shown in the table except as they affect the df for the other terms. The MS_{tcs} has four components: residual error (σ_e^2), a component of variance due to the interaction of member with time ($\sigma_{mt:g:cs}^2$), a weighted component of variance due to the interaction of time with group ($m\sigma_{tg:cs}^2$), and a weighted component of variance due to the intervention ($mg\sigma_{tcs}^2$). The test of the null hypothesis is $MS_{tcs}/MS_{tg:cs}$.

For each fixed covariate measured at the group level, df associated with that covariate (x_{gf}) are lost from $MS_{g:cs}$. For each fixed covariate measured at the member level, df associated with that covariate (X_{mf}) are lost from $MS_{m:g:cs}$. For each time-varying covariate measured at the group level, df associated with that covariate (x_{gv}) are lost from $MS_{g:cs}$ and $MS_{tg:cs}$. For each time-varying covariate measured at the member level, df associated with that covariate (x_{mv}) are lost from $MS_{m:g:cs}$ and $MS_{mt:g:cs}$.

Table 6.4. Expected Mean Squares for the Adjusted Time $\times$ Condition Analysis of Data From a Nested Cohort Pretest-Posttest Control Group Design With *A Priori* Stratification and With Stratum as a Fixed Effect

Source	df	E(MS)	MS
Condition	$c-1$	$\sigma_e^2 + t\sigma_{m:g:cs}^2 + mt\sigma_{g:cs}^2 + mtgs\sigma_c^2$	MS_c
Strata	$s-1$	$\sigma_e^2 + t\sigma_{m:g:cs}^2 + mt\sigma_{g:cs}^2 + mtgc\sigma_s^2$	MS_s
CS	$(c-1)(s-1)$	$\sigma_e^2 + t\sigma_{m:g:cs}^2 + mt\sigma_{g:cs}^2 + mtg\sigma_{cs}^2$	MS_{cs}
Group:CS	$cs(g-1)-x_{gf}-x_{gv}$	$\sigma_e^2 + t\sigma_{m:g:cs}^2 + mt\sigma_{g:cs}^2$	$MS_{g:cs}$
M:G:CS	$gcs(m-1)-x_{mf}-x_{mv}$	$\sigma_e^2 + t\sigma_{m:g:cs}^2$	$MS_{m:g:cs}$
Time	$t-1$	$\sigma_e^2 + \sigma_{mt:g:cs}^2 + m\sigma_{tg:cs}^2 + mgcs\sigma_t^2$	MS_t
TC	$(t-1)(c-1)$	$\sigma_e^2 + \sigma_{mt:g:cs}^2 + m\sigma_{tg:cs}^2 + mgs\sigma_{tc}^2$	MS_{tc}
TS	$(t-1)(s-1)$	$\sigma_e^2 + \sigma_{mt:g:cs}^2 + m\sigma_{tg:cs}^2 + mgc\sigma_{ts}^2$	MS_{ts}
TCS	$(t-1)(c-1)(s-1)$	$\sigma_e^2 + \sigma_{mt:g:cs}^2 + m\sigma_{tg:cs}^2 + mg\sigma_{tcs}^2$	MS_{tcs}
TG:CS	$(t-1)cs(g-1)-x_{gv}$	$\sigma_e^2 + \sigma_{mt:g:cs}^2 + m\sigma_{tg:cs}^2$	$MS_{tg:cs}$
MT:G:CS	$gcs(m-1)(t-1)-x_{mv}$	$\sigma_e^2 + \sigma_{mt:g:cs}^2$	MS_e

The Variance of the Intervention Effect

When the intervention effect is defined as the contrast between two strata in their net difference over two time intervals between two conditions, the variance of that intervention effect under the null hypothesis is:

$$\sigma_\Delta^2 = 2 * 2 * 2 \left(\frac{MS_{tg:cs}}{mg} \right) \tag{6.11}$$

Here m is the number of observations in each time $\times$ group survey and g is the number of groups in each condition $\times$ stratum cell. The $MS_{tg:cs}$ reflects the stratification, the repeat observations on the same groups and members, and the regression adjustment for covariates; details are provided in Chapter 9.

Assumptions

This analysis provides for five sources of random variation. If there are additional sources in the data, the model is misspecified and the true Type I and II error rates are unknown.

Under the General Linear Mixed Model, the random effects are assumed to be independent and distributed as $G_{k:lp} \approx N(0, \sigma_{g:cs}^2)$, $M_{i:k:lp} \approx N(0, \sigma_{m:g:cs}^2)$, $TG_{jk:lp} \approx N(0, \sigma_{tg:cs}^2)$, $MT_{ij:k:lp} \approx N(0, \sigma_{mt:g:cs}^2)$, and $\varepsilon_{ij:k:lp} \approx N(0, \sigma_e^2)$. With the important caveats noted in Chapter 5, the analysis can be extended to non-Gaussian data by assuming a different distribution for $\varepsilon_{ij:k:lp}$ and a different link function. The analysis would then represent an application of the Generalized Linear Mixed Model.

Even without reliance on the Generalized Linear Mixed Model, this analysis appears to be robust to violation of the normality assumption for the residual error distribution, given a moderate number of groups and members (Hannan and Murray, 1996). It also provides substantial protection against violations of the independence assumption as the most likely forms of dependence are modeled via $G_{k:lp}$, $TG_{jk:lp}$, and $M_{i:k:lp}$.

Stratification adds an additional between-member grouping factor, thereby increasing the number of within-member covariance matrices that are assumed homogeneous and circular in the traditional repeated-measures approach. This analysis also makes the assumptions related to the regression adjustment for covariates presented in Chapter 5. Violations have effects as described in those sections. In addition, this analysis assumes that the regression coefficients for each covariate are the same when estimated within members as between members. That assumption is reasonable so long as the intervention cannot affect the value of the covariate (Winer, 1971, p. 801).

The stratified analysis carries the additional assumption that the relationships among the covariates and endpoints are constant across the strata. Violations reduce power by reducing the precision of the intervention effect. This assumption may be tested by inclusion of interaction terms involving the strata and the covariates of concern in the analysis.

Strengths and Weaknesses

The strengths and weaknesses related to *a priori* stratification that were presented in Chapter 5 apply equally here. The major additional weakness derives from the assumption that the within-member random-effects covariance matrices remain homogeneous and circular even though their number has been increased as a result of the stratification. As the number of such matrices increases, the possibility for heterogeneity and noncircularity increases. If the investigator is not careful to test those assumptions, the threat to the validity of the analysis also increases. This adds another reason that the stratified analysis should be reserved for situations in which the investigator has a critical interest in the test of the homogeneity of the intervention effect across the strata.

Post Hoc Stratification in the Adjusted Time × Condition Analysis

With *post hoc* stratification, the investigator is interested only in the levels of the stratification factor that are included in the analysis, so that stratum is a fixed effect.

The Model

The model for the Pretest-Posttest Control Group Design that includes *post hoc* stratification on a characteristic measured at the member level and regression adjustment for baseline values is:

$$Y_{ij:kp:l} = \mu + C_l + S_p + CS_{lp} + T_j + TC_{jl} + TS_{jp} + TCS_{jlp}$$
$$+ \sum_{o=1}^{x} \beta_o (X_{oij:kp:l} - \overline{X}_{o\cdot\dots\dots}) + G_{k:l} + TG_{jk:l} + M_{i:kp:l} \qquad (6.12)$$
$$+ GS_{kp:l} + TGS_{jkp:l} + MT_{ij:kp:l} + \varepsilon_{ij:kp:l}$$

Stratum is added both as a main effect and as a series of interactions with the other fixed effects. This adds four fixed effects and two random effects to the unstratified model for this analysis. The notation $G_{k:l}$ reflects the nesting of the groups within the cells defined by the condition but not within strata. Instead, groups are crossed with strata, as evidenced by the $GS_{kp:l}$ term.

In most group-randomized trials, condition, time, and their interaction are fixed effects. With *post hoc* stratification, the investigator is interested only in the levels of the stratification factor that are included in the analysis, so stratum is a fixed effect, as are its interactions with the other fixed effects. In order to account for the positive intraclass correlation expected in the data, $G_{k:l}$, $GS_{kp:l}$, $TG_{jk:l}$, and $TGS_{jkp:l}$ must be included in the analysis as random effects. The five random effects carried over from the nested cross-sectional version of this design allow for correlation among members within a group $(G_{k:l})$, for correlation among members within a group specific to a stratum $(GS_{kp:l})$, for correlation among members within a time $\times$ group survey $(TG_{jk:l})$, for correlation among members within a time $\times$ group survey specific to a stratum $(TGS_{jkp:l})$, and for random variation among the members $(\varepsilon_{ij:kp:l})$. The $M_{i:kp:l}$ term allows for correlation among the repeat observations taken on the same member. The $MT_{ij:kp:l}$ allows for correlation among replicate measurements on the same member during a single survey. If such replicates are available, $MT_{ij:kp:l}$ is estimable apart from $\varepsilon_{ij:kp:l}$. If no replicate measures are taken on the same member during a single survey, those components cannot be estimated separately.

The Intervention Effect

In the ANCOVA, the *F*-statistic assesses the variation among the adjusted time $\times$ condition $\times$ stratum means against the variation among the adjusted time $\times$ group $\times$ stratum means. The null hypothesis is that the variation due to conditions over time and across strata is zero. When there are only two conditions, two time intervals, and two strata, the numerator of the *F*-statistic is based on a single *df* and it is more convenient to use the *t*-statistic. In that case, the intervention effect is defined as the difference between the two strata in their adjusted net differences. The null hypothesis is that the difference is zero.

The Expected Mean Squares

The expected mean squares for this analysis are shown in Table 6.5. Note that the covariates are not shown in the table except as they affect the *df* for the other terms. The MS_{tcs} has four components: residual error (σ_e^2), a component of variance due to the interaction of member with time $(\sigma_{mt:gs:c}^2)$, a weighted component of variance due to the interaction of time with group and strata

Table 6.5. Expected Mean Squares for the Adjusted Time × Condition Analysis of Data From a Nested Cohort Pretest-Posttest Control Group Design With *Post Hoc* Stratification

Source	df	E(MS)	MS
Condition	$c-1$	$\sigma_e^2 + t\sigma_{m:gs:c}^2 + mts\sigma_{g:c}^2 + mtgs\sigma_c^2$	MS_c
Group:C	$c(g-1)-x_{gf}-x_{gv}$	$\sigma_e^2 + t\sigma_{m:gs:c}^2 + mts\sigma_{g:c}^2$	$MS_{g:c}$
Strata	$(s-1)$	$\sigma_e^2 + t\sigma_{m:gs:c}^2 + mto_{gs:c}^2 + mtgc\sigma_s^2$	MS_s
CS	$(c-1)(s-1)$	$\sigma_e^2 + t\sigma_{m:gs:c}^2 + mt\sigma_{gs:c}^2 + mtg\sigma_{cs}^2$	MS_{cs}
GS:C	$c(g-1)(s-1)-x_{gf}-x_{gv}$	$\sigma_e^2 + t\sigma_{m:gs:c}^2 + mt\sigma_{gs:c}^2$	$MS_{gs:c}$
M:GS:C	$gsc(m-1)-x_{mf}-x_{mv}$	$\sigma_e^2 + t\sigma_{m:gs:c}^2$	$MS_{m:gs:c}$
Time	$t-1$	$\sigma_e^2 + \sigma_{mt:gs:c}^2 + ms\sigma_{tg:c}^2 + mgsc\sigma_t^2$	MS_t
TC	$(t-1)(c-1)$	$\sigma_e^2 + \sigma_{mt:gs:c}^2 + ms\sigma_{tg:c}^2 + mgs\sigma_{tc}^2$	MS_{tc}
TG:C	$(t-1)c(g-1)-x_{gv}$	$\sigma_e^2 + \sigma_{mt:gs:c}^2 + ms\sigma_{tg:c}^2$	$MS_{tg:c}$
TS	$(t-1)(s-1)$	$\sigma_e^2 + \sigma_{mt:gs:c}^2 + m\sigma_{tgs:c}^2 + mgc\sigma_{ts}^2$	MS_{ts}
TCS	$(t-1)(c-1)(s-1)$	$\sigma_e^2 + \sigma_{mt:gs:c}^2 + m\sigma_{tgs:c}^2 + mg\sigma_{tcs}^2$	MS_{tcs}
TGS:C	$(t-1)c(g-1)(s-1)-x_{gv}$	$\sigma_e^2 + \sigma_{mt:gs:c}^2 + m\sigma_{tgs:c}^2$	$MS_{tgs:c}$
MT:GS:C	$gsc(m-1)(t-1)-x_{mv}$	$\sigma_e^2 + \sigma_{mt:gs:c}^2$	MS_e

$(m\sigma_{tgs:c}^2)$, and a weighted component of variance due to the intervention $(mg\sigma_{tcs}^2)$. The test of the null hypothesis is $MS_{tcs}/MS_{tgs:c}$.

For each fixed covariate measured at the group level, *df* associated with that covariate (x_{gf}) are lost from $MS_{g:c}$ and from $MS_{gs:c}$. For each fixed covariate measured at the member level, *df* associated with that covariate (x_{mf}) are lost from $MS_{m:gs:c}$. For each time-varying covariate measured at the group level, *df* associated with that covariate (x_{gv}) are lost from $MS_{g:c}$, $MS_{gs:c}$, $MS_{tg:c}$ and $MS_{tgs:c}$. For each time-varying covariate measured at the member level, *df* associated with that covariate (x_{mv}) are lost from $MS_{m:gs:c}$ and MS_e.

The Variance of the Intervention Effect

When the intervention effect is defined as the contrast between two strata in their adjusted net difference over two time intervals between two conditions, the variance of that intervention effect under the null hypothesis is:

$$\sigma_\Delta^2 = 2*2*2\left(\frac{MS_{tgs:c}}{mg}\right) \tag{6.13}$$

Here *m* is the number of members in each time × group × stratum survey and *g* is the number of groups in each condition. The $MS_{tgs:c}$ reflects the stratification, the repeat observations on the same groups and members, and the regression adjustment for covariates; details are provided in Chapter 9.

Assumptions

This analysis provides for seven sources of random variation. If there are additional sources in the data, the model is misspecified and the true Type I and II error rates are unknown.

Under the General Linear Mixed Model, the random effects are assumed to be independent and distributed as $G_{k:l} \approx N(0, \sigma_{g:c}^2)$, $TG_{jk:l} \approx N(0, \sigma_{tg:c}^2)$, $M_{i:kp:l} \approx N(0, \sigma_{m:gs:c}^2)$, $GS_{kp:l} \approx N(0, \sigma_{gs:c}^2)$, $TGS_{jkp:l} \approx N(0, \sigma_{tgs:c}^2)$, $MT_{ij:kp:l} \approx N(0, \sigma_{mt:gs:c}^2)$, and $\varepsilon_{ij:kp:l} \approx N(0, \sigma_e^2)$. With the important caveats noted in Chapter 5, the analysis can be extended to non-Gaussian data by assuming a different distribution for $\varepsilon_{ij:kp:l}$ and a different link function. The analysis would then represent an application of the Generalized Linear Mixed Model.

Even without reliance on the Generalized Linear Mixed Model, this analysis appears to be robust to violation of the normality assumption for the residual-error distribution, given a moderate number of groups and members (Hannan and Murray, 1996). It also provides substantial protection against violations of the independence assumption as the most likely forms of dependence are modeled via $G_{k:l}$, $GS_{kp:l}$, $TG_{jk:l}$, $TGS_{jkp:l}$, and $M_{i:kp:l}$.

Post hoc stratification adds an additional between-member grouping factor, and so increases the number of within-member covariance matrices that are assumed homogeneous and circular in the traditional repeated-measures approach.

The stratified analysis carries the additional assumption that the relationships among the covariates and outcome are constant across the strata. Violations reduce power by reducing the precision of the intervention effect. This assumption may be tested by inclusion of interaction terms involving the strata and the covariates.

Strengths and Weaknesses

This analysis combines the strengths and weaknesses of the adjusted time $\times$ condition analysis presented earlier in this chapter and the *post hoc* stratified analysis described in Chapter 5.

A Priori Stratification in the Analysis of Posttest Data With Regression Adjustment for Baseline Values

The analysis of posttest data with regression adjustment for baseline values can be modified to reflect *a priori* stratification. In this instance stratum is a fixed effect, presuming that the strata included in the design are the only strata of interest.

The Model

The model for this analysis is written as:

$$Y_{i:k:lp} = \mu + C_l + S_p + CS_{lp} + \sum_{o=1}^{x} \beta_o(X_{oi:k:lp} - \overline{X}_{o\cdot\ldots})$$
$$+ G_{k:lp} + \varepsilon_{i:k:lp} \qquad (6.14)$$

Stratum is added to the analysis both as a main effect and as an interaction with the other fixed effect, condition. No additional random effects are added, though the notation for the random effects changes to reflect the nesting of groups within the CS_{lp} cells.

In most group-randomized trials, condition is a fixed effect. In this design, stratum is also a fixed effect, as is its interaction with condition. In order to account for the positive intraclass correlation expected in the data, $G_{k:lp}$ must be included in the analysis as a random effect; simulation studies have shown that failure to do so, in the presence of measurable intraclass correlation, will result in a Type I error rate that is inflated, often badly (Zucker, 1990; Murray and Wolfinger, 1994; Murray et al., 1996). The two random effects allow for correlation among members within a group ($G_{k:lp}$) and for random variation among the members ($\varepsilon_{i:k:lp}$).

The Intervention Effect

In the ANCOVA, the F-statistic assesses the variation among the adjusted condition $\times$ stratum means against the variation among the group means. The null hypothesis is that the variation due to conditions over strata is zero. When there are only two conditions and two strata, the numerator of the F-statistic is based on a single df and it is more convenient to use the t-statistic. In that case, the intervention effect is the adjusted net difference and the null hypothesis is that the adjusted net difference is zero.

The Expected Mean Squares

The expected mean squares for this analysis are shown in Table 6.6. Note that the covariates are not shown in the table except as they affect the df for the other terms. The MS_{cs} has three components: residual error (σ_e^2), a weighted component of variance due to the groups ($m\sigma_{g:cs}^2$), and a weighted component of variance due to the intervention effect ($mg\sigma_{cs}^2$). The test of the null hypothesis is $MS_{cs}/MS_{g:cs}$.

For each covariate measured at the group level (x_g), degrees of freedom associated with that covariate are lost from $MS_{g:cs}$. For each covariate mea-

Table 6.6 Expected Mean Squares for the Analysis of Posttest Data
With Regression Adjustment for Covariates for Data From a Nested
Cohort Pretest-Posttest Control Group Design With *A Priori*
Stratification and With Stratum as a Fixed Effect

Source	df	E(MS)	MS
Condition	$c - 1$	$\sigma_e^2 + m\sigma_{g:cs}^2 + mgs\sigma_c^2$	MS_c
Strata	$s - 1$	$\sigma_e^2 + m\sigma_{g:cs}^2 + mgc\sigma_s^2$	MS_s
CS	$(c-1)(s-1)$	$\sigma_e^2 + m\sigma_{g:cs}^2 + mg\sigma_{cs}^2$	MS_{cs}
Group:CS	$cs(g-1) - x_g$	$\sigma_e^2 + m\sigma_{g:cs}^2$	$MS_{g:cs}$
Member:G:CS	$gcs(m-1) - x_m$	σ_e^2	MS_e

sured at the member level (x_m), degrees of freedom associated with that covariate are lost from $MS_{m:g:cs}$.

The Variance of the Intervention Effect

When the intervention effect is defined as the adjusted net difference between two conditions over two strata, the variance of that intervention effect under the null hypothesis is:

$$\sigma_\Delta^2 = 2 * 2\left(\frac{MS_{g:cs}}{mg}\right) \tag{6.15}$$

Here m is the number of observations in each group and g is the number of observations in each condition $\times$ stratum cell. The $M_{g:cs}$ reflects the stratification and the regression adjustment for covariates; details are provided in Chapter 9.

Assumptions

This analysis provides for two sources of random variation. If there are additional sources in the data, the model is misspecified and the true Type I and II error rates are unknown.

Under the General Linear Mixed Model, the random effects are assumed to be independent and distributed $G_{k:lp} \approx N(0, \sigma_{g:cs}^2)$ and $\varepsilon_{i:k:lp} \approx N(0, \sigma_e^2)$. With the important caveats noted in Chapter 5, the analysis can be extended to non-Gaussian data by assuming a different distribution for $\varepsilon_{i:k:lp}$ and a different link function. The analysis would then represent an application of the Generalized Linear Mixed Model.

Even without reliance on the Generalized Linear Mixed Model, this analysis appears to be robust to violation of the normality assumption for the residual-error distribution, given a moderate number of groups and members (Hannan and Murray, 1996). It also provides substantial protection against violations of the independence assumption as the most likely form of dependence is modeled explicitly via $G_{k:lp}$.

The assumptions associated with regression adjustment for covariates that were presented in Chapter 5 and those associated with stratification that were presented earlier in this chapter apply equally here. Violations have effects as described in those earlier sections.

Strengths and Weaknesses

The advantages over the repeated-measures analyses apply equally here. Most of the weaknesses associated with regression adjustment for covariates also apply here. Finally, the strengths and weaknesses associated with *a priori* stratification apply here as well.

Post Hoc Stratification in the Analysis of Posttest Data With Regression Adjustment for Baseline Values

The analysis of posttest data with regression adjustment for baseline values also can be modified to reflect *post hoc* stratification. Again, stratum is a fixed effect, presuming that the strata used in the analysis are the only strata of interest.

The Model

The model for this analysis is written as:

$$Y_{i:kp:l} = \mu + C_l + S_p + CS_{lp} + \sum_{o=1}^{x} \beta_o(X_{oi:kp:l} - \bar{X}_{o\cdot\ldots}) $$
$$+ G_{k:l} + GS_{kp:l} + \varepsilon_{i:kp:l} \tag{6.16}$$

In most group-randomized trials, condition is a fixed effect. With *post hoc* stratification, stratum is also a fixed effect. In order to account for the positive intraclass correlation expected in the data, $G_{k:l}$ and $GS_{kp:l}$ must be included in the analysis as random effects. The three random effects in the model allow for correlation among members within a group $(G_{k:l})$, for correlation among members within a group in a particular stratum $(GS_{kp:l})$, and for random variation among the members $(\varepsilon_{i:kp:l})$.

The Intervention Effect

In the ANCOVA, the F-statistic assesses the variation among the adjusted condition $\times$ stratum means against the variation among the adjusted group $\times$ stratum means. The null hypothesis is that the variation due to conditions over strata is zero. When there are only two conditions and two strata, the numerator of the F-statistic is based on a single df and it is more convenient to use the t-statistic. In that case, the intervention effect is the adjusted net difference and the null hypothesis is that the adjusted net difference is zero.

The Expected Mean Squares

The expected mean squares for this analysis are shown in Table 6.7. Note that the covariates are not shown in the table except as they affect the df for the other terms. The MS_{cs} has three components: residual error (σ_e^2), a weighted component of variance due to the groups $(m\sigma_{gs:c}^2)$, and a weighted component of variance due to the intervention $(mg\sigma_{cs}^2)$. The test of the null hypothesis is $MS_{cs}/MS_{gs:c}$.

For each covariate measured at the group level (x_g), df associated with that covariate are lost from $MS_{gs:c}$. For each covariate measured at the member level (x_m), df associated with that covariate are lost from MS_e.

Table 6.7. Expected Mean Squares for the Analysis of Posttest Data With Regression Adjustment for Covariates for Data From a Nested Cohort Pretest-Posttest Control Group Design With *Post Hoc* Stratification

Source	df	E(MS)	MS
Condition	$c-1$	$\sigma_e^2 + ms\sigma_{g:c}^2 + mgs\sigma_c^2$	MS_c
Group:C	$c(g-1)$	$\sigma_e^2 + ms\sigma_{g:c}^2$	$MS_{g:c}$
Strata	$s-1$	$\sigma_e^2 + m\sigma_{gs:c}^2 + mgc\sigma_s^2$	MS_s
CS	$(c-1)(s-1)$	$\sigma_e^2 + m\sigma_{gs:c}^2 + mg\sigma_{cs}^2$	MS_{cs}
GS:C	$c(g-1)(s-1)-x_g$	$\sigma_e^2 + m\sigma_{gs:c}^2$	$MS_{gs:c}$
M:GS:C	$gcs(m-1)-x_m$	σ_e^2	MS_e

The Variance of the Intervention Effect

When the intervention effect is defined as the net difference between two conditions over two strata, the variance of the intervention effect under the null hypothesis is:

$$\sigma_\Delta^2 = 2 * 2 \left(\frac{MS_{gs:c}}{mg} \right) \qquad (6.17)$$

Here m is the number of members per group and g is the number of groups. $MS_{gs:c}$ reflects the regression adjustment for covariates as well as the stratification; details are provided in Chapter 9.

Assumptions

This analysis provides for three sources of random variation. If there are additional sources in the data, the model is misspecified and the true Type I and II error rates are unknown.

Under the General Linear Mixed Model, the random effects are assumed to be independent and distributed $G_{k:l} \approx N(0, \sigma_{g:c}^2)$, $GS_{kp:l} \approx N(0, \sigma_{gs:c}^2)$, and $\varepsilon_{i:kp:l} \approx N(0, \sigma_e^2)$. With the important caveats noted in Chapter 5, the analysis can be extended to non-Gaussian data by assuming a different distribution for $\varepsilon_{i:kp:l}$ and a different link function. The analysis would then represent an application of the Generalized Linear Mixed Model.

Even without reliance on the Generalized Linear Mixed Model, this analysis appears to be robust to violation of the normality assumption for the residual-error distribution, given a moderate number of groups and members (Hannan and Murray, 1996). It also provides substantial protection against violations of the independence assumption as the most likely forms of dependence are modeled explicitly via $G_{k:l}$ and $GS_{kp:l}$.

The assumptions associated with regression adjustment for covariates presented in Chapter 5 apply equally here. Violations have effects as described in that earlier section.

Strengths and Weaknesses

The advantages of the ANCOVA over the repeated-measures approach apply equally here. The strengths and weaknesses associated with regression adjustment for covariates also apply here. Finally, the strengths and weaknesses associated with *post hoc* stratification apply here as well.

Matching in the Analysis

As discussed in Chapter 5, matching is a simplified version of *a priori* stratification where there is only one group per stratum. There is no interest in the
matched sets per se, but the investigator wants to generalize to other sets like
those used in the study. As a result, the matched sets are levels of a random
effect. The term stratum is used to refer to the matched sets instead of introducing additional notation.

Matching serves the same purpose in a nested cohort design as in a nested
cross-sectional design. It provides a very effective method to control confounding when the investigator can create well-matched sets. The relative
strengths and weaknesses of matching were discussed in Chapter 3.

The Model

The model for the matched analysis of posttest data with regression adjustment
for baseline values is:

$$Y_{i:lp} = \mu + C_l + \sum_{o=1}^{x} \beta_o (X_{oi:lp} - \bar{X}_{o\cdot\cdot\cdot}) + S_p + CS_{lp} + \varepsilon_{i:lp} \qquad (6.18)$$

In most group-randomized trials, condition is a fixed effect. To provide a
statistical basis for generalization to other matched sets like those employed
in the study, stratum must be included as a random effect. Note that there is
no $G_{k:l}$ term in the model. This is because it cannot be estimated in the
matched design apart from CS_{lp} because there is only one group in each condition × stratum cell. In order to account for the positive intraclass correlation
expected in the data, CS_{lp} must be included in the analysis as a random effect.
The three random effects allow for correlation among members within the
matched sets (S_p), correlation among the members within the condition ×
stratum cells (CS_{lp}), and for random variation among the members $(\varepsilon_{i:lp})$.

The Intervention Effect

In the ANOVA, the *F*-statistic assesses the variation among the adjusted condition means against the variation among the adjusted group means. The null
hypothesis is that the variation due to the conditions is zero. When there are
only two conditions, the numerator of the *F*-statistic is based on a single *df*
and it is more convenient to use the *t*-statistic. In that case, the intervention
effect is the difference between the two adjusted condition means and the

null hypothesis is that the difference is zero. For the intervention and control conditions, the intervention effect is:

$$\Delta = (\bar{Y}_{..I} - \bar{Y}_{..C}) - \sum_{o=1}^{x} \beta_o (\bar{X}_{o..I} - \bar{X}_{o..C}) \qquad (6.19)$$

The Expected Mean Squares

The expected mean squares for this analysis are shown in Table 6.8. Note that the covariates are not shown in the table except as they affect the df for the other terms. The MS_c has three components: residual error (σ_e^2), a weighted component of variance due to the strata ($m\sigma_{cs}^2$), and a weighted component of variance due to the intervention ($ms\sigma_c^2$). The test of the null hypothesis is MS_c/MS_{cs}.

For each covariate measured at the group level (x_g), df associated with that covariate are lost from MS_{cs}. For each covariate measured at the member level (x_m), df associated with that covariate are lost from MS_e.

The Variance of the Intervention Effect

When the intervention effect is defined as the difference between two conditions, the variance of that intervention effect under the null hypothesis is:

$$\sigma_\Delta^2 = 2\left(\frac{MS_{cs}}{ms}\right) \qquad (6.20)$$

Here m is the number of observations in each condition $\times$ stratum cell and s is the number of strata. The MS_{cs} reflects the matching and the regression adjustment for covariates; details are provided in Chapter 9.

Table 6.8. Expected Mean Squares for the Analysis of Posttest Data With Regression Adjustment for Covariates for Data From a Nested Cohort Pretest-Posttest Control Group Design With A Priori Matching

Source	df	E(MS)	MS
Condition	$c-1$	$\sigma_e^2 + m\sigma_{cs}^2 + ms\sigma_c^2$	MS_c
Strata	$s-1$	$\sigma_e^2 + mc\sigma_s^2$	MS_s
CS	$(c-1)(s-1) - x_g$	$\sigma_e^2 + m\sigma_{cs}^2$	MS_{cs}
Member:CS	$cs(m-1) - x_m$	σ_e^2	MS_e

Assumptions

This analysis provides for three sources of random variation. If there are additional sources in the data, the model is misspecified and the true Type I and II error rates are unknown.

Under the General Linear Mixed Model, the three random effects are assumed to be independent and distributed $S_p \approx N(0, \sigma_s^2)$, $CS_{lp} \approx N(0, \sigma_{cs}^2)$, and $\varepsilon_{i:lp} \approx N(0, \sigma_e^2)$. With the important caveats noted in Chapter 5, the analysis can be extended to non-Gaussian data by assuming a different distribution for $\varepsilon_{i:lp}$ and a different link function. The analysis would then represent an application of the Generalized Linear Mixed Model.

Even without reliance on the Generalized Linear Mixed Model, this analysis appears to be robust to violation of the normality assumption for the residual error distribution, given a moderate number of groups and members (Hannan and Murray, 1996). It also provides substantial protection against violations of the independence assumption as the most likely forms of dependence are modeled explicitly via S_p and CS_{lp}.

The assumptions for this analysis include those related to regression adjustment for covariates; violations have the same effect as described in Chapter 5. Unlike the stratified analysis, the matched analysis does not provide a test of whether the intervention effect is homogeneous across the matched sets. That is simply assumed and is usually untestable in the matched analysis. Violations reduce power by reducing the precision of the estimate of the intervention effect. The matched analysis also assumes that the relationships among the covariates and endpoint are constant across the matched sets. Violations reduce power by reducing the precision of the estimate of the intervention effect. Of course, this assumption may be tested by including interaction terms involving the strata and the covariates of concern in the analysis.

Strengths and Weaknesses

The strengths and weaknesses of the matched analysis were presented in Chapter 5. Those points apply equally to this cohort analysis.

A Priori Stratification With Stratum as a Random Effect: Multicenter Group-Randomized Trials

As in nested cross-sectional studies, there are occasions in nested cohort studies in which stratum is a random effect. The best example is the multicenter group-randomized trial in which the investigators wish to generalize their findings to other centers like those in the trial.

To illustrate the development of an analysis plan for such a trial, consider as an example the Pathways study. This study was funded by the National Heart Lung and Blood Institute in 1993 as a three-year Phase I planning study with four field centers (University of Minnesota, University of New Mexico, Johns Hopkins University, Gila River Community) and a coordinating center (University of North Carolina). The purpose of the Phase I study was to develop the design, analysis plan, intervention materials, and evaluation protocols for a Phase II study to evaluate an intervention to prevent obesity among American Indian children. Phase II was funded in 1996 for five years to allow the investigators to conduct the trial planned during Phase I.[5]

The Phase II study design is described by Davis et al. (under review). At each field center, schools that met the study's eligibility requirements were recruited for Phase II. Each school completed a baseline survey of second-grade students in the spring of 1997. Using the results of that survey, schools were rank ordered on median predicted percent body fat (PBF) based on a regression equation developed in Phase I (Lohman et al., under review). Schools in the upper half of the distribution in a center were placed into one block, while schools in the lower half of the distribution in that center were placed in a second block. Schools within each block were assigned at random to the intervention condition or to the control condition. Posttest measures will be taken at the end of the fifth grade. This design is similar to that employed previously in the Child and Adolescent Trial for Cardiovascular Health (CATCH) (Zucker et al., 1995).

The research question is whether the children in the intervention and control conditions will differ at the end of the study in their level of obesity. The null hypothesis is that they will not. The alternative hypothesis is that the children in the intervention condition will display a lower average level of obesity than the children in the control condition at the end of the fifth grade. The primary endpoint is the value for predicted PBF. The prediction equation relies on measures of height, weight, bioelectric impedance, and several skinfold thicknesses for each child. The values obtained from the prediction equation have been shown to have good agreement with a criterion measure based on assessment of total body water (Lohman et al., under review).

The analysis of the primary endpoint must accommodate several features of the design. First, it is a group-randomized trial. Second, the study involves a cohort. Third, it includes both *a priori* stratification on field center and *a priori* stratification on the baseline school median predicted PBF. Finally, the investigators want to adjust for the child's baseline predicted PBF as an individual-level covariate. With these considerations, the analysis requires an extension of the mixed-model ANCOVA presented above to include two random-effect stratification factors.

Because two stratification factors are included in this example, the notation Blocks B_q ($q=1$ . . . b) is introduced to represent the strata defined by the baseline school median predicted PBF. Stratum S_p ($p=1$ . . . s) is used to represent the strata defined by field center.

The design has three main factors: Condition ($c=2$ levels), Stratum ($s=4$ centers), and Block ($b=2$ levels of median predicted PBF). Those factors are completely crossed, forming 16 cells in the design. Two of the field centers will contribute 12 schools each and two will contribute 8 schools each, providing 40 schools (i.e., groups) over the 16 cells. Half the cells will have three schools each and the other half will have two schools each. Individual children (i.e., members) within each school will be followed over time to assess the impact of the intervention program.

The Full Model

The full model for this analysis is:

$$Y_{i:k:lpq} = \mu + C_l + \sum_{o=1}^{x} \beta_o(X_{oi:k:lpq} - \overline{X}_{o. . . .}) + S_p + CS_{lp}$$
$$+ B_q + CB_{lq} + SB_{pq} + CSB_{lpq} + G_{k:lpq} + \varepsilon_{i:k:lpq} \qquad (6.21)$$

Condition and the covariate are the only fixed effects. The general form is used to represent the regression adjustment for covariates in the model, though in this study, $x=1$. Time is not included in the ANCOVA model, except through the inclusion of the baseline value for the primary endpoint. Both stratum and block must be included in the analysis as random effects, both as main effects and in their interactions with other variables, because the investigators want to generalize to other centers and blocks like those used in the study. Because the stratification was *a priori* on both stratum (center) and block (median school baseline PBF), groups (schools) are nested within the 16 cells defined by the condition (2) × stratum (4) × block (2) interaction. The notation $G_{k:lpq}$ reflects that nesting. Group must be included in the analysis as a nested random effect in order to account for the positive intraclass correlation expected in the data. The eight random effects allow for correlation within the strata defined by the field centers (S_p), correlation within the strata that is specific to each condition (CS_{lp}), correlation within the blocks defined by baseline school median predicted percent body fat (B_q), correlation within the blocks that is specific to each condition (CB_{lq}), correlation within the blocks that is specific to each stratum (SB_{pq}), correlation within the blocks that is specific to each stratum $\times$ condition combination (CSB_{lpq}), correlation within a group in a particular cell ($G_{k:lpq}$), and for random variation among members ($\varepsilon_{i:k:lpq}$).

The Intervention Effect

In the ANOVA, the F-statistic assesses the variation among the adjusted condition means against the variation among the adjusted group means. The null hypothesis is that the variation due to the conditions is zero. When there are only two conditions, the numerator of the F-statistic is based on a single df and it is more convenient to use the t-statistic. In that case, the intervention effect is the difference between the two adjusted condition means and the null hypothesis is that the difference is zero. For the intervention and control conditions, the intervention effect is:

$$\Delta = (\overline{Y}_{..I..} - \overline{Y}_{..C.}) - \sum_{o=1}^{x} \beta_o(X_{o\cdot\cdot I..} - \overline{X}_{o\cdot\cdot C.}) \qquad (6.22)$$

The Expected Mean Squares for the Full Model

The expected mean squares for this analysis are shown in Table 6.9. Note that the covariates are not shown in the table except as they affect the df for the other terms. If all the correlations allowed by the multiple random effects are nontrivial, there is no good test for the term of interest, condition. Even if condition were tested as MS_c/MS_s, the Type I error rate would be inflated to the extent that σ_{cs}^2 was greater than zero. This result underscores the need to

Table 6.9. Expected Mean Squares for the Full Model From the Pathways Study

Source	df	E(MS)
Condition	$c-1$	$\sigma_e^2 + m\sigma_{g:csb}^2 + mg\sigma_{csb}^2 + mgs\sigma_{cb}^2 + mgb\sigma_{cs}^2 + mgsb\sigma_c^2$
Strata	$s-1$	$\sigma_e^2 + m\sigma_{g:csb}^2 + mgc\sigma_{sb}^2 + mgcb\sigma_s^2$
CS	$(c-1)(s-1)$	$\sigma_e^2 + m\sigma_{g:csb}^2 + mg\sigma_{csb}^2 + mgb\sigma_{cs}^2$
Block	$b-1$	$\sigma_e^2 + m\sigma_{g:csb}^2 + mgc\sigma_{sb}^2 + mgcs\sigma_b^2$
CB	$(c-1)(b-1)$	$\sigma_e^2 + m\sigma_{g:csb}^2 + mg\sigma_{csb}^2 + mgs\sigma_{cb}^2$
SB	$(s-1)(b-1)$	$\sigma_e^2 + m\sigma_{g:csb}^2 + mgc\sigma_{sb}^2$
CSB	$(c-1)(s-1)(b-1)$	$\sigma_e^2 + m\sigma_{g:csb}^2 + mg\sigma_{csb}^2$
G:CSB	$csb(g-1)-x_g$	$\sigma_e^2 + m\sigma_{g:csb}^2$
M:G:CSB	$gcsb(m-1)-x_m$	σ_e^2

work out the expected mean squares for the primary analysis before collecting any data. It would be a pity to discover such an important problem only when it is too late to correct it.

The Reduced Model

The Pathways investigators were willing to assume several of these correlations to be zero (Davis et al., under review). In particular, they were willing to assume that $CSB = SB = CB = 0$. The reduced model is written as:

$$Y_{i:k:lpq} = \mu + C_l + \sum_{o=1}^{x} \beta_o(X_{oi:k:lpq} - \overline{X}_{o.....})$$
$$+ S_p + CS_{lp} + B_q + G_{k:lpq} + \varepsilon_{i:k:lpq} \qquad (6.23)$$

The Expected Mean Squares for the Reduced Model

The expected mean squares for this analysis are shown in Table 6.10. Note that the covariates are not shown in the table except as they affect the *df* for the other terms. With this simpler model, there is now a valid test for condition, though it has only $(c-1)(s-1)$ *ddf*.

The investigators plan a preliminary test of the *CS* interaction. If it is significant, it will mean that the intervention effects varied across the strata and the investigators will report center-specific results. If the *CS* interaction is not significant, the investigators can drop that term from the model. The term of interest will be condition and the null hypothesis will be that the difference between the posttest adjusted means for the two conditions is zero. The expected mean squares for the resulting doubly reduced analysis are shown in Table 6.11.

In the doubly reduced model, the MS_c has three components: residual error (σ_e^2), a weighted component of variance due to the groups ($m\sigma_{g:csb}^2$), and a

Table 6.10. Expected Mean Squares for the Reduced Model From the Pathways Study

Source	df	E(MS)	MS
Condition	$c-1$	$\sigma_e^2 + m\sigma_{g:csb}^2 + mgb\sigma_{cs}^2 + mgsb\sigma_c^2$	MS_c
Strata	$s-1$	$\sigma_e^2 + m\sigma_{g:csb}^2 + mgcb\sigma_s^2$	MS_s
Block	$b-1$	$\sigma_e^2 + m\sigma_{g:csb}^2 + mgcs\sigma_b^2$	MS_b
CS	$(c-1)(s-1)$	$\sigma_e^2 + m\sigma_{g:csb}^2 + mgb\sigma_{cs}^2$	MS_{cs}
G:CSB	$csb(g-1) - x_g$	$\sigma_e^2 + m\sigma_{g:csb}^2$	$MS_{g:csb}$
M:G:CSB	$gcsb(m-1) - x_m$	σ_e^2	MS_e

Table 6.11. Expected Mean Squares for the Doubly Reduced Model
From the Pathways Study

Source	df	E(MS)	MS
Condition	$c-1$	$\sigma_e^2 + m\sigma_{g:csb}^2 + mgsb\sigma_c^2$	MS_c
Strata	$s-1$	$\sigma_e^2 + m\sigma_{g:csb}^2 + mgcb\sigma_s^2$	MS_s
Block	$b-1$	$\sigma_e^2 + m\sigma_{g:csb}^2 + mgcs\sigma_b^2$	MS_b
Group:CSB	$csb(g-1) - x_g$	$\sigma_e^2 + m\sigma_{g:csb}^2$	$MS_{g:csb}$
M:G:CSB	$gcsb(m-1) - x_m$	σ_e^2	MS_e

weighted component of variance due to the intervention effect ($mgsb\sigma_c^2$). The test of the null hypothesis is $MS_c/MS_{g:csb}$.

For each covariate measured at the group level (x_g), df associated with that covariate are lost from $MS_{g:csb}$. For each covariate measured at the member level (x_m), df associated with that covariate are lost from MS_e. In this instance, no group-level covariates are planned, as the only covariate proposed is measured at the level of the member.

The Variance of the Intervention Effect

When the intervention effect is defined as the difference between two conditions, the variance of that intervention effect under the null hypothesis is:

$$\sigma_\Delta^2 = 2\left(\frac{MS_{g:csb}}{mgsb}\right) \tag{6.24}$$

Here m is the number of members observed in each group, g is the number of groups observed in each stratum $\times$ block cell, and s and b are the numbers of strata and blocks, respectively. The $M_{g:csb}$ reflects the regression adjustment for the covariate as well as the *a priori* stratification on stratum and block; details are provided in Chapter 9.

Assumptions

The doubly reduced analysis provides for four sources of random variation. If there are additional sources in the data, the model is misspecified and the true Type I and II error rates are unknown. This assumption is particularly important in this study, as the investigators have assumed several possible sources of random variation to be zero and plan no test of their assumption (Davis et al., under review). In particular, they have assumed that **CSB = SB = CB = 0**.

When the investigators assume that $CB = 0$, they assume that the intervention effect is the same in schools above and below the midpoint on predicted percent body fat. Given limited variation in the school midpoints, that would seem a reasonable assumption. Given substantial variation in the school midpoints, this assumption requires that children who are in schools that are high or low on median predicted percent body fat respond in the same way to the intervention. Without the regression adjustment for the baseline value, that assumption could easily be questioned. With the regression adjustment, it becomes less likely, but remains plausible. The investigators decided to forgo a test of that assumption because it would have required a study four times larger than that proposed. They also recognized that they could employ a *post hoc* stratification on the students' baseline predicted percent body fat in a secondary analysis to explore that issue.

When the investigators assume that $SB = 0$, they assume that differences among the high and low blocks for median predicted percent body fat are the same across the four field centers. That assumption also seems reasonable, as there is no reason to expect that schools above the midpoint in one center will be different from schools above the midpoint in another center.

When the investigators assume that $CSB = 0$, they assume that any differential intervention effect associated with the school median predicted percent body fact is the same across the four field centers. That assumption appears reasonable as long as $SB = CB = 0$.

Note that the investigators did not assume that $CS = 0$ and will conduct a preliminary test of that hypothesis.

Under the General Linear Mixed Model, the random effects are assumed to be independent and distributed $S_p \approx N(0, \sigma_s^2)$, $B_q \approx N(0, \sigma_b^2)$, $G_{k:lpq} \approx N(0, \sigma_{g:csb}^2)$ and $\varepsilon_{i:k:lpq} \approx N(0, \sigma_e^2)$. Preliminary work with predicted PBF indicates that it will meet these assumptions.

The assumptions associated with regression adjustment for covariates and those associated with stratification apply equally here. Violations have effects as described earlier.

Strengths and Weaknesses

The strengths and weaknesses associated with *a priori* stratification apply here. Stratification on field center and on a baseline school median for the primary endpoint provides considerable assurance that the two study conditions will be comparable at baseline. By also employing a regression adjustment for the baseline value on the primary endpoint, the investigators should reduce any residual nonequivalence between the two study conditions. By modeling the two stratification factors as random effects, the investigators will have the statistical basis for generalizing any findings to other strata like those used in the study. It would be inappropriate to generalize to other strata if the stratification factors had been included in the analysis as fixed effects.

Additional Baseline or Follow-up Intervals

As with nested cross-sectional designs, additional baseline and/or follow-up intervals may be included in the nested cohort design, extending the Pretest-Posttest Control Group Design. Chapters 2 and 3 review the general benefits of such an extension to the validity of the design. This section presents analysis methods for these Extended Designs.

As noted in Chapter 5, it is appropriate to treat time as a categorical variable when the data are collected during a few short and discrete intervals. And when there are only two time intervals, there are no alternatives to compound symmetry for the structure of the within-member random-effects covariance matrix. When additional intervals are added to the design the investigator can model time as a continuous variable. And whether time is treated as a continuous or as a categorical variable, the investigator can fit a variety of structures to the data in an effort to more accurately represent the pattern of within-member correlation over time.

The Traditional Mixed-Model ANOVA/ANCOVA

Two changes are required to extend the analyses presented for the Pretest-Posttest Control Group Design to incorporate additional levels of time. First, the definition and interpretation of the intervention effect must be generalized to reflect $t > 2$. Second, the investigator must consider alternative structures for the within-member random-effects covariance matrix.

The Model

The model for the Extended Design is the same as for the Pretest-Posttest Control Group Design (cf. Equations 6.1 and 6.4). The addition of more intervals increases the value of t in the T_j ($j = 1 \ldots t$) notation, but has no other effect on the model.

The Intervention Effect

In the familiar ANOVA, the F-statistic assesses the variation among the time $\times$ condition means against the variation among the time $\times$ group means. The null hypothesis is that the variation due to conditions over time is zero. With more than two time intervals, the intervention effect can no longer be reduced to a net difference over time even if there are only two conditions.

The Expected Mean Squares and the Variance of the Intervention Effect

As long as the within-member random-effects covariance structure is assumed compound symmetric, the expected mean squares and the variance of the intervention effect for this model are unchanged from those presented for the time × condition analysis of the nested cohort Pretest-Posttest Control Group Design. Those expected mean squares were presented in Tables 6.1 and 6.2 and the variances in Equations 6.3 and 6.6. Note that the null hypothesis is now that $TC_{jl} = 0$ for all j and l.

ddf for Fixed Effects

The discussion in Chapter 5 concerning the computation of *ddf* for fixed effects in more complex nested cross-sectional designs is also relevant here. The methods presented in Chapter 5 are easily generalized to the nested cohort design and are illustrated in Chapter 8.

Assumptions

Because the model for this analysis is the same as that for the Pretest-Posttest Control Group Design, the assumptions are also the same. The reader is referred to the presentation earlier in this chapter for a review of the assumptions and the effect of their violation.

When more than two time intervals are included in the design, two assumptions that were quite safe given only two time intervals must be considered more carefully. As noted in Chapter 5, the mixed-model ANOVA/ANCOVA assumes that each group in a condition shares a common time trend or slope that is unique to that condition. As long as there is no measurable deviation of the group-specific slopes from that common slope and the other assumptions are met, the mixed-model ANOVA/ANCOVA has a nominal Type I error rate for the test of the intervention effect, regardless of the number of time intervals included in the design and in the analysis (Murray et al., in press). However, if there is any measurable deviation among the group-specific slopes relative to the common slope, the variance of the intervention effect is too small and the Type I error rate is inflated (Murray et al., in press). Murray et al. (in press) demonstrated that the inflation in the Type I error rate increases as the component of variance for the group slopes represents a larger and larger fraction of the total variation in the data. Though the Murray et al. (in press) study focused exclusively on the nested cross-sectional design, there is every reason to expect that similar results would obtain for nested cohort designs.

The second assumption that must be considered as soon as there are additional time intervals in the design concerns the structure of the within-member covariance matrix. In a nested cohort design, there are both between-member and within-member random effects, as members may be measured more than once. Throughout the examples in this chapter, the random effects covariance matrix has been assumed to have a compound symmetry structure. This structure assumes that the lag between two measurements on the same member is unrelated to the magnitude of the correlation between those measurements. Phrased another way, compound symmetry assumes constant correlation over time within members. When there are only two measurements for each member and the lag between them is approximately the same, compound symmetry is a safe assumption. However, when there are more than two measurements on some of the members and when the lag between measurements varies across those members, compound symmetry is no longer a safe assumption. Moreover, violations may inflate the Type I error rate.

There are several options available to the analyst concerned about possible misspecification of the structure of the within-member random-effects covariance matrix. One alternative, suggested by Zeger and Liang (1986), is to employ an analysis that does not make a strong assumption about the structure of that matrix in the first place. That is the basis of the "empirical-sandwich" estimation of variances for fixed effects in their generalized estimating equations, described in Chapter 4. Recall from that discussion that the empirical-sandwich formula is asymptotically robust against misspecification of the within-member random-effects covariance matrix. However, results from a recent simulation study suggest that the desirable asymptotic properties associated with this method do not hold when the number of groups per condition is less than 20 (Murray et al., in press). As a result, this option is not recommended for group-randomized trials involving fewer than 20 groups per condition.

Another approach to the problem of questionable assumptions about the structure of the random-effects covariance matrix is to assess the fit of the assumed structure and select a more appropriate structure if necessary (Wolfinger, 1993). The analyst can begin by fitting an unstructured within-member random-effects covariance matrix that allows each variance and covariance to be estimated separately and to take on a different value if that is what the data dictate. The pattern in the unstructured matrix may suggest a structure, such as compound symmetry, autoregressive, etc. If so, the analyst can fit that structure to the data. Objective criteria such as the Schwarz Bayesian Information Criterion can be used to gauge the adequacy of the various structures and to select the one that best fits the data (Kass and Raftery, 1995; Kass and Wasserman, 1995; Littell et al., 1996; Wolfinger, 1993). Having established the appropriate structure for the random effects, the analyst can then move to test the fixed effects of interest.

There are three structures for the within-member covariance matrix that are particularly plausible for data from an Extended Design. The compound symmetry structure presumes constant correlation between repeat observations on the same member, regardless of the time elapsed between the two observations. This model is the simplest of the three, as it requires estimation of only a single correlation.

The first-order autoregressive structure accommodates correlations that reflect exponential decline over time. For $k > k'$, the correlation between observations on the same member at times k and k' is given as:

$$r_{yy(m)}^{|k-k'|}$$

The correlation between measurements taken in any two adjacent intervals would be $r_{yy(m)}$, while the correlation between any two measurements taken with one intervening interval would be $r_{yy(m)}^2$, with two intervening intervals, $r_{yy(m)}^3$, etc.

The Toeplitz structure provides for variances on the main diagonal and covariances on each of the other diagonals, constrained such that all the elements in the same diagonal have the same value. This pattern can accommodate correlation that declines over time but not necessarily with the exponential form of the first-order autoregressive structure.

Several of these alternative structures, together with methods to compare their fit to the data, are presented as part of the examples provided in Chapter 8.

Other assumptions may apply to this analysis as well. For example, if regression adjustment for covariates is included, then the assumptions associated with that procedure apply. Similarly, if stratification or matching is included in the analysis, the assumptions associated with those procedures apply. Violations have effects as described in earlier sections.

Strengths and Weaknesses

If the assumptions underlying the traditional mixed-model ANOVA/ANCOVA are met, it has two advantages. First, it makes no assumption about the pattern of the intervention effect over time. Second, the *ddf* increase as the number of time intervals increases, thereby increasing power, other factors constant.

The major weakness of the traditional mixed-model ANOVA/ANCOVA is that it has an inflated Type I error rate in the presence of measurable heterogeneity among the group-specific slopes when there are more than two time intervals included in the design. Another major weakness is that it may have an inflated Type I error rate if the structure of the within-member random-effects covariance matrix is misspecified. For these reasons, the analyst should take care to evaluate the assumptions underlying the traditional mixed-model ANOVA/ANCOVA when using that method with an Extended Design.

The fact that the traditional mixed-model ANOVA/ANCOVA makes no assumption about the pattern of the intervention effect over time is both a strength and a weakness. It was listed above as a strength because it puts no constraints on the pattern to be detected. However, this is also a weakness, for the power to detect such a diffuse and general intervention effect is poor if that effect in fact can be predicted. In that case, a more targeted analysis has better power.

Trend Analysis in the Mixed-Model ANOVA/ANCOVA

The trend analysis in the mixed-model ANOVA/ANCOVA represents an alternate parameterization of the fixed-effects portion of the traditional mixed-model ANOVA/ANCOVA. It allows the analyst, for example, to specify a particular pattern for the intervention effect in the fixed-effects portion of the analysis. As such, it can provide a much more targeted and hence more powerful test of the intervention effect when that effect is well described by the specified pattern. The nested cross-sectional version of the trend analysis in the mixed-model ANOVA/ANCOVA was presented in some detail in Chapter 5. Because the nested cohort version raises no new issues for other analyses in this chapter, it is not considered further here.

The Random-Coefficients Analysis

The random-coefficients analysis was introduced in Chapter 4. It is a mixed-model regression analysis that allows both a random intercept and a random slope in each group. In addition, the slope and intercept in a group may covary. In the nested cohort version of this analysis, the random intercepts and slopes exist both for members and for groups.

The Model

The random-coefficients model focuses on time trends, both in the fixed- and the random-effects portions of the model. A random-coefficients analysis that focuses on the linear time trends is written as:

$$Y_{ij:k:l} = \mu + C_l + T_{(\text{lin})}t_j + T_{(\text{lin})}t_j C_l +$$
$$G_{k:l} + M_{i:k:l} + T_{(\text{lin})}t_j G_{k:l} + M_{i:k:l}T_{(\text{lin})}t_j + \varepsilon_{i:jk:l} \qquad (6.25)$$

This model extends the linear random-coefficients analysis presented in Chapter 5 with the addition of two new terms. The $M_{i:k:l}$ term represents the random intercept for the member. The $M_{i:k:l}T_{(\text{lin})}$ term represents the random linear slope fit to the repeat observations available for the ith member in the kth group in the lth condition.

In most group-randomized trials, condition, time, and their interaction are fixed effects. The five random effects allow for heterogeneity among the group-specific mean intercepts $(G_{k:l})$, for heterogeneity among the group-specific mean slopes $(T_{(\text{lin})}G_{k:l})$, for heterogeneity in the member-specific intercepts $(M_{i:k:l})$, for heterogeneity among the member-specific slopes $(M_{i:k:l}T_{(\text{lin})})$, and for random variation among the members $(\varepsilon_{i:jk:l})$. Though not yet established via simulation studies, it is expected that failure to include the first four random effects in the model, if they are present in the data, would result in an inflated Type I error rate, with the magnitude of the inflation dependent upon the magnitude of those variance components relative to the total variation in the data. That expectation is based on findings from the parallel analysis as applied to a nested cross-sectional design (Murray et al., in press).

The Intervention Effect

In this analysis, the F-statistic assesses the variation among the condition mean slopes against the variation among the group-specific mean slopes. The null hypothesis is that the variation due to the conditions is zero. When there are only two conditions, the numerator of the F-statistic is based on a single df and it is more convenient to use the t-statistic. In that case, the intervention effect is the difference between the condition mean slopes and the null hypothesis is that the difference is zero.

The Expected Mean Squares

The expected mean squares for the random-coefficients analysis are shown in Table 6.12. The $MS_{t(\text{lin})c}$ has four components: residual error for the member-specific slope $\left[\dfrac{\sigma^2_{e(y)}}{\sigma^2_{e(t)}(t-f-1)}\right]$, a component of variance due to the heterogeneity among the member-specific slopes $(\sigma^2_{mt(\text{lin}):g:c})$, a weighted component of variance due to the heterogeneity among the group-specific mean slopes $(m\sigma^2_{t(\text{lin})g:c})$, and a weighted component of variance due to the intervention $(mg\sigma^2_{t(\text{lin})c})$. The test of the null hypothesis is $MS_{t(\text{lin})c}/MS_{t(\text{lin})g:c}$.

Table 6.12. Expected Mean Squares for a Random-Coefficients Analysis of Data From an Extended Nested Cohort Design in Which Time is Modeled as a Linear Term in Both the Fixed and Random Effects

Source	df	E(MS)	MS
Condition	$c-1$	$\sigma^2_{e(y)}\left(\dfrac{t-1}{t(t-f-1)}+\dfrac{\bar{t}^2}{\sigma^2_{e(t)}(t-f-1)}\right)+\sigma^2_{m:g:c}+m\sigma^2_{g:c}+mg\sigma^2_c$	MS_c
Group:C	$c(g-1)$	$\sigma^2_{e(y)}\left(\dfrac{t-1}{t(t-f-1)}+\dfrac{\bar{t}^2}{\sigma^2_{e(t)}(t-f-1)}\right)+\sigma^2_{m:g:c}+m\sigma^2_{g:c}$	$MS_{g:c}$
M:G:C	$gc(m-1)$	$\sigma^2_{e(y)}\left(\dfrac{t-1}{t(t-f-1)}+\dfrac{\bar{t}^2}{\sigma^2_{e(t)}(t-f-1)}\right)+\sigma^2_{m:g:c}$	$MS_{m:g:c}$
Time(lin)	1	$\dfrac{\sigma^2_{e(y)}}{\sigma^2_{e(t)}(t-f-1)}+\sigma^2_{mt(\text{lin}):g:c}+m\sigma^2_{t(\text{lin})g:c}+mgc\sigma^2_{t(\text{lin})}$	$MS_{t(\text{lin})}$
T(lin)C	$c-1$	$\dfrac{\sigma^2_{e(y)}}{\sigma^2_{e(t)}(t-f-1)}+\sigma^2_{mt(\text{lin}):g:c}+m\sigma^2_{t(\text{lin})g:c}+mg\sigma^2_{t(\text{lin})c}$	$MS_{t(\text{lin})c}$
T(lin)G:C	$c(g-1)$	$\dfrac{\sigma^2_{e(y)}}{\sigma^2_{e(t)}(t-f-1)}+\sigma^2_{mt(\text{lin}):g:c}+m\sigma^2_{t(\text{lin})g:c}$	$MS_{t(\text{lin})g:c}$
MT(lin):G:C	$gc(m-1)$	$\dfrac{\sigma^2_{e(y)}}{\sigma^2_{e(t)}(t-f-1)}+\sigma^2_{mt(\text{lin}):g:c}$	$MS_{mt(\text{lin}):g:.}$
MT:G:C	$(t-2)gc(m-1)$	$\sigma^2_{e(y)}$	MS_e

Though no covariates were included in this analysis, they certainly could be. For each covariate measured at the group level (x_g), df associated with that covariate are lost from $MS_{g:c}$ and from $MS_{t(\text{lin})g:c}$. For each covariate measured at the member level (x_m), df are lost from MS_e.

The Variance of the Intervention Effect

When the intervention effect is defined as the difference between two condition mean slopes, the variance of that intervention effect under the null hypothesis is:

$$\sigma^2_\Delta = 2\left(\frac{MS_{t(\text{lin})g:c}}{mg}\right) \qquad (6.26)$$

Here m is the number of members in each group and g is the number of groups in each condition. The $MS_{t(\text{lin})g:c}$ reflects any reduction due to repeat measurements on the same members and groups as well as the modeling of the linear time trend in each group and in each member; details are provided in Chapter 9.

Assumptions

The analysis provides for five sources of random variation. If there are additional sources in the data, the model is misspecified and the true Type I and II error rates are unknown.

Under the General Linear Mixed Model, the random effects are assumed to be distributed as $G_{k:l} \approx N(0, \sigma^2_{g:c})$, $M_{i:k:l} \approx N(0, \sigma^2_{m:g:c})$, $T_{(\text{lin})}G_{k:l} \approx N(0, \sigma^2_{t(\text{lin})g:c})$, $M_{i:k:l}T_{(\text{lin})} \approx N(0, \sigma^2_{mt(\text{lin}):g:c})$, and $\varepsilon_{i:jk:l} \approx N(0, \sigma^2_e)$. Both $G_{k:l}$ and $T_{(\text{lin})}G_{k:l}$ are assumed to be independent of $\varepsilon_{i:jk:l}$; however, $G_{k:l}$ and $T_{(\text{lin})}G_{k:l}$ are allowed to covary. Similarly, both $M_{i:k:l}$ and $M_{i:k:l}T_{(\text{lin})}$ are assumed to be independent of $\varepsilon_{i:jk:l}$; however, $M_{i:k:l}$ and $M_{i:k:l}T_{(\text{lin})}$ are allowed to covary. With the important caveats noted in Chapter 5, the analysis can be extended to non-Gaussian data by assuming a different distribution for $\varepsilon_{i:jk:l}$ and a different link function. The analysis would then represent an application of the Generalized Linear Mixed Model.

It is unclear whether the random-coefficients analysis is robust to violation of the normality assumption for the residual error given a moderate number of groups and members. However, the Central Limit Theorem suggests that it would be, as do the results by Hannan and Murray (1996) reported for the mixed-model ANOVA. The recent report by Murray et al. (in press) suggests that the random-coefficients analysis provides good protection against violation of the independence assumption as the most likely forms of dependence are modeled via $G_{k:l}$, $M_{i:k:l}$, $T_{(\text{lin})}G_{k:l}$, and $M_{i:k:l}T_{(\text{lin})}$.

This analysis also assumes that the nonlinear components of time and its interactions in the fixed- and random-effects portions of the model are zero; their df are pooled with the df for MS_e.

Strengths and Weaknesses

The major strength of this analysis is that it accommodates whatever level of heterogeneity among the member- and group-specific slopes and intercepts exists in the data. As a result, it is expected to have the nominal Type I error rate whatever that level of heterogeneity might be, even if it is zero.

Another strength of the random-coefficients analysis is that it can accommodate nonlinear trends over time as well. The analysis presented above included only linear components for time, but nonlinear terms could certainly be added.

Another strength of the random-coefficients analysis is that it provides a test of whether there is measurable heterogeneity among the member- or group-specific slopes. That test is available for the null hypotheses $\sigma^2_{mt(\text{lin}):g:c} = 0$ and $\sigma^2_{t(\text{lin})g:c} = 0$, and many of the programs that provide estimates of the variance components also provide information to assess those null hypotheses.[6]

The major weakness of the random-coefficients analysis is that it is less efficient and therefore less powerful for assessing intervention effects than the mixed-model ANOVA/ANCOVA analyses when the assumptions underlying the ANOVA/ANCOVA models are satisfied. However, the loss of efficiency appears to be modest and may well prove a fair price to pay for the protection against inflation in the Type I error rate expected with the mixed-model ANOVA/ANCOVA analyses when there is measurable heterogeneity among the member- or group-specific slopes.

Summary

This chapter reviewed analytic methods for the nested cohort designs that are most likely to be used in group-randomized trials. Most of these methods are based on mixed-model ANOVA/ANCOVA and stand as extensions of the familiar ANOVA/ANCOVA methods used in comparative trials that do not involve group randomization. All reflect the additional components of variance due to the nested designs that characterize group-randomized trials. Several simulation studies have demonstrated that these analyses have the nominal Type I error rate across a wide range of characteristics common to group-randomized trials, as long as only one or two time intervals are included in the analysis (Zucker, 1990; Murray and Wolfinger, 1994; Murray et al., 1996).

When more than two time intervals are included in the design, analysts must consider the possibility that there is heterogeneity among the time trends for members and groups within conditions. Where no measurable heterogeneity exists, the mixed-model ANOVA/ANCOVA methods still have the nominal Type I error rate (Murray et al., in press). However, in the presence of measurable heterogeneity among the group- or member-specific slopes, the mixed-model ANOVA/ANCOVA methods are expected to have an inflated Type I error rate, and the degree of inflation is expected to be directly related to the degree of heterogeneity.

Given measurable heterogeneity among the group-specific slopes, the random-coefficients model will still have the nominal Type I error rate. Such models accommodate whatever degree of heterogeneity exists among the member- or group-specific slopes and are recommended when more than two time intervals are included in the analysis of data from a group-randomized trial.

Endnotes

1. A circular covariance matrix is one in which the sum of any two variances minus twice their covariance yields a constant value across the entire matrix. A circular covariance matrix is sometimes called a spherical matrix because it is spherical after a normalized orthogonal transformation. A spherical matrix has the constant value on the main diagonal and all zeros elsewhere.

2. Violation of the circularity assumption is not an issue when there are only two time intervals included in the design. In this case, there is only a single over-time correlation within members, so there is no risk of misrepresenting the pattern of within-member correlation over time.

3. Any analysis involves some assumptions. The recent advances simply allow the analyst greater control over the assumptions that are made rather than eliminating assumptions altogether. The analyst must still take care to ensure that the assumptions involved in the analysis are justified.

4. This sentence fell short of a complete rejection of fixed covariates. Under some conditions, they can effect the intervention effect, though usually to such a minor degree as to make little difference. If the cohort is kept intact, or if cases missing an observation at any time are dropped from the analysis entirely, addition of fixed covariates has no effect whatever. However, software based on maximum-likelihood estimation makes use of whatever observations are available. To the extent that occasional missing observations result in slight differences over time in the marginal distribution of the covariates, those covariates can have a subtle effect on the intervention-effect estimates. If their effect is great, it is likely due to substantial missing data and the entire analysis becomes suspect.

5. The author is a member of the Design and Analysis Committee for this trial and is also Co–Principal Investigator for the University of Minnesota Field Center.

6. Significance tests for variance components are illustrated in Chapter 7. That chapter also provides a discussion of alternative methods and problems associated with such tests.

7

Applications of Analyses for Nested Cross-Sectional Designs

Organization of the Chapter

This chapter illustrates the analyses appropriate for data from nested cross-sectional designs, including examples for most of the analyses presented in Chapter 5. The analyses are illustrated with data from the cross-sectional survey of the Minnesota Heart Health Program (MHHP). The MHHP was a 10-year research and demonstration project designed to reduce morbidity and mortality due to coronary heart disease in three upper-midwestern communities during the 1980s. Its design supports most of the analyses presented in Chapter 5.

The design of the MHHP is described by Jacobs et al. (1986). Three pairs of communities were selected for the study, each pair having one education and one comparison site. Communities were matched for size, community type (small and agricultural, independent and urban, or metropolitan), and distance from the Minneapolis–St. Paul metropolitan area. Assignment to conditions from within the matched pairs was not random, but was completed before collection of any data and structured to optimize the baseline comparability of the two conditions. Following a 16-month baseline period used for study planning, community analysis, and baseline data collection, a 5–6-year intervention program was introduced in November 1981 in Mankato, a small community in southern Minnesota. Twenty-two and 28 months later, respectively, the intervention program was introduced in Fargo-Moorhead, an urban area along the North Dakota–Minnesota border, and in Bloomington, a large Twin Cities suburb. This staggered entry allowed for gradual development of the intervention program and strengthened the design through replication; it also provided two, three, and four baseline surveys in the first, second, and third community pairs, respectively. The three pairs and their assignment to intervention *(I)* and comparison *(C)* conditions are shown in Figure 7.1.

Periodic cross-sectional surveys of 300–500 randomly selected 25–74-year-old adults were conducted in each community based on a two-stage cluster-sampling design (Kish, 1965). Discrete sequential surveys were implemented throughout the study and each community was assigned to a two-month survey window; paired communities were assigned to adjacent windows to maximize seasonal comparability. This plan resulted in the staggered series of cross-sectional surveys in each community shown in Figure 7.1.

Cast in terms of the notation used in this book, the MHHP design had two conditions (intervention vs. control), three groups (whole communities) per condition, and several hundred different members (community residents) observed during each time × group (year × community) cross-sectional survey. Different fractions of the data are used to illustrate the analyses presented in Chapter 5. The full data set has 2–4 baseline observations on each group, 4–5 intervention observations on those same groups, and more than 17,000 individual observations.

The results from the MHHP are published elsewhere, both for risk factors (Luepker et al., 1994) and for morbidity and mortality (Luepker, Rastam et

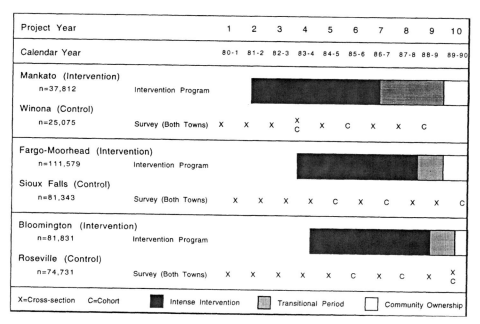

Figure 7.1. Research design of the Minnesota Heart Health Program.

al., 1996). The analyses presented here are based on the same risk-factor data reported in Luepker et al. (1994). Though they may shed some further light on the results from the MHHP, that is not the primary purpose of this presentation. Instead, the primary purpose is to illustrate the analysis methods presented in Chapter 5.

The analysis methods for the MHHP risk-factor data were developed during the early 1990s (Murray, Hannan et al., 1994). While the basic approach to the published analysis of the risk-factor data remains sound, the implementation of that approach was hindered by the lack of suitable software. As a result, the analysis was conducted in two stages. In a first stage, adjusted means were generated for each community in each survey year after stratifying by gender, educational attainment, and age; adjustments were made for confounding variables by standardizing all subjects to the population average within strata for each covariate. A second stage employed those adjusted strata-specific community-year means as the unit of analysis in a series of regressions to evaluate the main and stratum-specific effects of the intervention program. As such, the published risk-factor analysis illustrates the two-stage mixed-model ANCOVA described in Chapter 4.

With the availability today of better software, this two-stage approach is no longer required. Indeed, the analysis of the MHHP morbidity and mortality data, conducted during 1993–94, implemented the same basic analysis but did so in a single stage (Luepker, Rastam et al., 1996). As such, the morbidity and mortality analysis illustrates the one-stage mixed-model ANCOVA described in Chapter 4. The analyses presented in this chapter also illustrate the one-stage approach, though for both mixed-model ANOVA/ANCOVA and for random-coefficients models.

The Software: SAS PROC MIXED and the GLIMMIX Macro

The analyses based on the General Linear Mixed Model are implemented with SAS PROC MIXED, Version 6.11 (SAS Institute Inc., 1996). Analyses based on the Generalized Linear Mixed Model are carried out with the 06-APR-96 version of the GLIMMIX macro (Littell et al., 1996).[1] SAS PROC MIXED implements the General Linear Mixed Model quite broadly and uses REML estimation as the default. The GLIMMIX macro implements the Generalized Linear Mixed Model quite broadly and uses PQL+ estimation as the default. Both programs employ model-based standard errors as the default and compare the observed test statistics against the t-, F-, or chi-square distributions.

The selection of these SAS procedures should not be seen as an endorsement of SAS programs over the alternatives. Indeed, there are many situations in which other programs may be more appropriate or easier to use depending on the nature of the question, the variables, the experience of the investigator, and the existing resources. There are now a number of alternative programs that can provide a valid analysis for data from a group-randomized trial, as summarized in Chapter 4.

The SAS programs were chosen to illustrate analyses in this book because of my familiarity with them. Quite apart from my work on community and other group-randomized trials, SAS has for some time been the primary analysis package in the Division of Epidemiology at the University of Minnesota. Since it is always easier to learn to use a new component within a familiar package, and to use data files created for that package, it was an easy decision to explore MIXED and GLIMMIX when they became available in 1992 and 1993.

Like any software, the SAS programs have their own quirks and limitations. Several persist in Version 6.11 and are identified as this chapter unfolds. Fortunately, like any good software, these programs have improved with each new release and Version 6.11 represents a substantial improvement over the initial offering in Version 6.07.

The PROC MIXED developer, Russell Wolfinger, has contributed substantively to the literature on mixed-model regression (e.g., Wolfinger, 1993, 1996; Wolfinger and O'Connell, 1993). He has also collaborated with me on two papers analyzing data from group-randomized trials (Murray and Wolfinger, 1994; Murray et al., in press). Wolfinger's work has made PROC MIXED a powerful and flexible tool with broad application to the analysis of data that have multiple sources of random variation (e.g., Littell et al., 1996). It is well suited to the analysis of data from group-randomized trials.

The Computer

All analyses were run on a Digital Equipment Corporation Alpha 2000 4/275, equipped with the 21064 RISC processor chip and operating at 275 MHz. This Alpha has a total of 512 Mb of RAM, but operates as a virtual memory machine and so can allot large blocks of memory to simultaneous users. The account used for the analyses presented in this book had a quota of 512 Mb of virtual memory.

Notation

The notation introduced in Chapters 5 and 6 continues in Chapter 7. In addition, the font courier is used to distinguish SAS code and output from other parts of the text. Some abbreviations are used—for example, cond for condition. Nesting is often shown with parentheses—for example, group(cond) to reflect the nesting of groups within conditions—consistent with the syntax used in SAS.

Considerable attention is given to the SAS code because it has a direct bearing on the structure and assumptions of the analysis. Indeed, some issues are best raised in the context of an example and so are raised for the first time in Chapters 7 and 8 instead of Chapters 5 and 6. Readers who employ other software should develop a good understanding of the code employed in that software to ensure that their analysis is implemented as intended.

Posttest-Only Control Group Design

The original MHHP design can be reduced to a Posttest-Only Control Group Design by limiting the analysis to the data collected during the first year after the introduction of the intervention. With this restriction, MHHP provides two conditions ($c = 2$), three communities per condition ($g = 3$), and observations on several hundred persons per community ($m \approx 300$).

Unadjusted Analysis of Posttest Data

Implementation for Gaussian Data

Diastolic blood pressure is used to illustrate the unadjusted analysis of posttest data based on the General Linear Mixed Model. The code is shown in Table 7.1.

MIXED is called with the `proc mixed` statement. The `info` option adds details on the model to the output that can help the user confirm that the SAS code generated the desired model. The `order = internal` option controls the order in which the levels of the variables in the `class` statement are listed. The default order in MIXED is alphabetical based on the values assigned to the levels in the `format` statement. The `order = internal` op-

Table 7.1. SAS PROC MIXED Code for the Unadjusted Analysis of Diastolic Blood Pressure in the Posttest-Only Control Group Design

```
proc mixed info order = internal;
  class cond group;
  model dbp = cond/ddf = 4 ddfm = res;
  random group(cond);
  lsmeans cond/pdiff cl;
run;
```

tion orders the values numerically. Either may be preferred, and other options are also available (SAS Institute Inc., 1996).

The `class` statement identifies discrete variables, here `cond` and `group`. The `model` statement identifies all fixed effects to be included in the model, here only `cond`.

From its inception, MIXED has employed approximate methods to compute *ddf* for fixed effects. Unfortunately, MIXED does not always compute the *ddf* correctly, even in Version 6.11. As a result, the analyst should compute the *ddf* based on the table of expected mean squares for the design and the partitioning of the total *df* among the sources in that table. The analyst can then specify the correct *ddf* using the `ddf=` option in the `model` statement.[2] In this example, the table of expected mean squares in Chapter 5 gives the *ddf* for condition as $c(g-1)$; with $c=2$ and $g=3$, $ddf=4$.

The `ddfm=res` option specifies the *df* associated with the residual error as the *ddf* for all fixed effects not specified in the `ddf=` option. Strictly speaking, it is not necessary in this example, as there are no other fixed effects in the model. However, it often reduces processing time and so is included for that reason.[3]

The `random` statement is used to model variation between members. In this analysis, `group(cond)` is the only random effect in the model aside from residual error, and so is the only term listed in the `random` statement. The major options available for the `random` statement allow the user to specify a structure for the between-member random-effects covariance matrix (`type=`), to specify heterogeneity in that structure across levels of a between-member grouping factor (`group=`), and to specify repeat observations on a between-member grouping factor (`subject=`). In addition, the user can print the between-member random-effects covariance matrix if desired.

Because no `type=` option is included in the `random` statement, the default structure provides a separate variance component for each of the random effects with no covariances among them. Because no `subject=` option was included, it is assumed that there are no repeat observations on any between-member factors. Because no `group=` option was included, the random-effects covariance structure is assumed homogeneous across all between-member grouping factors.

Least-squares means and their standard errors are requested with the `lsmeans` statement. In this example, those means are the unadjusted means, as no covariates were included in the analysis. The `pdiff` option requests *t*-tests for pairwise differences among the least-squares means.[4] The `cl` option requests confidence bounds around both the least-squares means and their pairwise differences.

Table 7.2 summarizes the model fit to the data as a result of the `info`

Table 7.2. Model Information From the Unadjusted Analysis of Diastolic Blood Pressure in the Posttest-Only Control Group Design

Description	Value
Data Set	WORK.CROSS
Dependent Variable	DBP
Covariance Structure	Variance Components
Residual Variance Method	Profile
Fixed Effects SE Method	Model-Based
Degrees of Freedom Method	Residual
Estimation Method	REML

option in the `model` statement. Table 7.3 identifies each variable included in the `class` statement, the number of levels for each variable, and their values. The labels are established via an earlier `format` statement to make the printout more readily interpretable; otherwise, numeric values are printed.

Table 7.4 summarizes the structure of the model for the analysis and the data set. It reports the number of random-effects covariance parameters, here two. It indicates that three columns have been created in the fixed-effects design matrix *(X)*, representing the intercept and the two levels of condition.[5] Similarly, six columns have been created in the random-effects design matrix *(Z)*, representing the six groups. The output indicates that the analysis involved only one subject with 1726 observations used in the analysis. In reality, the analysis was based on 1726 members with 1 observation each. This may seem inconsistent, but it is not. Because the code for this analysis was structured around the `random` statement with no `subject=` option, the code defines a single between-member "subject" or population and all the "observations" are from that population.

Table 7.5 presents the iteration history from the analysis. In this case, estimation converged after two iterations; most analyses using MIXED converge

Table 7.3. Class Level Information From the Unadjusted Analysis of Diastolic Blood Pressure in the Posttest-Only Control Group Design

Class	Levels	Values
COND	2	I C
GROUP	6	MANKATO WINONA FARGO/MOORHD SIOUX FALLS BLOOMINGTON ROSEVILLE

Table 7.4. Dimensions of the
Unadjusted Analysis of Diastolic Blood
Pressure in the Posttest-Only Control
Group Design

Description	Value
Covariance Parameters	2
Columns in X	3
Columns in Z	6
Subjects	1
Max Obs Per Subject	1741
Observations Used	1726
Observations Not Used	15
Total Observations	1741

in less than five iterations. If the number of iterations exceeds the number of parameters, the program is having trouble estimating the parameters and the investigator should try to simplify the model.[6]

Table 7.6 presents the variance-component estimates and their asymptotic standard errors. In this example, the residual-error variance for diastolic blood pressure is estimated as 107. The variance component for group is estimated as 2.82.

The variance components can be used to estimate the mean squares for the random effects in the model, drawing on the table of expected mean squares given in Chapter 5. Given 1726 observations and $g = 3$ groups in each of $c = 2$ conditions, the average $m = 288$. Using these values, the mean squares are estimated in Table 7.7

Given 919 as the estimate for $MS_{g:c}$, the standard error of the intervention effect is estimated using Equation 5.3:

$$\hat{\sigma}_\Delta = \sqrt{2\left(\frac{M\hat{S}_{g:c}}{mg}\right)} = \sqrt{2\left(\frac{919}{288 * 3}\right)} = 1.46$$

Table 7.5. REML Estimation Iteration History From the Unadjusted Analysis of Diastolic Blood Pressure in the Posttest-Only Control Group Design

Iteration	Evaluations	Objective	Criterion
0	1	9822.5614685	
1	2	9802.0581351	0.00000002
2	1	9802.0580307	0.00000000

Table 7.6. Covariance-Parameter Estimates (REML) From the Unadjusted Analysis of Diastolic Blood Pressure in the Posttest-Only Control Group Design

Cov Parm	Ratio	Estimate	SE	Z	Pr>|Z|
GROUP(COND)	0.02634	2.81897	2.26618	1.24	0.2135
Residual	1.00000	106.99941	3.64868	29.33	0.0001

The $ICC_{m:g:c}$ is estimated using Equation 1.5:

$$I\hat{C}C_{m:g:c} = \frac{\hat{\sigma}^2_{g:c}}{\hat{\sigma}^2_e + \hat{\sigma}^2_{g:c}} = \frac{2.82}{107 + 2.82} = 0.0257$$

The $VIF_{m:g:c}$ is estimated as shown in Chapter 1:

$$V\hat{I}F_{m:g:c} = \left(1 + (m-1)I\hat{C}C_{m:g:c}\right) = \left(1 + (288 - 1)0.0257\right) = 8.38$$

Even though the $ICC_{m:g:c}$ is modest, the VIF is substantial. It indicates that the variance of the intervention effect is 8.38 times as large as it would have been with random assignment of individual members to study conditions.

Table 7.6 includes a two-tailed z-test and p-value for each variance component. Those z-tests and their p-values should be interpreted cautiously, because the z-test is valid only asymptotically. In this case, the df for group(cond) are only 4 and the z-test is inappropriate.

An alternative approach is described by Self and Liang (1987). They suggest fitting REML models with and without the covariance parameter of interest and testing the difference in the -2 Log Likelihood ($-2LL$) from the two models as a Likelihood Ratio (LR) chi-square. The df are based on the difference in the number of covariance parameters between the two models. The LR chi-square test is a two-tailed test; for a one-tailed test, the usual p-value must be divided by two (Self and Liang, 1987).[7]

The $-2LL$ for this model was 12970.56. An analysis that deleted

Table 7.7. Selected Mean-Square Estimates for the Unadjusted Analysis of Diastolic Blood Pressure in the Posttest-Only Control Group Design

Source	E(MS)	Estimate
Group:C	$\sigma^2_e + m\sigma^2_{g:c}$	$107 + 288*2.82 = 919$
Member:G:C	σ^2_e	107

group(cond) from the random statement produced a $-2LL$ of 12991.06. The resulting LR chi-square of 20.5 with 1 *df* is highly significant, whether one- or two-tailed, confirming the need to retain group(cond) in the analysis. It also demonstrates the inappropriateness of the z-test.

Even if a covariance parameter is judged not statistically different from zero on the basis of the LR chi-square test, investigators and analysts should be very cautious about removing the term from the model, and especially if that term represents the unit of assignment. Both the z-test and the LR chi-square test are sensitive to departures from the normality assumption, and so may give misleading results if the component of variance in question is not distributed Gaussian. In addition, these tests will often have little power in a group-randomized trial because they are based on the number of groups in the design and that number is usually quite small. Simulation studies have shown that the Type I error rate can be substantially inflated, even in the presence of modest variation due to groups, if that variation is ignored (Murray and Wolfinger, 1994; Murray et al., 1996; Zucker, 1990). Given the high probability of a Type II error for the test of the group component of variance and the high probability of a Type I error for an intervention effect in an analysis that improperly ignores that component of variance, the prudent approach is to retain the group as a factor in the analysis and accept the penalty imposed by whatever level of variance inflation is estimated in the data. If the group component of variance is estimated close to zero, the variance inflation penalty will be quite small.[8]

Table 7.8 presents information that can be helpful when comparing models that differ in their random effects. The REML Log Likelihood, Akaike's Information Criterion, Schwarz's Bayesian Information Criterion, and the -2 REML Log Likelihood can be used to assess improvement in fit due to the addition of one or more random effects. They can also be used to compare analyses

Table 7.8. Model-Fitting Information From the Unadjusted Analysis of Diastolic Blood Pressure in the Posttest-Only Control Group Design

Description	Value
Observations	1726.000
Variance Estimate	106.9994
Standard Deviation Estimate	10.3441
REML Log Likelihood	-6485.28
Akaike's Information Criterion	-6487.28
Schwarz's Bayesian Criterion	-6492.73
-2 REML Log Likelihood	12970.56

Table 7.9. Tests of Fixed Effects From the Unadjusted Analysis of Diastolic Blood Pressure in the Posttest-Only Control Group Design

Source	NDF	DDF	Type III F	Pr > F
COND	1	4	0.09	0.7810

based on the same random effects but having different covariance structures. Details are provided in the MIXED documentation (Littell et al., 1996; SAS Institute Inc., 1996). These methods are also illustrated later in this chapter.

Table 7.9 presents the Type III F-tests for the fixed effects. Experience has shown that these F-tests are accurate under a wide variety of conditions commonly encountered in group-randomized trials. However, experience has also shown that the default *ddf* are often wrong. This is why the ddf= option is recommended for general use and why it was used in this example.

Table 7.10 presents the least-squares means for each level of the specified fixed effect, here cond. Since there are no covariates included in this analysis, these least-squares means are simply the unadjusted condition means. Each *t*-test assesses the null hypothesis that a single mean is zero; that null hypothesis may or may not be of interest, depending on the circumstances of the trial.

Of considerable interest is the difference between the two condition means, since that is the estimate of the intervention effect. The intervention-effect estimate is 0.434, as shown in Table 7.11, indicating that the average diastolic blood pressure in the intervention condition was 0.434 mm Hg higher than in the control condition. The standard error for that estimate is 1.46, exactly the value estimated earlier using the variance components. The *t*-test for the difference is the square root of the F-test for condition reported in Table 7.9. Neither offers any evidence of a significant intervention effect.

Table 7.10. Least-Squares Means From the Unadjusted Analysis of Diastolic Blood Pressure in the Posttest-Only Control Group Design

Level	LSMEAN	SE	DDF	T	Pr > |T|
COND I	75.20230	1.03164	4	72.90	0.0001
COND C	74.76851	1.03133	4	72.50	0.0001
Level			Alpha	Lower	Upper
COND I			0.05	72.3380	78.0666
COND C			0.05	71.9051	77.6320

234 Design and Analysis of Group-Randomized Trials

Table 7.11. Differences in Least-Squares Means From the Unadjusted Analysis of Diastolic Blood Pressure in the Posttest-Only Control Group Design

Level 1	Level 2	Diff	SE	DDF	T	Pr>|T|
COND I	COND C	0.43378	1.45874	4	0.30	0.7810

	Alpha		Lower	Upper
	0.05		−3.6163	4.4839

Implementation for Dichotomous Data

Smoking status is used to illustrate the unadjusted analysis of posttest data for the Posttest-Only Comparison Group Design. To implement the analysis in MIXED, the code shown in the upper panel of Table 7.12 is appropriate. To implement this analysis in GLIMMIX, the code shown in the lower panel of Table 7.12 is appropriate.

The code for the MIXED analysis is identical to that presented above for diastolic blood pressure, except that the endpoint has been changed to smkstat. In contrast, the GLIMMIX macro requires a different syntax. The

Table 7.12. SAS PROC MIXED and GLIMMIX Code for the Unadjusted Analysis of Smoking Status in the Posttest-Only Control Group Design

MIXED
```
proc mixed info order=internal;
  class cond group;
  model smkstat=cond/ddf=4 ddfm=res;
  random group(cond);
  lsmeans cond/pdiff cl;
run;
```

GLIMMIX
```
%include 'glimmix.sas';
%glimmix(
  procopt=info order=internal,
  data=cross,
  stmts=%str(
    class cond group;
    model smkstat=cond/ddf=4 ddfm=res;
    random group(cond);
    lsmeans cond/pdiff cl;
    ),
  error=binomial,
  link=logit);
run;
```

macro is called with the statement %include 'filename.sas', where filename.sas refers to the name of the GLIMMIX macro file.[9] The macro compiler generates the job-specific code based on the parameters contained within the parentheses in the %glimmix() statement. GLIMMIX then iteratively calls MIXED until convergence.

Within the %glimmix() specification, each keyword is followed by an = sign, after which the keywords, names, or options are entered; a comma is used to end each statement instead of a semicolon. In the example, proc-opt = info adds the info option to the proc mixed statement, the data set is identified by data = cross, the error distribution is identified by error = binomial, and the link function is identified by link = logit.

The stmts = statement introduces a second macro nested within %glimmix(). The %str() macro allows the user to write the class, model, random and several other statements just as they would be written in MIXED. A benefit of this syntax is that the analyst can debug the class, model, random and other statements in a preliminary MIXED job on a sample of the data, then transfer the code to GLIMMIX.

GLIMMIX supports a number of link and variance functions under the Generalized Linear Mixed Model, and these are designated in the error = and link = statements. The variance function must be specified in the error statement; if not specified separately, the program assumes the default link for the specified variance function. The default links are the canonical links shown in Table 7.13 (cf., Littell et al., 1996).

A summary of the GLIMMIX analysis is printed in the .log file together with a summary of the iteration history. Both summaries are shown in Table 7.14. Note that the number of iterations is the number of times that the macro called MIXED, not the number of iterations within a single MIXED call. The macro may call MIXED many times and so the CPU time for the macro may be many times greater than for MIXED. In addition, any convergence problems are exacerbated in GLIMMIX, as the model must converge both within and across the iterations of MIXED.[10]

Table 7.13. Canonical Links for the Variance and Link Functions

Variance Function	Link Function
Binomial	Logit
Poisson	Log
Normal	Identity
Gamma	Reciprocal
Inverse Gaussian	Power(-2)

Table 7.14. Excerpts From the GLIMMIX .log File From the
Unadjusted Analysis of Smoking Status in the Posttest-Only
Control Group Design

Description		*Value*
Data Set	:	Work.Cross
Error Distribution	:	Binomial
Link Function	:	LOGIT
Response Variable	:	SMKSTAT
Iteration		Convergence Criterion
1		0.1192835058
2		0.0535728244
3		0.0013382124
4		9.2722909E-7
5		4.76631E-13

The information in Table 7.15 is printed at the top of the .lis file as a result of the procopt = info statement. With GLIMMIX, the variable and data set names won't match the names used in the SAS code, but the other components of the information table are the same as in the MIXED analysis.

Because the variables in the class statement are the same, the class-level information from the GLIMMIX analysis of smoking status (not shown) is identical to that presented above from the MIXED analysis of diastolic blood pressure. The dimensions of the analysis (not shown) in GLIMMIX are also the same as for diastolic blood pressure, except that fewer members were missing data so that 1758 observations were available for the analysis.

Table 7.16 presents the covariance-parameter estimates from MIXED and

Table 7.15. GLIMMIX Model Information From the
Unadjusted Analysis of Smoking Status in the Posttest-Only
Control Group Design

Description	*Value*
Data Set	Work._DS
Dependent Variable	_Z
Weight Variable	_W
Covariance Structure	Variance Components
Residual Variance Method	Profile
Fixed Effects SE Method	Model-Based
Degrees of Freedom Method	Residual
Estimation Method	REML

Table 7.16. MIXED and GLIMMIX Covariance-Parameter Estimates (REML) From the Unadjusted Analysis of Smoking Status in the Posttest-Only Control Group Design

| MIXED
Cov Parm	Ratio	Estimate	SE	Z	Pr>|Z|
GROUP(COND)	0.00000	0.00000	.	.	.
Residual	1.00000	0.21103	0.00712	29.63	0.0001
GLIMMIX
Cov Parm		Estimate			
GROUP(COND)		0.00000			

GLIMMIX. The default GLIMMIX output does not include the `Ratio`, `Std Error`, `Z` or `Pr>Z` columns, nor the `Residual` row, leaving only the `Cov Parm` and `Estimate` columns for the other random effects, here only `GROUP(COND)`. The omission of the `Residual` row reflects the fact that the residual error is defined in GLIMMIX *a priori* as the theoretical variance for the distribution named in the `error=` statement. Once the `Residual` row is omitted, there is no place for the `Ratio` column. The `Std Error`, `Z` and `Pr>Z` columns are omitted from the GLIMMIX output because they are quite sensitive to departures from normality and so have little place in a macro designed for non-Gaussian data. They are included in the MIXED output because that program is designed for Gaussian data.

In this example, the `GROUP(COND)` component of variance was fixed at zero in both MIXED and GLIMMIX. This happens under the default whenever a variance component estimate drops below zero. This default illustrates the non-negativity constraint described in Chapter 4. Because the non-negativity constraint artificially depresses the Type I error rate, it is recommended that analyses of group-randomized trials permit estimation of negative variance components (Murray et al., 1996).

MIXED allows estimation of negative variance components through the `nobound` option in the `proc mixed` statement. In the macro, this option is added to the `procopt=` statement. Unfortunately, the analysis runs much more slowly when the `nobound` option is invoked and the difference in processing time can be substantial for complex analyses.

Fortunately, MIXED offers the minimum-variance quadratic unbiased estimation method, MIVQUE(0), as an alternative to REML and ML. MIVQUE(0) estimators are the first-step REML estimators with *a priori* values of 1 for residual error and 0 for all other variance components; in fact, MIXED computes the MIVQUE(0) estimators as the starting values prior to REML or ML iteration. MIVQUE(0) estimators have the advantage of requiring no iteration and so are computed more rapidly than ML or REML estimators. They also have the advantage of easily accommodating negative estimates of variance components. At the same time, they have the disadvantage of being increasingly inefficient and biased as the proportion of the total variance attributed to residual error declines (Swallow and Monahan, 1984). But because their performance is adequate when the residual error accounts for >90% of the total variation, they can be used effectively when that condition holds, as it often does when one or more variance components is estimated as negative.[11]

To examine the impact of these options, the analysis was rerun using the nobound option alone and again using the method=mivque0 and nobound options together. These analyses were run in both MIXED and GLIMMIX. Table 7.17 summarizes the results of those six analyses.

The point estimates for the smoking-prevalence rates were virtually identical across the six analyses.[12] The p-value for the test comparing the two conditions was 0.225 under the defaults, whether by MIXED or GLIMMIX; those defaults include REML estimation and the non-negativity constraint. Consistent with the report by Murray et al. (1996), the p-value was smaller, at $p = 0.15$, when the non-negativity constraint was removed via the noboundoption, whether in MIXED or GLIMMIX and whether by REML or MIVQUE(0) estimation. There was also close agreement between MIVQUE(0) and REML in the estimate of the GROUP(COND) variance under the nobound option. Readers should note that the nobound analysis required in excess of 15 hours CPU time using GLIMMIX with REML estimation, but

Table 7.17. Least-Squares Means, the P-Value for Their Difference, the Estimate of the GROUP(COND) Component of Variance, and CPU Time From Six Unadjusted Analyses of the Same Smoking-Status Data in the Posttest-Only Control Group Design

Program	Options	Cond=I LSMEAN	Cond=C LSMEAN	p-value	GROUP (COND)	cpu time h:m:s
	default	0.3184	0.2870	0.2251	0.00000	00:00:13
	nobound	0.3190	0.2871	0.1557	−0.00501	15:16:49
GLIMMIX						
	nobound, MIVQUE(0)	0.3190	0.2871	0.1513	−0.00530	01:11:35
	default	0.3184	0.2870	0.2247	0.00000	00:00:01
	nobound	0.3191	0.2871	0.1509	−0.00023	03:09:46
MIXED						
	nobound, MIVQUE(0)	0.3191	0.2871	0.1487	−0.00024	00:09:25

less than 10 minutes using MIXED and MIVQUE(0) estimation. So while the results from the four analyses that included the nobound option were equivalent, the processing time was not, with the advantage clearly to the combination of MIXED and MIVQUE(0) estimation.

The variance-component estimate for GROUP (COND) included in the GLIMMIX output is scaled in terms of the variance function:

$$\sigma^2_{\text{scaled}} \cong \frac{\sigma^2_{\text{unscaled}}}{(\text{variance function})^2} \tag{7.1}$$

In this example, where the variance function is binomial, the GROUP (COND) variance component as presented in GLIMMIX is related to the GROUP (COND) variance in the original scale approximately as:

$$\sigma^2_{\text{scaled}} \cong \frac{\sigma^2_{\text{unscaled}}}{(\overline{p}(1 - \overline{p}))^2} \tag{7.2}$$

where $\overline{p}$ is the average prevalence rate for smoking in the sample. To return the scaled estimate to the original scale,

$$\sigma^2_{\text{unscaled}} \cong \sigma^2_{\text{scaled}}(\overline{p}(1 - \overline{p}))^2 \tag{7.3}$$

In this example, the scaled estimate of the GROUP (COND) variance from GLIMMIX under the nobound and method=mivque0 options was -0.000501. With an average prevalence rate of 30.3%, the unscaled estimate is computed as:

$$\hat{\sigma}^2_{\text{unscaled}} \cong -0.00530 * (0.303 * (1-0.303))^2 = -0.00024$$

The unscaled estimate from MIXED under the nobound and method= mivque0 options was -0.00024, so that the GROUP (COND) variance-component estimates agree once the difference in scaling is removed.

Note that the factor $\overline{p}(1 - \overline{p})$ is also the variance function under the binomial distribution. GLIMMIX reports an extra-dispersion scale *(EDS)* and this value represents the ratio of the observed residual variance to the variance function (see Table 7.19). As such, the observed residual variance is estimated as:

$$\sigma^2_{\text{residual}} \cong EDS \times \sigma^2_{\text{theoretical}} = EDS \times \overline{p}(1 - \overline{p}) \tag{7.4}$$

Here, the reported value was $EDS = 1.003$, so that the residual variance is estimated as:

$$\hat{\sigma}^2_{residual} \cong 1.0030 * (0.303 * (1 - 0.303)) = 0.212$$

The MIXED estimate (shown above) was 0.211. Once again, the results from the two analyses agree when the difference in scaling is removed.

The covariance-parameter estimates can be used to construct the mean squares for the random effects in the model, drawing on the table of expected mean squares given in Chapter 5. Given 1758 observations and $g = 3$ groups in each of $c = 2$ conditions, the average $m = 293$. Using these values, the mean squares are estimated in Table 7.18.

Given 0.141 as the estimate for $MS_{g:c}$, the standard error of the intervention effect is estimated as:

$$\hat{\sigma}_\Delta = \sqrt{2\left(\frac{\hat{MS}_{g:c}}{mg}\right)} = \sqrt{2\left(\frac{0.141}{293 * 3}\right)} = 0.0179$$

The $ICC_{m:g:c}$ is estimated as:

$$I\hat{C}C_{m:g:c} = \frac{\hat{\sigma}^2_{g:c}}{\hat{\sigma}^2_e + \hat{\sigma}^2_{g:c}} = \frac{-0.00024}{0.211 + (-0.00024)} = -0.00114$$

The $VIF_{m:g:c}$ is estimated as:

$$V\hat{I}F_{m:g:c} = \left(1 + (m-1)I\hat{C}C_{m:g:c}\right) = \left(1 + (293 - 1)(-0.00114)\right) = 0.667$$

With a negative correlation, the $VIF_{m:g:c}$ is fractional.

GLIMMIX does not report a model-fitting table. Instead, the GLIMMIX macro provides the raw and scaled deviance and the Pearson chi-square score (Table 7.19). The deviance is two times the difference in the log-likelihoods between the observed data and the values predicted by the model for the analysis. The scaled deviance reflects the extra variation in the data beyond what is expected given the specified error distribution; it is preferred when the extra-dispersion factor is large. The Pearson chi-square compares the sum of the

Table 7.18. Selected Mean-Square Estimates for the Unadjusted Analysis of Smoking Status in the Posttest-Only Control Group Design

Source	E(MS)	Estimate
Group:C	$\sigma^2_e + m\sigma^2_{g:c}$	$0.211 + 293*(-0.00024) = 0.141$
Member:G:C	σ^2_e	0.211

Table 7.19. GLIMMIX Model Statistics From the Unadjusted Analysis of Smoking Status in the Posttest-Only Control Group Design

Description	Value
Deviance	2156.7960
Scaled Deviance	2150.3474
Pearson Chi-Square	1763.2794
Scaled Pearson Chi-Square	1758.0074
Extra-Dispersion Scale	1.0030

squared deviations between the observed data and the mean against the variance function. The extra-dispersion scale is the ratio of the observed residual variance to the theoretical variance under the variance function.

The deviance and scaled deviance statistics can be interpreted as goodness-of-fit chi-square statistics for the conditional model given the random effects (Littell et al., 1996). In addition, nested models can be compared in terms of their deviance or scaled deviance to compute an improvement-in-fit chi-square with *df* equal to the difference in the number of random effects in the two models. McCullagh and Nelder (1989, pp. 33–36) warn that testing procedures based on the deviance statistics are not well studied in the context of the Generalized Linear Model and should be interpreted cautiously. They are even less well studied in the context of the Generalized Linear Mixed Model, so analysts should treat them accordingly.[13]

Table 7.20 presents the *F*-test for condition from GLIMMIX and MIXED. The *F*-tests and *p*-values from the two analyses are in close agreement and provide no evidence that condition was related to smoking status.

Table 7.21 introduces a new parameter from the GLIMMIX output, labeled MU. Quite generally, MU is an estimate after it has been subject to the inverse link function. Given the error = binomial and link = logit statements,

Table 7.20. GLIMMIX and MIXED Tests of Fixed Effects From the Unadjusted Analysis of Smoking Status in the Posttest-Only Control Group Design

GLIMMIX Source	NDF	DDF	Type III F	Pr > F
COND	1	4	3.14	0.1513

MIXED Source	NDF	DDF	Type III F	Pr > F
COND	1	4	3.19	0.1487

Table 7.21. GLIMMIX and MIXED Least-Squares Means From the Unadjusted Analysis of Smoking Status in the Posttest-Only Control Group Design

GLIMMIX Level	LSMEAN	SE	DDF	T	Pr>|T|
COND I	−0.7584	0.0594	4	−12.77	0.0002
COND C	−0.9097	0.0614	4	−14.82	0.0001
Alpha	Lower	Upper	MU	Lower MU	Upper MU
0.05	−0.9234	−0.5935	0.3190	0.2843	0.3558
0.05	−1.0802	−0.7393	0.2871	0.2535	0.3232
MIXED Level	LSMEAN	SE	DDF	T	Pr>|T|
COND I	0.31909	0.01274	4	25.04	0.0001
COND C	0.28707	0.01262	4	22.74	0.0001
Level			Alpha	Lower	Upper
COND I			0.05	0.2837	0.3545
COND C			0.05	0.2520	0.3221

the analyst might expect the least-squares means and the MU that accompany them to be the log odds and probabilities of smoking at posttest, respectively. That is the interpretation given in Littell et al. (1996), and the close agreement between the GLIMMIX MU and the MIXED LSMEAN in Table 7.21 also supports that view.

Even so, that interpretation is valid only in the simplest case where calculation of the estimate of interest requires only the summation of unweighted parameter estimates. Under those limited conditions, the GLIMMIX LSMEAN and MU are interpretable as estimates in the scale defined by the link function and in the original scale, respectively.

That interpretation is not necessarily valid in a more complex situation. In general, the GLIMMIX LSMEAN and MU are interpretable as estimates in the scale defined by the link function and in the original scale, respectively, if and only if the arithmetic operations involved in the computation of the LSMEAN and MU are commutative across the link function. Unfortunately, the arithmetic operations involved in computing means and other estimates are not commutative across all link functions for all estimates. As a result, interpretation of the results generated by the lsmeans statement in a complex analysis is hazardous at best and often not possible. The action message is that analysts must be very cautious in the use of the lsmeans statement in GLIMMIX.[14]

The preferred point estimate from GLIMMIX is the parameter estimate, as it is interpretable regardless of the `link=` and `error=` statements. When `error=binomial` and `link=logit`, the parameter estimates are mixed-model logistic regression coefficients. In a two-condition design such as this, the coefficient for condition is the log odds ratio reflecting the relative difference in the odds of smoking between the two conditions. In more complex designs that include interactions involving condition, the parameter estimates can be more difficult to interpret. In that case, it may be easier is to combine the parameter estimates to compute log odds ratios for the cells in the design, choosing one cell as the reference level.

In a two-condition design such as this, it is also easy to combine the parameter estimates to compute log odds for the two conditions. The log odds can then be converted to probabilities using the inverse link function for the logit link:

$$\text{probability} = \text{invlink}\big(\ln(\text{odds})\big) = \frac{\exp\big(\ln(\text{odds})\big)}{1 + \exp\big(\ln(\text{odds})\big)}$$

Table 7.22 presents the parameter estimates from the GLIMMIX analysis. The estimate for the `INTERCEPT` is the log odds of smoking among persons at the zero level of the other terms in the model. In this case, the only other term in the model is condition and the zero level corresponds to the control condition. Exponentiating -0.9097 gives 0.4026 as the odds of smoking among members in the control condition. Application of the inverse link function gives 0.287 as the probability of smoking among members in the control condition. The log odds of smoking among members in the intervention condition are computed as $-0.9097 + 0.1513 = -0.7584$. Exponentiating gives 0.4684 as the odds of smoking, and application of the inverse link function gives 0.319 as the probability of smoking. These results agree with the least-squares means computed by MIXED shown in Table 7.21. Because the arithmetic operations involved in the computation of the LSMEAN and MU are commutative across the link function, the results also agree with the MU computed by GLIMMIX.

Table 7.23 provides the results from the `pdiff` option in the `lsmeans`

Table 7.22. GLIMMIX Parameter Estimates From the Unadjusted Analysis of Smoking Status in the Posttest-Only Control Group Design

Parameter	Estimate	SE	DDF	T	Pr>|T|
INTERCEPT	−0.9097	0.0614	1756	−14.82	0.0001
COND I	0.1513	0.0854	4	1.77	0.1513
COND C	0.0000	.	.	.	.

Table 7.23. GLIMMIX and MIXED Differences of Least-Squares Means From the Unadjusted Analysis of Smoking Status in the Posttest-Only Control Group Design

GLIMMIX Level 1	Level 2	Diff	SE	DDF	T	Pr>|T|
COND I	COND C	0.1513	0.0854	4	1.77	0.1513
			Alpha		Lower	Upper
			0.05		−0.0859	0.3884
MIXED Level 1	Level 2	Diff	SE	DDF	T	Pr>|T|
COND I	COND C	0.03202	0.01793	4	1.79	0.1487
			Alpha		Lower	Upper
			0.05		−0.0178	0.0818

statement in GLIMMIX and MIXED. The `Diff` value from the GLIMMIX analysis is computed simply as the difference between the least-squares means for the two conditions: $0.1513 = -0.7584 - (-0.9097)$. In this case, the original means were in the logit scale and so were log odds. As a result, the `Diff` value is a difference in the log odds of smoking between the two conditions, or a log odds ratio. As a result, it has the same value as the parameter estimate for the intervention condition shown in Table 7.22. Exponentiating 0.1513 gives $OR = 1.16$, suggesting that the odds of smoking among members in the intervention condition were 16% greater than for members in the control condition. The confidence bounds on the *ln(OR)* are based on the *t*-distribution and the *ddf* specified in the `ddf =` option; exponentiating the upper and lower bounds gives bounds around the odds ratio.

In MIXED, the difference estimate is a difference between the two condition means in their original scale and has a different value and meaning than the difference computed in GLIMMIX. Note, however, the close agreement between the *t*-tests and *p*-values for the two analyses, as the two *t*-tests are evaluating the same null hypothesis of no intervention effect.

The results of GLIMMIX and MIXED applied to the same dichotomous endpoint agree quite closely in many respects. The *F*-test and *p*-values are quite similar for the same null hypothesis. The least squares means from MIXED and computed probabilities based on the parameter estimates from GLIMMIX are in close agreement when used correctly. So, too, are the variance components after correcting for the scale defined by the link function. These results illustrate the major finding reported by Hannan and Murray (1996), that analyses based on the General Linear Mixed Model (e.g., MIXED) and the Generalized Linear Mixed Model (e.g., GLIMMIX) give comparable results so long as there are even just a few groups per condition and a modest number of members in each group.

Given the close agreement between MIXED and GLIMMIX when used properly in the analysis of data from group-randomized trials, and the potential for misinterpretation of the GLIMMIX results, MIXED is preferred over GLIMMIX for the analysis of data from most group-randomized trials.[15] As a result, though all subsequent analyses of dichotomous endpoints presented in Chapters 7 and 8 were run in both GLIMMIX and MIXED, only the MIXED results are presented as long as the two programs gave equivalent results.

Adjusted Analysis of Posttest Data

Implementation for Gaussian Data

The analysis of diastolic blood pressure is easily expanded to include regression adjustment for covariates. In the published report (Luepker et al., 1994), the MHHP investigators adjusted diastolic blood pressure for age, sex, educational attainment (eight levels), seasonal trend, cuff size, observer, and location of measurement (home vs. clinic vs. other). The code shown in Table 7.24 is appropriate for this analysis in MIXED.[16]

Categorical covariates are listed in the `class` statement. Categorical and continuous covariates are listed in the `model` statement.

Because covariates measured at the member level are crossed with the groups, they are tested against the residual error. The addition of the `ddfm = res` option ensures that all fixed effects other than those named in the `ddf =` option are tested using residual *ddf*. Covariates measured at the group level would be tested against $MS_{g:c}$ and the *df* for that term would be reduced for each *df* allocated to those covariates. Because there are no covariates at that level in this example, the *ddf* for the test of `cond` remain at 4.[17]

The *ddf* for condition are very limited at 4, and any decrease due to the addition of a covariate measured at the group level would exact a measurable

Table 7.24. SAS PROC MIXED Code for the Adjusted Analysis of Diastolic Blood Pressure in the Posttest-Only Control Group Design

```
proc mixed info order = internal;
  class cond group sex educlvl bpobsrvr bplocatn;
  model dbp = cond age sex educlvl bpobsrvr bplocatn
    /ddf = 4 ddfm = res;
  random group(cond);
  lsmeans cond/om pdiff cl;
run;
```

price in terms of the power of the test for the intervention effect. Unless this price is offset by a sufficient reduction in the variance of the intervention effect, the adjusted analysis will have less power than the unadjusted analysis. No loss in the *ddf* for condition results from the covariates included in this analysis, as they are measured at the member level.

The default method for computing least-squares means in MIXED computes them as though the observations were balanced on all fixed effects in the `class` statement that are not included in the `lsmeans` effect. In this example, the `lsmeans` effect is `cond` and there are three other fixed effects in the `class` statement, `educlvl`, `bpobsrvr`, and `bplocatn`. As a result, the default method would compute adjusted means for `cond` as though there had been an equal number of observations at every level of `educlvl`, `bpobsrvr`, and `bplocatn`. This would be appropriate if the design of the study intended for the observations to be balanced on those factors. However, group-randomized trials rarely are structured that way, and so the default option is rarely appropriate. Moreover, it can generate very odd results.

Prior to SAS 6.10, the only solution was to replace each offending variable with a set of dummy-coded indicator variables. By putting the indicator variables in the `model` statement but not in the `class` statement, the adjusted means were computed based on the means of the indicator variables. Those means correspond to the observed marginal distribution of the variables in question regardless of the imbalance in the data. Unfortunately, this solution was an extra burden and did not work in every case.[18]

The `om` option was introduced in SAS 6.10 to solve this problem. Where adjusted means could be obtained with the dummy-coded indicator variables, the `om` option gives the same results without the extra work. More important, the `om` option gives adjusted means based on the observed marginal distribution of the variables in the `class` statement even where the dummy-coded indicator variable solution would not. Because adjustments should be made based on the observed marginals in most group-randomized trials, the `om` option has broad application in these studies.[19]

Table 7.25 shows the three categorical covariates in addition to the design variables `cond` and `group`. Table 7.26 confirms the number of variance components at two. The number of columns in the fixed-effects design matrix (X) is larger than that in the previous section, reflecting the new categorical covariates. The number of columns in the random-effects design matrix (Z) is unchanged. The number of observations remains the same, indicating that no additional observations were lost due to missing data on the covariates. The model converged in one iteration (not shown).

Table 7.27 presents the covariance-parameter estimates and can be used to construct the mean squares for the random effects. Given 1726 observations

Table 7.25. Class-Level Information From the Adjusted Analysis of Diastolic Blood Pressure in the Posttest-Only Control Group Design

Class	Levels	Values
COND	2	I C
GROUP	6	MANKATO WINONA FARGO/MOORHD SIOUX FALLS BLOOMINGTON ROSEVILLE
SEX	2	FEMALE MALE
EDUCLVL	8	<7th GRADE 7TH-9TH GRADE 10-11TH GRADE HS GRADUATE VOCAT/BUSINESS SOME COLL. COLL.GRAD. POST.GRAD.
BPOBSRVR	23	002 003 005 006 007 009 010 016 030 031 032 034 052 079 081 083 098 101 102 309 623 927 999
BPLOCATN	3	CLINIC HOME OTHER

distributed over $g = 3$ groups in each of $c = 2$ conditions, the average $m = 288$. Using these values, the mean squares are estimated as shown in Table 7.28.

Given 1000 as the estimate for $MS_{g:c}$, the standard error for the intervention effect is estimated using Equation 5.6:

$$\hat{\sigma}_\Delta = \sqrt{2\left(\frac{\hat{MS}_{g:c}}{mg}\right)} = \sqrt{2\left(\frac{1000}{288*3}\right)} = 1.52$$

Table 7.26. Dimensions of the Adjusted Analysis of Diastolic Blood Pressure in the Posttest-Only Control Group Design

Description	Value
Covariance Parameters	2
Columns in X	40
Columns in Z	6
Subjects	1
Max Obs Per Subject	1741
Observations Used	1726
Observations Not Used	15
Total Observations	1741

Table 7.27. Covariance-Parameter Estimates (REML) From the Adjusted Analysis of Diastolic Blood Pressure in the Posttest-Only Control Group Design

Cov Parm	Ratio	Estimate	SE	Z	Pr>|Z|
GROUP(COND)	0.03288	3.14000	2.51753	1.25	0.2123
Residual	1.00000	95.48340	3.28757	29.04	0.0001

This standard error is slightly larger than that in the unadjusted analysis; that can and does happen. A reduction in the residual error improves precision, but an increase in the group component of variance decreases precision. This underscores the need to select covariates carefully. In the MHHP, the investigators chose the covariates *a priori,* knowing that they would likely act as confounders in the data. Adjustment should always be made in the presence of measurable confounding, even if there are adverse consequences for precision. Confounding due to covariates was substantial in this instance, and so the adjustments are appropriate even if they have an adverse effect on power.

The adjusted $ICC_{m:g:c}$ is estimated as:

$$I\hat{C}C_{m:g:c} = \frac{\hat{\sigma}^2_{g:c}}{\hat{\sigma}^2_e + \hat{\sigma}^2_{g:c}} = \frac{3.14}{95.5 + 3.14} = 0.0318$$

The adjusted $VIF_{m:g:c}$ is estimated as:

$$V\hat{I}F_{m:g:c} = \left(1 + (m-1)I\hat{C}C_{m:g:c}\right) = \left(1 + (288-1)0.0318\right) = 10.1$$

Table 7.29 confirms that each of the fixed covariates is significantly related to diastolic blood pressure. However, there is still no evidence of an intervention effect.

The use of the om option is confirmed by the inclusion of the margins column in Table 7.30.[20]

Table 7.28. Selected Mean-Square Estimates for the Adjusted Analysis of Diastolic Blood Pressure in the Posttest-Only Control Group Design

Source	E(MS)	Estimate
Group:C	$\sigma^2_e + m\sigma^2_{g:c}$	$95.5 + 288*3.14 = 1000$
Member:G:C	σ^2_e	95.5

Table 7.29. Tests of Fixed Effects From the Adjusted Analysis of Diastolic Blood Pressure in the Posttest-Only Control Group Design

Source	NDF	DDF	Type III F	Pr>F
COND	1	4	0.19	0.6849
AGE	1	1691	57.20	0.0001
SEX	1	1691	151.03	0.0001
EDUCLVL	7	1691	3.55	0.0009
BPOBSRVR	22	1691	1.62	0.0346
BPLOCATN	2	1691	3.85	0.0215

The estimated intervention effect was appreciably larger in the adjusted analysis (Table 7.31) than in the unadjusted analysis (Table 7.11).[21] Note that the standard error of the intervention effect is almost identical to the value estimated from variance components.

Implementation for Dichotomous Data

The analysis of smoking status in the MHHP data also can be expanded to include regression adjustment for covariates. In the published report (Luepker et al., 1994), the MHHP investigators adjusted for age, sex, educational attainment (eight levels), and marital status.

To implement the analysis in SAS PROC MIXED, the code shown in the upper panel of Table 7.32 is appropriate. To implement the analysis in the GLIMMIX macro, the code shown in the lower panel of Table 7.32 is appropriate.

The results from the MIXED and GLIMMIX analyses were again quite similar. Given their familiar format and easier interpretation, only selected results from the MIXED analysis are presented.

Table 7.30. Least-Squares Means From the Adjusted Analysis of Diastolic Blood Pressure in the Posttest-Only Control Group Design

Level	Margins	LSMEAN	SE	DDF	T	Pr>|T|
COND I	WORK.CROSS	75.33008	1.07906	4	69.81	0.0001
COND C	WORK.CROSS	74.66189	1.07910	4	69.19	0.0001
Level			Alpha		Lower	Upper
COND I			0.05		72.3341	78.3260
COND C			0.05		71.6658	77.6580

Table 7.31. Differences of Least-Squares Means From the Adjusted Analysis of Diastolic Blood Pressure in the Posttest-Only Control Group Design

Level 1	Level 2	Margins	Diff	SE	DDF	T
COND I	COND C	WORK.CROSS	0.66818	1.53040	4	0.44
Pr>|T|				*Alpha*	*Lower*	*Upper*
0.6849				0.05	−3.5809	4.9173

As in the unadjusted analysis, the variance estimate for GROUP(COND) was fixed at zero in the initial analysis (not shown). As a result, the analysis was rerun using MIXED with the nobound and method=mivque0 options. Table 7.33 presents the covariance-parameter estimates from that analysis.

These covariance-parameter estimates can be used to construct the mean squares for the random effects in the model. Given 1758 observations and $g = 3$ groups in each of $c = 2$ conditions, the average $m = 293$. Using these values, the mean squares are estimated as shown in Table 7.34.

Table 7.32. SAS PROC MIXED and GLIMMIX Code for the Adjusted Analysis of Smoking Status in the Posttest-Only Control Group Design

MIXED
```
proc mixed info order=internal;
  class cond group sex educlvl maritals;
  model smkstat=cond age sex educlvl maritals
    /ddf=4 ddfm=res;
  random group(cond);
  lsmeans cond/om pdiff cl;
run;
```

GLIMMIX
```
%include 'glimmix.sas';
%glimmix(
  procopt=info order=internal,
  data=cross,
  stmts=%str(
    class cond group sex educlvl maritals;
    model smkstat=cond age sex educlvl maritals
      /ddf=4 ddfm=res solution;
    random group(cond);
    ),
  error=binomial,
  link=logit);
run;
```

Table 7.33. Covariance-Parameter Estimates (MIVQUE(0)) for the Adjusted Analysis of Smoking Status in the Posttest-Only Control Group Design

Cov Parm	Estimate
GROUP(COND)	−0.0003388
Residual	0.1975241

Given 0.0987 as the estimate for $MS_{g:c}$, the standard error for the intervention effect is estimated using Equation 5.6:

$$\hat{\sigma}_\Delta = \sqrt{2\left(\frac{\hat{MS}_{g:c}}{mg}\right)} = \sqrt{2\left(\frac{0.0987}{293*3}\right)} = 0.0150$$

This standard error is considerably smaller than that in the unadjusted analysis. This is the more common result of regression adjustment for covariates, in contrast to the slight increase observed in the analysis of diastolic blood pressure.

The adjusted $ICC_{m:g:c}$ is estimated as:

$$I\hat{C}C_{m:g:c} = \frac{\hat{\sigma}^2_{g:c}}{\hat{\sigma}^2_e + \hat{\sigma}^2_{g:c}} = \frac{-0.000339}{0.198 + (-0.000339)} = -0.00172$$

The adjusted $VIF_{m:g:c}$ is estimated as:

$$V\hat{I}F_{m:g:c} = \left(1 + (m-1)I\hat{C}C_{m:g:c}\right) = \left(1 + (293-1)(-0.00172)\right) = 0.50$$

With the adjustment, the $VIF_{m:g:c}$ was reduced from 0.667 to 0.50.

Table 7.35 confirms the strong relationship between all of the covariates and smoking status, except for sex. Were there no further interest in this variable, it could be deleted from the model and the analysis rerun. However, because the MHHP investigators had an *a priori* interest in sex-specific intervention

Table 7.34. Selected Mean-Square Estimates for the Adjusted Analysis of Smoking Status in the Posttest-Only Control Group Design

Source	E(MS)	Estimate
Group:C	$\sigma^2_e + m\sigma^2_{g:c}$	$0.198 + 293*(-0.000339) = 0.0987$
Member:G:C	σ^2_e	0.198

Table 7.35. Tests of Fixed Effects for the Adjusted Analysis of
Smoking Status in the Posttest-Only Control Group Design

Source	NDF	DDF	Type III F	Pr > F
COND	1	4	8.03	0.0471
AGE	1	1743	31.96	0.0001
SEX	1	1743	0.15	0.7004
EDUCLVL	7	1743	13.22	0.0001
MARITALS	4	1743	5.32	0.0003

effects, that issue will be pursued further. Note that the test of the intervention effect is marginally significant after adjustment for the covariates measured at the member level. Note as well that under the non-negativity constraint, this test would have been reported as 3.77 with a p-value of 0.1243. This demonstrates the impact of the non-negativity constraint, which serves to inflate the variance components, deflate the Type I error rate, and in so doing, to deflate power. Indeed, because the true Type I and II error rates are unknown under the non-negativity constraint, interpretation of the test result and p-values generated under that constraint is quite difficult. In contrast, the test based on the nobound option has Type I and II error rates at the nominal levels and can be interpreted on that basis.

Pretest-Posttest Comparison Group Design

The MHHP design can be reduced to a Pretest-Posttest Control Group Design by limiting the analysis to the data collected during the surveys just prior to and during the first year after the introduction of the intervention. With this restriction, MHHP provides $c = 2$ conditions, $g = 3$ communities per condition, $t = 2$ time intervals for each community, and observations on several hundred members per community per time interval.

Unadjusted Time × Condition Analysis

Implementation for Gaussian Data

To implement this analysis for diastolic blood pressure, the code shown in the upper panel of Table 7.36 is appropriate.

In this analysis, time is treated as a categorical variable with two levels, and so is added to the class statement. In addition, it is added to the model statement, both as a main effect and as an interaction with cond. The

Table 7.36. SAS PROC MIXED Code for the Unadjusted Analysis of Diastolic Blood Pressure in the Pretest-Posttest Control Group Design

```
NO SUBJECT=OPTION IN THE RANDOM STATEMENT
proc mixed info order=internal;
  class cond group time;
  model dbp=cond time cond*time/ddf=4,4,4 ddfm=res;
  random group(cond) time*group(cond);
  lsmeans cond*time/om e slice=time slice=cond;
  estimate '(I1-10)-(C1-C0)' cond*time -1 1 1 -1/cl e;
run;

SUBJECT=OPTION IN THE RANDOM STATEMENT
proc mixed info order=internal;
  class cond group time;
  model dbp=cond time cond*time/ddf=4,4,4 ddfm=res;
  random int time/subject=group(cond);
  lsmeans cond*time/om e slice=time slice=cond;
  estimate '(I1-I0)-(C1-C0)' cond*time -1 1 1 -1/cl e;
run;
```

expected-mean-squares table in Chapter 5 shows that the *ddf* for the first fixed effect are $c(g\text{-}1)=4$ and for the second and third fixed effects are $(t\text{-}1)c(g\text{-}1)=4$. As a result, the `ddf=4,4,4` option is included in the `model` statement.

The `random` statement now includes two terms: a main effect for `group(cond)` and the interaction `time*group(cond)`. This specification provides the correct analysis and corresponds to the table of expected mean squares. However, it often runs more slowly and requires more memory than an alternative specification for the `random` statement, shown in the lower panel of Table 7.36.

In the alternative specification, the element `group(cond)` is factored out of the terms `group(cond)` and `time*group(cond)` to give the result `int time/subject=group(cond)`. The program interprets the random statement as crossing the effect of the `subject=` option with all other terms listed in the `random` statement. Crossing `int` with `group(cond)` gives `group(cond)`. Crossing `time` with `group(cond)` gives `time*group-(cond)`. So the two specifications generate the same terms, but the latter often allows a more efficient analysis.[22] For that reason, this "factorization" method is used whenever possible.

The `lsmeans` statement requests the interaction means rather than the main-effect means, because the intervention effect is represented by the interaction. In this analysis, the `slice=time` option provides tests of simple main effects, here testing the effect of condition at each level of time. In addition, `slice=cond` provides a test of whether the linear time trend in each condition was zero. Generally, the `slice=` option is more useful than the `pdiff` option when the `lsmeans` effect is an interaction.

The `estimate` statement requests that an estimate representing the intervention effect be computed. The particular values assigned in the `estimate` statement correspond to the weights to be applied to the regression coefficients for the variables included in the `estimate` statement. In this case, the only variable included is `cond*time`, which has four coefficients.

An easy way to construct `estimate` statements in MIXED is to conduct a preliminary analysis to obtain the weights used to construct least-squares means for the corresponding effect with the e option in the `lsmeans` statement. The output from the e option is presented in Table 7.37. The row numbers that define the columns correspond to the rows in the least-squares-means table (Table 7.42); they also follow the same order as that shown for the interaction terms in the coefficients table (Table 7.37). Here they correspond to the four means `I0`, `I1`, `C0`, and `C1`.

To generate any estimate of interest involving these four means, the analyst need only write down the estimate of interest and then reorder the terms to correspond to the order of these columns. The + and − values then define the coefficients for the estimate. In this case, the desired contrast is `(I1−I0)−(C1−C0)`. Rearranging those terms to match the order of the columns gives:

$$-I0 \ +I1 \ +C0 \ -I1$$
This defines the coefficients for the estimate as:

$$-1 \ +1 \ +1 \ -1$$

Table 7.37. Coefficients for COND*TIME Least-Squares Means From the Unadjusted Analysis of Diastolic Blood Pressure in the Pretest-Posttest Control Group Design

Parameter	Row 1	Row 2	Row 3	Row 4
INTERCEPT	1	1	1	1
COND I	1	1	0	0
COND C	0	0	1	1
TIME 0	1	0	1	0
TIME 1	0	1	0	1
COND*TIME I 0	1	0	0	0
COND*TIME I 1	0	1	0	0
COND*TIME C 0	0	0	1	0
COND*TIME C 1	0	0	0	1

Each value in the column marked Row 1 is multiplied by -1, each value in the column marked Row 2 is multiplied by $+1$, etc. Then the four products in each row are summed. Variables whose rows sum to zero do not contribute to the estimate and may be omitted from the `estimate` statement. Variables whose rows sum to a nonzero value must be included, using the sum as the coefficient in the `estimate` statement.

Applying those rules here, the first two rows each sum to zero, indicating that the variable `COND` need not be included in the `estimate` statement. The same is true for `TIME`. However, the four rows representing the interaction term sum to -1, 1, 1, and -1, respectively. As a result, the `estimate` statement is written as:

```
estimate '(I1-I0) - (C1-C0)' cond*time  -1 1 1  -1/cl e
```

The e option in the `estimate` statement generates the table of coefficients used to compute the estimate and allows the analyst to confirm that the estimate was constructed properly.

The information table (not shown) confirms the use of the `subject =` option in the `random` statement, noting the effect in that option as `group(cond)`. The class table (not shown) includes the time variable, with two levels.

Table 7.38 reflects the larger design with more than twice the number of observations. It also reflects the use of the `subject =` option in the `random` statement, as the table now identifies 6 subjects. The three covariance parameters are the three variance components in the model. The 9 columns in the fixed-effects design matrix are the intercept, `cond` (2), `time` (2), and `cond* time` (4). The 3 columns in the random-effects design matrix for each `group(cond)` are `int` (1) and `time` (2). This analysis converged in 3

Table 7.38. Dimensions of the Unadjusted Analysis of Diastolic Blood Pressure in the Pretest-Posttest Control Group Design

Description	Value
Covariance Parameters	3
Columns in X	9
Columns in Z	3
Subjects	6
Max Obs Per Subject	836
Observations Used	3936
Observations Not Used	29
Total Observations	3965

Table 7.39. Covariance-Parameter Estimates (REML) From
the Unadjusted Analysis of Diastolic Blood Pressure in
the Pretest-Posttest Control Group Design

Cov Parm	Estimate
INTERCEPT	3.61318
TIME	2.77915
Residual	112.41756

iterations (not shown). The maximum number of observations per
group(cond) is 836.

Table 7.39 presents the covariance-parameter estimates. Under the factorization method, INTERCEPT is GROUP(COND) and TIME is TIME*GROUP
(COND).

The covariance-parameter estimates can be used to construct the mean
squares for the random effects in the model. Given 3936 observations and
$g=3$ groups in each of $c=2$ conditions observed at each of $t=2$ time intervals, the average $m=328$. Using these values, the mean squares are estimated
in Table 7.40.

Given 1024 as the estimate for $MS_{tg:c}$, the standard error for the intervention
effect is estimated using Equation 5.9:

$$\hat{\sigma}_\Delta = \sqrt{2*2\left(\frac{\hat{MS}_{tg:c}}{mg}\right)} = \sqrt{2*2\left(\frac{1024}{328*3}\right)} = 2.04$$

This standard error is considerably larger than that for the simpler Posttest-
Only Control Group Design. It reflects the greater complexity of the intervention effect, which is now a net difference involving four means rather than a
simple difference involving only two means.

Note that the *ICC* of interest here is a different correlation than the *ICC* of
interest for the simpler Posttest-Only Control Group Design. That *ICC* reflected the correlation among members within a group and so was labeled

Table 7.40. Selected Mean-Square Estimates for the
Unadjusted Analysis of Diastolic Blood Pressure in the
Pretest-Posttest Control Group Design

Source	E(MS)	Estimate
TG:C	$\sigma_e^2 + m\sigma_{tg:c}^2$	$112 + 328*2.78 = 1024$
Member:TG:C	σ_e^2	112

$ICC_{m:g:c}$. Here, the ICC of interest reflects the correlation among members within a time $\times$ group survey, and so is labeled $ICC_{m:tg:c}$.

This is a very general point and one that should be emphasized: there is no such thing as a universal ICC that is applicable across all endpoints, designs, and analyses. The ICC of interest depends on the endpoint, the design, and the analysis under consideration. That point is particularly relevant to power analysis (Chapter 9) and to *post hoc* adjustments for variance inflation (Chapter 4).

The ICC of interest in this analysis is estimated as:

$$I\hat{C}C_{m:tg:c} = \frac{\hat{\sigma}^2_{tg:c}}{\hat{\sigma}^2_e + \hat{\sigma}^2_{tg:c}} = \frac{2.78}{112 + 2.78} = 0.0242$$

The $VIF_{m:tg:c}$ is estimated as

$$V\hat{I}F_{m:tg:c} = \left(1 + (m-1)I\hat{C}C_{m:tg:c}\right) = \left(1 + (328-1)0.0242\right) = 8.91$$

Table 7.41 presents F-tests for the two main effects of COND and TIME, and for the interaction COND*TIME. The test of interest is the test for COND *TIME, as it is the test of the intervention effect. Indeed, the tests listed for COND and TIME are generally of little interest in this analysis.[23] In this case, the F-test for COND*TIME is 0.68 and is clearly not significant.

Table 7.42 presents the least-squares means. The label COND*TIME I 0 refers to the intervention condition at Time 0 (the pretest). The label COND *TIME C 1 refers to the control condition at Time 1 (the posttest). The other labels follow the same general pattern. The means suggest a decline of nearly 2 mm Hg in the control condition but only a slight decline in the intervention condition.

The results of the slice= options can be helpful for interpreting intervention effects when they are present and supported by the omnibus F-test. Those results are summarized in Table 7.43. In the absence of a significant F-test, they should be interpreted cautiously. In the example, the first effect slice tests the difference between the two conditions at Time 0. The last effect slice tests

Table 7.41. Tests of Fixed Effects From the Unadjusted Analysis of Diastolic Blood Pressure in the Pretest-Posttest Control Goup Design

Source	NDF	DDF	Type III F	Pr > F
COND	1	4	0.05	0.8382
TIME	1	4	1.04	0.3661
COND*TIME	1	4	0.68	0.4555

Table 7.42. Least-Squares Means From the Unadjusted Analysis of Diastolic Blood Pressure in the Pretest-Posttest Control Group Design

Level	Margins	LSMEAN	SE
COND*TIME I 0	WORK.CROSS	75.40572	1.49607
COND*TIME I 1	WORK.CROSS	75.20844	1.50390
COND*TIME C 0	WORK.CROSS	76.65481	1.49656
COND*TIME C 1	WORK.CROSS	74.76935	1.50368

the difference between the Time 0 and Time 1 among members in the control condition. As such, the tests reported in the tests of effect slices are tests of simple main effects as defined, for example, by Winer et al. (1991).[24]

Table 7.44 confirms that the contrast computed with the estimate statement was constructed properly. The estimate itself is presented in Table 7.45. The *t*-test that accompanies it is the square root of the *F*-test for the COND*TIME interaction presented in the Table 7.41, and the *p*-values for the two tests are the same. The standard error for the intervention effect is exactly as computed above from the variance components. The positive value of the estimate confirms that the decline in diastolic blood pressure was greater in the control condition than in the intervention condition.

Adjusted Time × Condition Analysis

Implementation for Gaussian Data

To implement this analysis for diastolic blood pressure, the code shown in Table 7.46 is appropriate.

The slice= option is used instead of the pdiff option because the lsmeans effect is an interaction. The om option ensures that the adjusted means are computed based on the marginal distribution of the covariates. The e option generates the coefficients used to compute the least-squares means to

Table 7.43. Tests of Effect Slices From the Unadjusted Analysis of Diastolic Blood Pressure in the Pretest-Posttest Control Group Design

Effect	Slice	NDF	DDF	F	Pr>F
COND*TIME	TIME 0	1	4	0.35	0.5867
COND*TIME	TIME 1	1	4	0.04	0.8465
COND*TIME	COND I	1	4	0.02	0.8981
COND*TIME	COND C	1	4	1.70	0.2623

Table 7.44. Coefficients for (I1-I0)-(C1-C0) From the Unadjusted Analysis of Diastolic Blood Pressure in the Pretest-Posttest Control Group Design

Parameter			Row 1
INTERCEPT			0
COND I			0
COND C			0
TIME 0			0
TIME 1			0
COND*TIME I	0		-1
COND*TIME I	1		1
COND*TIME C	0		1
COND*TIME C	1		-1

aid in the construction of estimate statements. The estimate statement is again used to generate the estimate of the intervention effect.

Table 7.47 presents the covariance-parameter estimates. Given 3936 observations and $g=3$ groups in each of $c=2$ conditions observed at each of $t=2$ time intervals, the average $m=328$. Using these values, the mean squares are estimated in Table 7.48.

The estimated $MS_{tg:c}$ is considerably reduced compared to the unadjusted analysis. Given 590 as the estimate, the standard error for the intervention effect is estimated using Equation 5.12:

$$\hat{\sigma}_\Delta = \sqrt{2*2\left(\frac{\hat{MS}_{tg:c}}{mg}\right)} = \sqrt{2*2\left(\frac{590}{328*3}\right)} = 1.55$$

This standard error reflects any reduction due to repeat measurements on the same groups and to regression adjustment for covariates.

The results from the estimate statement are summarized in Table 7.49. With the regression adjustment for covariates, the estimate of the intervention

Table 7.45. Estimate for (I1-I0)-(C1-C0) From the Unadjusted Analysis of Diastolic Blood Pressure in the Pretest-Posttest Control Group Design

Parameter	Estimate	SE	DDF	T
(I1-I0)-(C1-C0)	1.68817	2.04524	4	0.83
	Pr>|T|	Alpha	Lower	Upper
	0.4555	0.05	-3.9903	7.3667

Table 7.46. SAS PROC MIXED Code for the Adjusted Analysis of Diastolic Blood Pressure in the Pretest-Posttest Control Group Design

```
proc mixed info order=internal;
  class cond group time sex educlvl bpobsrvr bplocatn;
  model dpb=cond time cond*time age sex educlvl bpobsrvr
    bplocatn/ddf=4,4,4 ddfm=res;
  random int time/subject=group(cond);
  lsmeans cond*time/om e slice=time slice=cond;
  estimate '(I1-I0)-(C1-C0)' cond*time -1 1 1 -1/cl e;
run;
```

Table 7.47. Covariance-Parameter Estimates (REML) From the Adjusted Analysis of Diastolic Blood Pressure in the Pretest-Posttest Control Group Design

Cov Parm	Estimate
INTERCEPT	4.00884
TIME	1.48721
Residual	100.86909

Table 7.48. Selected Mean-Square Estimates for the Adjusted Analysis of Diastolic Blood Pressure in the Pretest-Posttest Control Group Design

Source	E(MS)	Estimate
TG:C	$\sigma_e^2 + m\sigma_{tg:c}^2$	$101 + 328*1.49 = 590$
Member:TG:C	σ_e^2	101

Table 7.49. Estimate for (I1-I0)-(C1-C0) from the Adjusted Analysis of Diastolic Blood Pressure in the Pretest-Posttest Control Group Design

Parameter	Estimate	SE	DDF	T
(I1-I0)-(C1-C0)	2.03937	1.57374	4	1.30
	Pr>|T|	Alpha	Lower	Upper
	0.2647	0.05	-2.3300	6.4088

effect increased from 1.68 to 2.04. The standard error was reduced by 23.0%, reflecting a large improvement in precision. Even so, there was no evidence of a significant intervention effect.

Stratification or Matching in the Analysis

A Priori Stratification With Stratum as a Fixed Effect

SAS PROC MIXED and the GLIMMIX macro can be used to implement a stratified analysis for a design based on *a priori* stratification, following the presentation in Chapter 5. However, the MHHP did not employ *a priori* stratification and so the MHHP data cannot be used to illustrate that analysis. Indeed, *a priori* stratification was not possible for MHHP, given only three communities in each condition.

A Priori Stratification With Stratum as a Random Effect

SAS PROC MIXED and the GLIMMIX macro also can be used to implement a stratified analysis for a multicenter trial in which the center is considered to be a random effect. However, the MHHP was conducted in 'a single center and so the MHHP data cannot be used to illustrate that analysis either.

Matching in the Analysis

The communities in the MHHP were matched on size, type, and distance from Minneapolis–St. Paul. One city from each of the three pairs was assigned to the intervention condition and the other to the control condition. The primary analysis did not reflect the matching (Luepker et al., 1994), but a matched analysis is certainly possible, following the presentation in Chapter 5.

Implementation for Gaussian Data

To implement the matched analysis for diastolic blood pressure, the code shown in Table 7.50 is appropriate.

   In the matched analysis, `group` is left out of the `class` and `random` statements because it is completely confounded with `cond*strata`. `Strata` and its interactions are placed in the `random` statement. There is no nesting explicitly shown in the MIXED code, as none of the effects shown is a nested effect. The member is of course nested within the cells of the *TCS* interaction, but because Member:*TCS* is the residual error, it is not written into the code.

Table 7.50. SAS PROC MIXED Code for the Adjusted Analysis of Diastolic Blood Pressure in the Pretest-Posttest Control Group Design With *A Priori* Matching

```
proc mixed info order = internal;
  class cond strata time sex educlvl bpobsrvr bplocatn;
  model dbp = cond time cond*time sex age educlvl bpobsrvr
    bplocatn/ddf = 2,2,2 ddfm = res;
  random int cond time cond*time/subject = strata;
  lsmeans cond*time/om e slice = cond slice = time;
  estimate '(I1-I0)-(C1-C0)' cond*time -1 1 1 -1/cl e;
run;
```

One of the effects of the matching is clearly shown in the `ddf=` option, which specifies *ddf* for the first three fixed effects. Because the analysis is based on the number of pairs, which is only 3, the *ddf* are half what they would be in an unmatched analysis. From Table 5.7, the *ddf* for the first two fixed effects are computed as $(c-1)(s-1)-x_g=2$, and for the third fixed effect as $(t-1)(c-1)(s-1)-x_g=2$. Matching always reduces the *ddf* for the test of interest by half in the absence of covariates at the group level, exacting a large power penalty when the number of matched sets is small.

The `lsmeans` effect is the `cond*time` interaction. Because it is a two-way interaction, the two `slice=` statements can help guide the interpretation of those means if the `cond*time` effect is significant.

The REML covariance-parameter estimates (not shown) indicated that one of the parameters was fixed at zero. That meant that it was estimated as negative at some point during the REML estimation process. Use of the `nobound` option in combination with `method=mivque0` is a good solution as long as the residual error captures most of the variation in the data. In this case, the residual error accounted for about 93% of the variation in the data, and so MIVQUE(0) estimation was appropriate. Table 7.51 presents the MIVQUE(0) estimates.

Table 7.51. Covariance-Parameter Estimates (MIVQUE(0)) From the Adjusted Analysis of Diastolic Blood Pressure in the Pretest-Posttest Control Group Design With *A Priori* Matching

Cov Parm	Estimate
INTERCEPT	0.71426
COND	4.15011
TIME	1.54804
COND*TIME	−0.02051
Residual	100.68140

Table 7.52. Selected Mean-Square Estimates for the Adjusted Analysis of Diastolic Blood Pressure in the Pretest-Posttest Control Group Design With *A Priori* Matching

Source	E(MS)	Estimate
TCS	$\sigma_e^2 + m\sigma_{tcs}^2$	$101 + 328*(-0.02051) = 94.3$
Member:TCS	σ_e^2	101

Given 3936 observations in $c = 2$ conditions, $s = 3$ strata (pairs), and $t = 2$ time intervals, $m = 328$. Using these values, the mean squares are estimated in Table 7.52. The standard error of the intervention effect is then estimated via Equation 5.20:

$$\hat{\sigma}_\Delta = \sqrt{2*2\left(\frac{\hat{MS}_{tcs}}{ms}\right)} = \sqrt{2*2\left(\frac{94.3}{328*3}\right)} = 0.619$$

The intervention effect resulted in a Type III F-test of 8.63; with 1,2 df, $p = 0.0990$. Even so, there was a noticeable increase in the F-test for COND *TIME from the unmatched analysis. Because the residual error was little changed from that of the unmatched analysis, this increase in the F-test is almost entirely due to partialing out variation among the groups due to the pairs in this matched analysis.

Table 7.53 presents the estimate of the intervention effect. The parameter estimate is quite similar to that estimated in the adjusted but unmatched analysis (2.04). However, the benefit of the matching is apparent here, as the standard error in that analysis was 1.57, compared to 0.682 in the matched analysis.

Post Hoc Stratification

The MHHP investigators had *a priori* interest in stratum-specific intervention effects based on age, gender, and educational attainment. Even though their

Table 7.53. Estimate for (I1-I0)-(C1-C0) From the Adjusted Analysis of Diastolic Blood Pressure in the Pretest-Posttest Control Group Design With *A Priori* Matching

Parameter	Estimate	SE	DDF	T
(I1-I0)-(C1-C0)	2.00471	0.68244	2	2.94
	$Pr > \lvert T \rvert$	Alpha	Lower	Upper
	0.0990	0.05	-0.9316	4.9410

interest was *a priori,* communities could not easily be stratified on these factors prior to randomization, nor were there enough communities included in
the MHHP design to permit *a priori* stratification. As a result, the MHHP
investigators employed *post hoc* stratification on these factors as a part of their
primary analysis (Luepker et al., 1994).

Implementation for Gaussian Data

To implement the time × condition analysis with *post hoc* stratification on
sex, the code shown in Table 7.54 is appropriate.

Three fixed-effect interactions involving `sex` must be included in the
`model` statement, along with the main effect of `sex`, which was already
there. The three-way interaction is the term of interest in the stratified analysis.

Two random-effect interactions must be added to the `random` statement.
The nesting structure in the code reflects the nesting structure of the model for
the *post hoc* stratified analysis.

The *ddf* for each fixed effect are computed based on the formulae shown in
the table of expected mean squares, Table 5.8. The *ddf* for `cond` are $c(g-1)$
$-x_g$, here $2(3-1)-0=4$. The *ddf* for `sex` and for `cond*sex` are $c(g-1)$
$(s-1)-x_g$ here $2(3-1)(2-1)-0=4$. The *ddf* for `time` and `time*cond` are
$(t-1)c(g-1)-x_g$ here $(2-1)2(3-1)-0=4$. The *ddf* for `sex*time` and `cond`
`*sex*time` are $(t-1)c(g-1)(s-1)-x_g$, here $(2-1)2(3-1)(2-1)-0=4$. With additional strata or time intervals, these *ddf* will vary among the fixed effects.

The `lsmeans` effect is `cond*sex*time`, to provide the means that define the null hypothesis in this analysis. The `slice=` option cannot be used
to provide tests of simple interactions or simple main effects, because the
`lsmeans` effect is a three-way interaction. To ensure that the least-squares
means are computed based on the marginal distribution of the data, the `om`
option is included in the `lsmeans` statement.

Table 7.54. SAS PROC MIXED Code for the Adjusted Analysis of
Diastolic Blood Pressure in the Pretest-Posttest Control Group
Design With *Post Hoc* Stratification

```
proc mixed info order=internal;
  class cond group time sex educlvl bpobsrvr bplocatn;
  model dbp=cond sex cond*sex time cond*time sex*time
    cond*sex*time age educlvl bpobsrvr bplocatn
    /ddf=4,4,4,4,4,4,4 ddfm=res;
  random int sex time sex*time/subject=group(cond);
  lsmeans cond*sex*time/om cl e;
  estimate '(I1-I0)-(C1-C0) (m-w)'
    cond*sex*time 1 -1 -1 1 -1 1 1 -1/cl e;
run;
```

The estimate statement is complex in this analysis because the intervention effect is complex. It is a difference between two net differences and so involves 8 means. That requires 8 coefficients for the levels of the cond *sex*time interaction. The proper values for the coefficients are best determined by examination of the coefficients employed to construct the least-squares means.

The stratified analysis is a much more complex analysis, as is clear from the dimensions table (not shown). There are now 67 columns in the fixed-effects design matrix (2 each for cond, sex, and time; 1 each for the intercept and age; 4 each for cond*sex, cond*time, and sex*time; 3 for bplocatn; 8 each for cond*sex*time and educlvl; and 28 for bpobsrvr). There are now 54 columns in the random-effects design matrix (6 for group(cond), 12 each for sex*group(cond) and time*group(cond), and 24 for sex*time*group(cond)). Even so, the analysis converged after 4 iterations (not shown).

Table 7.55 presents the covariance-parameter estimates. Given 3936 observations and $g=3$ groups in each of $c=2$ conditions observed at each of $t=2$ time intervals and $s=2$ strata, the average $m=164$. Using these values, the mean squares are estimated in Table 7.56.

The estimated for $MS_{tgs:c}$ is considerably reduced compared to the unstratified analysis. However, it must be combined with a larger numerator and smaller denominator. As a result, the standard error for the intervention effect in this analysis is estimated using Equation 5.22 and is the largest of those estimated in this chapter:

$$\hat{\sigma}_\Delta = \sqrt{2*2*2\left(\frac{\hat{MS}_{tgs:c}}{mg}\right)} = \sqrt{2*2*2\left(\frac{349}{164*3}\right)} = 2.38$$

The *ICC* of interest in this analysis is the adjusted $ICC_{m:tgs:c}$:

Table 7.55. Covariance-Parameter Estimates (REML) From the Adjusted Analysis of Diastolic Blood Pressure in the Pretest-Posttest Control Group Design With *Post Hoc* Stratification

Cov Parm	Estimate
INTERCEPT	4.12600
SEX	0.03309
TIME	0.64841
TIME*SEX	1.51982
Residual	100.45989

Table 7.56. Selected Mean-Square Estimates for the Adjusted Analysis of Diastolic Blood Pressure in the Pretest-Posttest Control Group Design With *Post Hoc* Stratification

Source	E(MS)	Estimate
TGS:C	$\sigma_e^2 + m\sigma_{tgs:c}^2$	$100 + 164*1.52 = 349$
Member:TGS:C	σ_e^2	100

$$I\hat{C}C_{m:tgs:c} = \frac{\hat{\sigma}_{tgs:c}^2}{\hat{\sigma}_e^2 + \hat{\sigma}_{tgs:c}^2} = \frac{1.52}{100 + 1.52} = 0.0150$$

The adjusted $VIF_{m:tgs:c}$ is estimated as

$$V\hat{I}F_{m:tgs:c} = \left(1 + (m-1)I\hat{C}C_{m:tgs:c}\right) = \left(1 + (164-1)0.0150\right) = 3.45$$

The tests of fixed effects (not shown) provided no evidence to reject the null hypotheses of homogeneity of the intervention effect across the two strata. Given that result, the investigator and analyst would move back to the unstratified analysis.

Table 7.57 provides the desired contrast between men and women in terms of net change over time in diastolic blood pressure. The result of 0.065 indicates that the net change was 0.065 mm Hg larger in men than women. Relative to a standard error of 2.41, that change was trivial.

Additional Baseline or Follow-up Intervals

The full MHHP design involved 2–4 baseline observations on each community, plus 4–5 observations on those same communities after the intervention

Table 7.57. Estimate for (I1-I0)-(C1-C0) (m-w) from the Adjusted Analysis of Diastolic Blood Pressure in the Pretest-Posttest Control Group Design With *Post Hoc* Stratification

Parameter	Estimate	SE	DDF	T
(I1-I0)-(C1-C0)	0.06516	2.40579	4	0.03
	Pr>|T|	Alpha	Lower	Upper
	0.9797	0.05	−6.6144	6.7447

program was introduced. This section illustrates analyses appropriate for nested cross-sectional designs involving additional baseline or follow-up intervals.

Analyses for Extended Designs are less developed than for the simpler Pretest-Posttest Control Group Design; readers should keep that in mind as they study the material in this section. There is much room for additional research to develop the methods presented in this section further, as well as to develop new methods.

The Traditional Mixed-Model ANOVA/ANCOVA

Chapter 5 noted two weaknesses in the traditional mixed-model ANOVA/ ANCOVA as applied to data from an Extended Design. First, when more than two time intervals are included in the design, the assumption that each group in a condition shares a common time slope may not be appropriate. Second, this analysis has less power for a predictable intervention effect than its alternatives because it casts a very broad net in the estimation of the intervention effect.

Given these considerations, this section illustrates the traditional mixed-model ANOVA/ANCOVA in the full MHHP cross-sectional data set, but only in a limited fashion. In particular, this section illustrates the definition of time, the computation of *ddf* for fixed effects, and the MIXED code for this analysis, but does not include any examples.

Defining Time

Figure 7.1 reflects the staggered start of intervention in the three MHHP intervention communities. That staggered start made it impossible to use calendar year as the index for time and suggested that time be measured from the pair-specific start of the intervention program. Because that start occurred just after the last baseline survey, the investigators defined the end of the last baseline survey as Time 0. Prior surveys were designated with negative numbers and subsequent surveys with positive numbers, where each number reflected the number of years prior to or following that Time 0 survey (Luepker et al., 1994).

Because it will be instructive to consider alternative representations for time, this presentation does not follow exactly the scheme employed by the MHHP investigators in their published analysis. Readers should understand, however, that the alternative schemes presented here are offered for pedagogical purposes only.

Alternative representations of time are possible because the survey date was recorded for each participant. As a result, it is possible to calculate the length of time between the survey date and the intervention start-up date. That measure can be computed in days, weeks, months, or years, with negative values for baseline surveys and positive values for intervention surveys. Under this coding scheme, members surveyed on the day the intervention began in a given pair are assigned a zero.

Categorization of this continuous time variable provides new variables scaled in terms of years (10 levels, -2 to $+7$), months (71 levels, -34 to $+83$), and weeks (222 levels, -148 to $+358$). With more than 17,000 observations in the cross-sectional data set, most of these levels have many observations, though there are also cells that are empty and a few that have only one observation.[25]

ddf for Fixed Effects

Chapter 5 includes a discussion on the calculation of *ddf* for fixed effects in the context of an Extended Design. To accurately determine the *ddf*, the investigator should create the multidimensional matrix defined by the number of groups per condition, and the number of times, conditions, and *post hoc* strata, if any. The investigator can then determine the number of cells in that matrix that have more than one observation. That figure represents the total *df* available at the group level. The *df* not allocated to other sources are available as the *ddf* for the intervention effect.

Absent *post hoc* stratification, the matrix is created simply by crossing group with time. To illustrate, the cross-tabulation for year $\times$ community for the MHHP data is shown in Table 7.58. Year has 10 levels and there are six communities, so that the upper limit on the group-level *df* is $10*6 = 60$; 10 of the cells have 1 or 0 observations, reducing the total *df* to 50.

Table 7.59 presents the partition of the *df* for the traditional mixed-model ANOVA/ANCOVA when time is scaled in years. One *df* is allocated for the intercept and another for condition ($c - 1 = 1$). Four are allocated for group (condition). Nine each are allocated for time and condition $\times$ time. Those *df* sum to 24; assuming that there are no group-level covariates, there are 26 *df* available for *TG:C*, the residual error at the group level. Note that the formula for $df_{tg:c} = (t-1)c(g-1) = 32$, which is larger than 26. This can and does happen, and the analyst has no choice, of course, but to work with the smaller number.

To further illustrate this point, consider the same analysis for the month and week time intervals, also presented in Table 7.59. In each case, a categorical representation of time in the fixed effects exhausts the total *df* at the group level, leaving no *df* for the group-level error term. As a result, the traditional mixed-model ANOVA/ANCOVA cannot be conducted at the level of the month or week if time is treated as a categorical variable.

Table 7.58. Cross-Tabulation of Survey Year and Community in the Minnesota Heart Health Program Cross-Sectional Data

Year			Community				
	M	W	F/M	SF	B	R	Total
−2	0	0	283	499	532	518	1832
−1	0	0	410	328	285	290	1313
0	879	452	335	293	304	283	2546
1	396	492	290	298	298	306	2080
2	490	305	46	0	267	273	1381
3	292	487	309	457	48	0	1593
4	66	304	173	33	326	458	1360
5	407	0	360	471	1	0	1239
6	537	494	229	476	483	476	2695
7	45	495	381	0	446	429	1796
Total	3112	3029	2816	2855	2990	3033	17,835

Implementation for Gaussian Data.

The SAS PROC MIXED code for this analysis is presented in Table 7.60. The code is similar to that for the time $\times$ condition analysis in the Pretest-Posttest Control Group Design (cf. Table 7.46). It substitutes `year` for the more generic `time`. It specifies *ddf* for the first three fixed effects based on the partition of the 50 total *df* available at the group level as shown in Table 7.59. In particular, the *ddf* for `cond` are computed as $c(g-1) = 2(3-1) = 4$. The *ddf* for `year` and `cond*year` are the residual *df* available at the group level, 26.

Note that the code does not include either an `lsmeans` statement or an

Table 7.59. Partition of the *df* for the Mixed-Model ANOVA/ANCOVA When Time is Scaled in Years, Months, and Weeks

Source	df	Year	Month	Week
Intercept	1	1	1	1
Condition	$c-1$	1	1	1
Group:C	$c(g-1)-x_g$	4	4	4
Time	$t-1$	9	70	221
TC	$(t-1)(c-1)$	9	—	—
TG:C	$(t-1)c(g-1)-x_g$	26	—	—
Total	tgc	50	119	315

Table 7.60. SAS PROC MIXED Code for the Mixed-Model ANCOVA of Diastolic Blood Pressure in the Extended Design

```
proc mixed info order=internal;
  class cond group year sex educlvl bpobsrvr bplocatn;
  model dbp=cond year cond*year age sex educlvl bpobsrvr
    bplocatn/ ddfm=res ddf=4,26,26;
  random int year/subject=group(cond);
run;
```

estimate statement. Given 10 time intervals and 2 conditions, there would be 20 least-squares means. They can be requested using the familiar lsmeans statement, but would be difficult to interpret due to their number. An estimate statement can help considerably here, as it directs the program to compute an estimate of a specific intervention effect and a standard error for that effect. This often is a more profitable course than simply requesting all possible least-squares means.

Trend Analysis in the Mixed-Model ANOVA/ANCOVA

Coding Time as a Continuous Variable

Having defined time in terms of years, months, and weeks from the introduction of the intervention program, those variables may be used to treat time as a continuous variable. All three measures are scaled in real time and each has an appropriate zero point.

Specifying an Intervention Pattern

Chapter 5 specified an intervention pattern for the MHHP in the context of the Extended Design. Time is treated as a continuous variable with linear and quadratic components. The secular trend is constructed using all the non-intervention observations, pooling data from the intervention and comparison communities. The intervention effect is modeled as a departure from the secular trend, also with linear and quadratic components. That model can be applied whether time is scaled in years, months, or weeks.

ddf for Fixed Effects

As noted in Table 7.59, the total *df* at the level of the group for these three levels of time were 50, 119, and 315. The partition of these *df* for trend analysis is shown in Table 7.61.

Table 7.61. Partition of the *df* for the Trend Analysis in the Extended Design When Time is Scaled in Years, Months, and Weeks

Source	Generic	Year	Month	Week
Intercept	1	1	1	1
Condition	$c-1$	1	1	1
Group:Condition	$c(g-1)$	4	4	4
Time	1	1	1	1
Time × Time	1	1	1	1
Time × Condition	$c-1$	1	1	1
Time × Time × Condition	$c-1$	1	1	1
Time × Group:Condition	res_{tgc}	40	109	305
Total	tgc	50	119	315

Because the total *df* at the group level in this analysis depends on the number of time intervals, the total *df* increases dramatically as the number of time intervals increases. Because the representation of the first seven effects is identical in each of the three analyses except for the time scale, their *df* are identical, and so the *df* available for the time × condition(group) term benefits directly from the additional time intervals.

Implementation for Gaussian Data

Prior to the MIXED code, a data step must be used to define the intervention effect and other variables specified in the model. The code for the analysis with time scaled in years is shown in Table 7.62.

The `yearcat` variable is set equal to `year` so that time can be represented as a categorical variable in the `random` statement. A quadratic term for time, `year2`, is also defined. The if/else statement creates a new variable, `iyear`, set equal to `year` for observations in the intervention condition (`cond=0`) after the baseline period and set equal to zero for all other observations. As

Table 7.62. SAS Code to Define the Intervention Effect and Other Variables for the Trend Analysis in the Extended Design

```
data cross;
  yearcat=year;
  year2=year*year;
  if year>0 and cond=0 then iyear=year;
  else iyear=o;
  iyear2=iyear*iyear;
run;
```

such, this term is a variant on the usual time × condition interaction, constrained to zero during the baseline period and linear thereafter.

The SAS PROC MIXED code for this analysis for diastolic blood pressure is shown in Table 7.63. The term `year` is defined as a continuous variable by leaving it out of the `class` statement. The quadratic term is included as `year2`. This combination of statements defines a common secular trend, with linear and quadratic components. The regression coefficients for these components are reported because the `solution` option is included in the `model` statement. Separate intercepts for the secular trend are allowed for the two conditions by putting `cond` into the `model` statement.

The term `iyear` is also defined as a continuous variable by leaving it out of the `class` statement. The quadratic term is included as `iyear2`. This combination of statements defines the intervention effect, with linear and quadratic components.

The *ddf* for `cond` are $c(g-1) = 4$ *df*. The *ddf* for `year`, `year2`, `iyear` and `iyear2` are the *ddf* left to res_{tgc}, here 40 *df*. The other variables in the `model` statement are covariates measured at the member level and so are tested against the residual *df* at that level via the `ddfm = res` option.

Note that `yearcat` is used in the `random` statement. This ensures that the *tgc* time × group surveys are represented as distinct entities so that the group-level error term is based on the variation among the time × group means.

Note that the `lsmeans` statement asks only for the adjusted means for condition. Those are of no interest in and of themselves, but by asking for them with the `e` option, the output will include the information needed to construct the `estimate` statements of interest, as shown below.

The code for the analyses by month and week is identical, except that `yearcat`, `year`, `year2`, `iyear`, and `iyear2` are replaced by terms for month or week, respectively. The *ddf* for the 2nd, 3rd, 4th, and 5th fixed effects listed in the `ddf =` option also change to 109 or 305.

Table 7.64 summarizes the dimensions for the three analyses. They differ

Table 7.63. SAS PROC MIXED Code for the Trend Analysis in the Extended Design

```
proc mixed info order = internal;
  class cond group yearcat sex educlvl bpobsrvr
    bplocatn;
  model dbp = cond year year2 iyear iyear2 age sex
    educlvl bpobsrvr bplocatn/ddf = 4,40,40,40,40 ddfm = res
    solution;
  random int yearcat/subject = group(cond);
  lsmeans cond/om e;
run;
```

Table 7.64. Dimensions of the Trend Analyses in the Extended
Design With Time Scaled in Years, Months, and Weeks

	Year	Month	Week
Covariance Parameters	3	3	3
Columns in X	101	101	101
Columns in Z	11	72	223
Subjects	6	6	6
Max Obs Per Subject	3090	3090	3090
Observations Used	17658	17658	17658
Observations Not Used	0	0	0
Total Observations	17658	17658	17658

only in the number of columns in the random-effects design matrix. This is
expected, because there is no difference in the fixed-effects structure among
the three analyses. The three analyses differ only in the time scale employed,
which translates into differences in the number of levels in the time*
group(cond) interaction, with more levels as time is more finely defined.
They also differ in the labels applied to represent time in the model statement.

The components of variance were of fairly similar magnitude across the
three analyses (Table 7.65). Prior to proceeding further with those estimates,
consideration should be given to the results in the model-fitting tables.

The model-fitting-information (Table 7.66), together with the dimensions of
the analyses, provide information to guide the selection of the best-fitting
model. In particular, the -2 REML Log Likelihood (-2 REML LL),
Schwarz's Bayesian Information Criterion (BIC), and Akaike's Information
Criterion (AIC) can be used to compare models.

The model that used monthly intervals resulted in the -2 REML LL, AIC,
and BIC values that were closest to zero. In general, a model with -2 REML
LL, AIC, or BIC values closer to zero is considered a better fit to the data. All
three of these criteria point to the model based on month as the best fitting of

Table 7.65. Covariance-Parameter Estimates (REML) From the
Trend Analyses in the Extended Design With Time Scaled in
Years, Months, and Weeks

Cov Parm	Year	Month	Week
INTERCEPT	0.13036	0.00000	0.18283
TIME	3.24351	3.26364	3.44319
Residual	102.28988	101.63493	101.25344

Table 7.66. Model-Fitting Information From the Trend Analyses in the Extended Design

Model Fitting Information	Year	Month	Week
−2 REML Log Likelihood	131623.2	131601.1	131682.9
Akaike's Information Criterion	−65814.6	−65803.5	−65844.4
Schwarz's Bayesian Criterion	−65826.3	−65815.2	−65856.1

the three. The three models can't be distinguished in terms of the number of observations or the number of parameters, as they are identical on both. They don't differ greatly on any of the three indicators in Table 7.66 either, but because all three indicators point toward the model based on month, only that model is pursued further.

A second inspection of the covariance-parameter estimates from the analysis by month indicates that the estimate for INTERCEPT was fixed at zero. Because the residual error captured 95% of the variation in the data, the analysis by month was rerun using the method=mivque0 and nobound options. The covariance-parameter estimates from that analysis are summarized in Table 7.67.

Given 17658 observations used in the analysis and distributed over $tgc = 119$ group × time surveys, the average $m = 148.4$ while $g = 3$ and the average $t = 19.83$. Using these values, the mean squares are estimated in Table 7.68.

Given 591.8 as the estimate of $MS_{tg:c}$, the standard error formula still requires an estimate for $\sigma_{e(tc)}^2$. For the quadratic component of the intervention effect, this is given in Chapter 9 as 75599. As a result, the standard error of the intervention effect is estimated using Equation 5.24:[26]

$$\hat{\sigma}_\Delta = \sqrt{\frac{\hat{MS}_{tg:c}}{\hat{\sigma}_{e(tc)}^2(mtgc - f - 1)}} = \sqrt{\frac{591.8}{75599(148.4*19.83*3*2* - 95 - 1)}}$$
$$= 0.000668$$

Table 7.67. Covariance-Parameter Estimates (MIVQUE(0)) From the Trend Analysis in the Extended Design With Time Scaled in Months

Cov Parm	Estimate
INTERCEPT	0.11482
MONCAT	3.30264
Residual	101.57511

Table 7.68. Selected Mean-Square Estimates for the Trend Analysis in the Extended Design With Time Scaled in Months

Source	E(MS)	Estimate
TG:C	$\sigma_e^2 + m\sigma_{tg:c}^2$	$101.6 + 148.4*3.303 = 591.8$
Member:TG:C	σ_e^2	101.6

The $ICC_{m:tg:c}$ is estimated as:

$$I\hat{C}C_{m:tg:c} = \frac{\hat{\sigma}_{tg:c}^2}{\hat{\sigma}_e^2 + \hat{\sigma}_{tg:c}^2} = \frac{3.303}{101.6 + 3.303} = 0.0315$$

The $VIF_{m:tg:c}$ is estimated as:

$$V\hat{I}F_{m:tg:c} = \left(1 + (m-1)I\hat{C}C_{m:tg:c}\right) = \left(1 + (148.4 - 1)(0.0315)\right) = 5.64$$

Table 7.69 presents the tests of fixed effects for the model based on months. The tests for the intervention effect, imonth and imonth2, provide evidence for a possible intervention effect, as the p-values are just larger than the nominal level.

The solution option was used to generate the regression coefficients for each of the terms in the model, including the two intervention-effect terms. Selected coefficients are shown in Table 7.70. The coefficients for the effects of interest are difficult to interpret given the quadratic terms. However, they

Table 7.69. Tests of Fixed Effects From the Trend Analysis in the Extended Design With Time Scaled in Months

Source	NDF	DDF	Type III F	Pr > F
COND	1	4	0.00	0.9644
MONTH	1	109	0.07	0.7926
MONTH2	1	109	1.17	0.2819
IMONTH	1	109	3.39	0.0682
IMONTH2	1	109	3.13	0.0798
AGE	1	18E3	382.31	0.0001
SEX	1	18E3	995.80	0.0001
EDUCLVL	7	18E3	3.71	0.0005
BPOBSRVR	79	18E3	3.94	0.0001
BPLOCATN	2	18E3	2.75	0.0642

Table 7.70. Fixed-Effect Regression Coefficients From the Trend Analysis in the Extended Design With Time Scaled in Months

Parameter	Estimate	SE	DDF	T	Pr>|T|
INTERCEPT	70.443390	3.726734	18E3	18.90	0.0001
COND I	−0.031923	0.673109	4	−0.05	0.9600
COND C	0.000000	.	.	.	.
MONTH	−0.003938	0.014942	109	−0.26	0.7926
MONTH2	−0.000280	0.000259	109	−1.08	0.2819
IMONTH	−0.088174	0.047869	109	−1.84	0.0682
IMONTH2	0.001172	0.000663	109	1.77	0.0798

Note: Coefficients for covariates are not shown.

can be used to estimate means for the study conditions at several time intervals over the course of the study, and a plot of those means will reflect the pattern over time. Note that the standard error for the IMONTH2 term is given as 0.000663, which is close to the earlier estimate of 0.000668.

Recall that an lsmeans statement was included in the analysis. The least-squares means themselves are of no particular interest, as they represent only the average diastolic blood pressure in each group over the full period of the study. However, the coefficients used to construct those means are valuable and the coefficients for many of the fixed effects are presented in Table 7.71. The two rows identified in the column headings of Table 7.71 refer to the rows in the least-squares means table in the output. As a result, Row 1 corresponds to the intervention condition and Row 2 corresponds to the control condition. The values listed for the rows are the sample means for continuous variables and sample fractions for categorical variables. The values in the two columns are the values applied to the regression coefficients to obtain the least-squares means for the intervention and control conditions, respectively.

Of interest are estimates of diastolic blood pressure for the two conditions at regular intervals over the course of the study as predicted by the model. Also of interest are the confidence bounds around the difference between the two conditions over time. These can be estimated in MIXED using the estimate statement together with the coefficients for the least-squares means.

Consider the mean for the intervention condition at the midpoint of the intervention period. The midpoint occurred at about 36 months. As a result, the estimate coefficient for month is set at 36, while that for month2 is set at 36*36 = 1296. All mean values include the intercept, so the estimate coefficient for the intercept is 1. The desired mean is for the average level on all covariates, so the values in Table 7.71, plus those for bpobsrvr, are used as the estimate coefficients for the covariates. The desired mean is for

Table 7.71. Coefficients Used to Estimate the Least-Squares Means for Condition From the Trend Analysis in the Extended Design With Time Scaled in Months

Parameter	Row 1 COND I	Row 2 COND C
INTERCEPT	1	1
COND I	1	0
COND C	0	1
MONTH	23.912334	23.912334
MONTH2	1809.865896	1809.865896
IMONTH	14.479442	14.479442
IMONTH2	841.129573	841.129573
AGE	44.974006	44.974006
SEX FEMALE	0.535507	0.535507
SEX MALE	0.464492	0.464492
EDUCLVL <7TH GRADE	0.005493	0.005493
EDUCLVL 7TH-9TH GRADE	0.063257	0.063257
EDUCLVL 10-11TH GRADE	0.044908	0.044908
EDUCLVL HS GRADUATE	0.291086	0.291086
EDUCLVL VOCAT/BUSINESS	0.111564	0.111564
EDUCLVL SOME COLL.	0.199569	0.199569
EDUCLVL COLL.GRAD.	0.195322	0.195322
EDUCLVL POST.GRAD.	0.088798	0.088798
BPLOCATN CLINIC	0.945633	0.945633
BPLOCATN HOME	0.052893	0.052893
BPLOCATN OTHER	0.001472	0.001472

Note: Coefficients for bpobsrvr are not shown.

the intervention condition, so the estimate coefficient for COND I is 1 and for COND C is 0. The estimate coefficients for IMONTH and IMONTH2 are 36 and 1296. Table 7.72 presents the code for the estimate for the mean in the intervention condition 36 months after the introduction of the intervention program.

The values listed in the estimate statement for a variable from the class statement must be in the same order as the levels for that variable so that they are applied to the proper regression coefficient. This is another benefit of using the solution option in the model statement or the lsmeans statement, as the order of the levels of each variable from the class statement is given in the output generated by those statements. It is easy to confirm that the proper coefficients have been assigned by examining the results generated by the e option in the estimate statement (not shown).

Table 7.72. SAS PROC MIXED Code to Estimate the Intervention Condition
Mean at +36 Months of Intervention

```
estimate 'I  at +36 Months'
  month 36 month2 1296
  intercept 1 age 44.974 sex 0.5355 0.4645
  educlvl  0.0055 0.0633 0.0449 0.2911 0.1116 0.1996 0.1953 0.0888
  bpobsrvr 0.0459 0.0334 0.0477 0.0351 0.0484 0.0651 0.0130 0.0416
           0.0001 0.0127 0.0174 0.0001 0.0008 0.0553 0.0001 0.0001
           0.0001 0.0001 0.0241 0.0008 0.0029 0.0018 0.0251 0.0213
           0.0019 0.0024 0.0070 0.0001 0.0324 0.0273 0.0026 0.0180
           0.0001 0.0001 0.0001 0.0251 0.0112 0.0007 0.0374 0.0144
           0.0163 0.0001 0.0132 0.0003 0.0002 0.0001 0.0002 0.0002
           0.0001 0.0001 0.0108 0.0001 0.0001 0.0887 0.0180 0.0209
           0.0001 0.0190 0.0157 0.0011 0.0017 0.0003 0.0003 0.0047
           0.0001 0.0001 0.0001 0.0001 0.0096 0.0001 0.0396 0.0177
           0.0007 0.0377 0.0016 0.0026 0.0020 0.0002 0.0016 0.0006
  bplocatn 0.9456 0.0529 0.0015
  imonth 36 imonth2 1296 cond 1 0;
```

The order of the variables in the estimate statement has no effect on the computation of the estimate. However, that order does determine the *ddf* for the estimate and therefore affects its *p*-value and confidence limits. MIXED assigns as the *ddf* for the estimate the *ddf* associated with the last variable in the estimate statement. In this example, the *ddf* for the estimate are the *ddf* for cond, as is appropriate.

To construct the mean in the control condition after 36 months of intervention, a similar estimate statement is used (not shown). This statement differs from that for the intervention condition only in the values assigned to cond (now cond 0 1 instead of cond 1 0) and in the values assigned to imonth and imonth2 (now 0 and 0 instead of 36 and 1296).

The difference of interest in MHHP and any other group-randomized trial based on such an Extended Design is the difference between the slopes estimated for the conditions. That difference is estimated using a third estimate statement:

```
estimate 'I-C at 36 months'
  imonth +36 imonth2 1296/e cl;
```

In this case, the contrast of interest is given in terms of the regression coefficients for the interaction terms imonth and imonth2 alone. It represents the difference between the two conditions 36 months after the introduction of the intervention condition, computed as though the conditions had the same distribution on all covariates and as if they had the same *y*-intercept. The results of all three estimate statements are shown in Table 7.73.

Table 7.73. Estimates at +36 Months From the Trend Analysis in the Mixed-Model ANCOVA of Diastolic Blood Pressure in the Extended Design With Time Scaled in Months

Parameter	Estimate	SE	DDF	T	Pr>|T|
I at +36 Months	73.328	0.5882	4	124.65	0.0001
C at +36 Months	75.015	0.4512	4	166.26	0.0001
I-C at +36 Months	−1.654	0.9326	109	−1.77	0.0789

Parameter			Alpha	Lower	Upper
I at +36 Months			0.05	71.695	74.962
C at +36 Months			0.05	73.762	76.267
I-C at +36 Months			0.05	−3.503	0.194

Through a series of such estimate statements, the means for the control condition were estimated at 12-month intervals. The means for the intervention condition, after subtracting out the difference in y-intercepts, were computed by adding the $I-C$ difference to the control-condition mean. The confidence bounds around the $I-C$ differences were taken directly from the results of the $I-C$ estimate statements. The results from those statements are plotted in Figure 7.2.

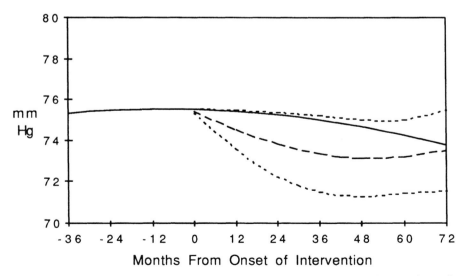

Figure 7.2. Predicted diastolic blood pressure in the intervention and control conditions, together with 95% confidence bounds on their difference, based on the trend analysis in the Extended Design.

This figure makes it easy to see that there was a downward trend in the control condition, after a very slight increase during the baseline period. It also makes it easy to see that there was a temporary acceleration of that downward trend in the intervention condition before the two conditions converged at the end of the study. Both the `imonth` and `imonth2` F-tests were at about the nominal level (p about 0.05), and the confidence bounds on the $I - C$ difference are consistent with those tests. The upper confidence bound is so close in value to the secular trend that it can barely be distinguished in the figure during the first two years of the intervention program. However, by the end of the study, the intervention effect had waned and the control condition had caught up, such that the curves for the two conditions came back together and the confidence bounds on the intervention effect clearly included the secular trend. This figure is consistent with that published in the original report by Luepker et al. (1994).

The Random-Coefficients Analysis

The random-coefficients model presented in Chapter 5 assumed that the condition and group mean slopes were strictly linear. Such a model is plausible for a design with a single baseline survey in each group. Indeed, that is exactly the model presumed in the REACT study, described in Chapter 1 and revisited in Chapter 10. Such a model also might be appropriate for the MHHP data, but only if the multiple baseline surveys were collapsed into a single baseline or if the analysis was restricted to data from just one of the baseline surveys plus any follow-up surveys.

In the context of the entire MHHP data set, that linear random-coefficients model is not appropriate. Given multiple baseline surveys in each condition, the investigators would expect at least one discontinuity in the mean slope for the intervention condition. It is also plausible that a second discontinuity might exist, especially if an initial intervention effect decayed over time.

This section presents results for two random-coefficients models applied to the MHHP data. The first is the linear model presented in Chapter 5, for it has wide application in designs that have a single baseline and multiple follow-up surveys. The second is patterned after the quadratic-trend analysis in the mixed-model ANCOVA presented in the previous section. It illustrates a more complex random-coefficients model that is applicable when there are multiple baseline and follow-up surveys. Both analyses are implemented with time scaled in months.

Linear Random-Coefficients Model

This model is appropriate when the investigator expects a linear slope in each group and wants to know whether the average linear slope is the same across the conditions. The linear model allows no change in slope in any group at any time. As a result, the MHHP observations prior to the last baseline survey were excluded from this analysis. The null hypothesis is that there is no difference in the average linear slopes estimated in the two conditions beginning at the last baseline survey.

To implement this analysis for diastolic blood pressure, the code shown in Table 7.74 is appropriate.

The method = mivque0 option is included in the proc mixed statement in anticipation that the variance components other than residual error will be small and in recognition of the fact that the data set is large. MIVQUE(0) estimation is much faster than either REML or ML whenever the data set is large or the problem is complex. As noted earlier, MIVQUE(0) estimators are valid as long as the residual error accounts for at least 90% of the variance (Swallow and Monahan, 1984).

The ddf = option is used to set the *ddf* for the first three fixed effects at 4, consistent with the formulae in the table of expected mean squares for this analysis (Table 5.10). Those formulae gave $c(g-1)$ as the *ddf* for the tests of cond, time, and cond*time. In this example, the generic time is replaced by month and the generic cond*time is replaced by imonth.

The intercept estimates the *y*-intercept in the control condition and cond estimates the difference between the *y*-intercepts for the two conditions. Month estimates the time trend in the control condition. Imonth is set equal to month for all observations in the intervention condition and to zero for all observations in the control condition; as a result, imonth estimates any difference in time trend between the intervention and control conditions.

The random statement structures the random-coefficients part of the analysis. The int and month terms provide different intercepts and slopes for each group, while the type = un allows them to covary.

Table 7.74. SAS PROC MIXED Code for the Linear Random-Coefficients Analysis of Diastolic Blood Pressure in the Extended Design

```
proc mixed info order = internal method = mivque0;
  class cond group sex educlvl bpobsrvr bplocatn;
  model dbp = cond month imonth age sex educlvl
    bpobsrvr bplocatn/ddf = 4,4,4 ddfm = res solution;
  random int month/subject = group(cond) type = un;
run;
```

Table 7.75. Covariance-Parameter Estimates (MIVQUE(0)) From the Linear Random-Coefficients Analysis of Diastolic Blood Pressure in the Extended Design With Time Scaled in Months

Cov Parm		Estimate
INTERCEPT UN(1,1)		5.29087938
UN(2,1)		−0.10226163
UN(2,2)		0.00198817
Residual		101.87119326

As seen in Table 7.75, the covariance parameters other than residual error were small. Residual error accounted for 94% of the variation in the data, confirming the appropriate use of the method=mivque0 option.

Given 12,945 observations in $tgc=86$ group × time surveys, the average $m=150.5$, while $g=3$ and the average $t=14.33$. From Chapter 9, the remaining parameter, $\sigma^2_{e(t)}$, is estimated as 162.0. Using these values, the mean squares are estimated in Table 7.76.

Given 0.00230 as the estimate of $MS_{t(quad)g:c}$, the standard error of the intervention effect is estimated using Equation 5.26:[27]

$$\hat{\sigma}_\Delta = \sqrt{2\left(\frac{\hat{MS}_{t(\text{lin})g:c}}{g}\right)} = \sqrt{2\left(\frac{0.00230}{3}\right)} = 0.0392$$

The solution option was used to generate the regression coefficients for each of the fixed effects in the model, including the intervention effect. The coefficient for month was −0.026, indicating a change per month of −0.026

Table 7.76. Selected Mean-Square Estimates for the Linear Random-Coefficients Analysis of Diastolic Blood Pressure in the Extended Design With Time Scaled in Months

Source	E(MS)
$T(\text{lin})G:C$	$\dfrac{\sigma^2_{e(y)}}{\sigma^2_{e(t)}(mt-f-1)} + \sigma^2_{t(\text{lin})g:c}$
$M:TG:C$	$\sigma^2_{e(t)}$

Source	Estimate
$T(\text{lin})G:C$	$\dfrac{102}{162(150.5*14.33-93-1)} + 0.00199 = 0.00230$
$M:TG:C$	102

Table 7.77. Tests of Fixed Effects From the Linear Random-Coefficients Analysis of Diastolic Blood Pressure in the Extended Design With Time Scaled in Months

Source	NDF	DDF	Type III F	Pr > F
COND	1	4	0.30	0.6125
MONTH	1	4	0.95	0.3844
IMONTH	1	4	0.05	0.8305
AGE	1	13E3	231.06	0.0001
SEX	1	13E3	664.17	0.0001
EDUCLVL	7	13E3	2.15	0.0358
BPOBSRVR	63	13E3	4.44	0.0001
BPLOCATN	2	13E3	1.97	0.1393

mm Hg in the control condition from the last baseline survey until the end of the study. The coefficient for IMONTH was +0.00847, indicating that the average decline was not as negative in the intervention condition. The mean change per month in diastolic blood pressure in the intervention condition is estimated as $(-0.0260 + 0.00847) = -0.0175$ mm Hg. The standard error for the IMONTH term was reported as 0.0371, which is in good agreement with value estimated from the variance components above.

Table 7.77 presents the F-tests for the fixed effects. The test for IMONTH was not significant and so provides no basis to reject the null hypothesis of no difference in the mean linear slopes between the two conditions.

These results are substantially consistent with the pattern seen in the trend analysis. They are based on the data collected after the last baseline, and so represent the time period -2 to 72 months. The trend analysis fit quadratic slopes to that period, where this analysis fit linear slopes. Given that the two conditions began at about the same mean level of diastolic blood pressure at -2 months, gradually diverged, but converged again at 72 months, it is not surprising that linear-trends fit to the same data would be so similar.[28]

Having examined the results from the linear random-coefficients analysis, it is of interest to determine whether there is evidence that the group-specific slopes are in fact heterogeneous. One approach to assessing the heterogeneity in the group-specific slopes is to compare the model-fitting criteria in the random-coefficients analysis to those in a parallel analysis that omits the random slopes and their covariances. The code for the reduced model is shown in Table 7.78.

The revised code deletes month and the type = un option from the first random statement. That eliminates both the component of variance for linear slopes and the covariance between the slope and the intercept.

Table 7.78. SAS PROC MIXED Code for a Reduced Model Patterned After the Linear Random-Coefficients Model

```
proc mixed info order=internal method=mivque0;
  class cond group sex educlvl bpobsrvr bplocatn;
  model dbp=cond month imonth age sex educlvl
    bpobsrvr bplocatn/ddf=4,4,4 ddfm=res solution;
  random int/subject=group(cond);
run;
```

Table 7.79 presents the model-fitting information from the random-coefficients model and from the reduced model. The random-coefficients analysis had values for the -2 REML Log Likelihood, AIC, and BIC that were closer to zero. All three of these criteria point toward the random-coefficients analysis as the better fitting of the two.

Another approach to assessing the heterogeneity in the group-specific slopes is to compute an LR chi-square test comparing the two models that differ only in the components related to the heterogeneity of the group-specific slopes. In this case, the two models are those represented in Table 7.79. Those models differ by 2 covariance parameters, and so the LR chi-square test has 2 *df*. However, its interpretation is complicated by the fact that the null hypothesis for the covariance is two-tailed and the null hypothesis for the slope component of variance is one-tailed. As a result, evaluation of the 2 *df* LR chi-square with the usual *p*-value is somewhat conservative. That LR chi-square is 98.03 and is highly significant, indicating that one of the two covariance parameters is nonzero and that the random-coefficients model fits the data better than does the reduced model.[29]

One problem with these approaches to assessing the heterogeneity of the group-specific slopes is that the reduced model makes no provision for within-group correlation over time. An alternative model would be the trend analysis in the mixed-model ANCOVA, which does allow for within-group correlation

Table 7.79 Model-Fitting Information From the Random-Coefficients Analysis of Diastolic Blood Pressure in the Extended Design and From a Reduced Model Fit to the Same Data

Description	Random-Coefficients Model	Reduced Model	Alternative Comparison Model
-2 REML Log Likelihood	96352.5	96450.5	96230.6
Akaike's Information Criterion	-48180.3	-48225.3	-48118.3
Schwarz's Bayesian Criterion	-48195.2	-48239.5	-48129.5

over time but not for heterogeneity among the group-specific slopes. The code for a model for linear trend in the ANCOVA is shown in Table 7.80.

In this code, the first `random` statement is changed by replacing `month` with `moncat`, as defined for the trend analysis in the mixed-model AN-COVA. This alternative model has four covariance parameters and allows within-group correlation over time but presumes that the group-specific slopes are homogeneous.

The model-fitting information from the alternative comparison model is also shown in Table 7.79. The alternative comparison model had values of the -2 REML Log Likelihood, AIC, and BIC that were the closest to zero of any of the three models under consideration in this section. Thus, all three of these criteria point toward the linear trend analysis, with four covariance parameters, as fitting the data better than either the random-coefficients analysis, with five covariance parameters, or the reduced model, with only three covariance parameters.[30]

Given this result, the investigator may choose to report the results of the linear trend analysis in the mixed-model ANCOVA, as there is good evidence that the ANCOVA model fits the data better than the linear random-coefficients model. However, where the evidence favors the random-coefficients model, the investigator should report the results based on that model.

Quadratic Random-Coefficients Model

The quadratic random-coefficients model allows some curvature in each group-specific pattern. Because the MHHP investigators expected a favorable change in the intervention communities relative to the control communities after the introduction of the intervention program, the quadratic model is more appropriate to the full MHHP design than is the linear model. The null hypothesis is that there is no difference in the average quadratic pattern between the two conditions.

In this analysis, `imonth` is set equal to `month` for observations from the intervention condition and to zero otherwise. Quadratic terms are defined as

Table 7.80. SAS PROC MIXED Code for an Alternative Comparison Model Patterned After the Trend Analysis

```
proc mixed info order=internal method=mivque0;
  class cond group moncat sex educlvl bpobsrvr
    bplocatn;
  model dbp=cond month imonth age sex educlvl
    bpobsrvr bplocatn/ddf=4,78,78 ddfm=res solution;
  random int moncat/subject=group(cond);
run;
```

Table 7.81. SAS PROC MIXED Code for the Quadratic Random-Coefficients Analysis of Diastolic Blood Pressure in the Extended Design With Time Scaled in Months

```
proc mixed info order=internal method=mivque0;
  class cond group sex educlvl bpobsrvr bplocatn;
  model dbp=cond month imonth month2 imonth2
    age sex educlvl bpobsrvr bplocatn
    /ddf=4,4,4,4,4 ddfm=res solution;
  random int month month2/subject=group(cond) type=un;
run;
```

month2 = month*month and imonth2 = imonth*imonth. Table 7.81 presents the code for the analysis of diastolic blood pressure.

This code includes the method=mivque0 option in the proc mixed statement, for the same reason as in the linear model.

To allow each group's slope to have some curvature, month2 is added to the random statement. To allow the mean slope estimated in the control condition to have some curvature, month2 is added to the model statement. To allow the mean slope in the intervention condition to have a different pattern, imonth and imonth2 are added to the model statement.

As seen in Table 7.82, the covariance parameters are small. Residual error accounted for >90% of the variation in the data, confirming the appropriateness of the MIVQUE(0) estimation.

The mean square for $T(\text{quad})G{:}C$ is identical to that shown in Chapter 5 for $T(\text{lin})G{:}C$, except that the second term in the mean square is the quadratic component of variance rather than the linear component. Given 17,658 observations in $tgc = 119$ group $\times$ time surveys, the average $m = 148.4$ while $g = 3$ and the average $t = 19.83$. The remaining parameter, $\sigma^2_{e(t)}$, is estimated as

Table 7.82. Covariance-Parameter Estimates (MIVQUE(0)) From the Quadratic Random-Coefficients Analysis of Diastolic Blood Pressure in the Extended Design With Time Scaled in Months

Cov Parm		Estimate
INTERCEPT	UN(1,1)	2.60652757
	UN(2,1)	−0.01234141
	UN(2,2)	0.00019589
	UN(3,1)	−0.00063889
	UN(3,2)	0.00000794
	UN(3,3)	0.00037150
Residual		103.73881866

Table 7.83. Selected Mean-Square Estimates for the Quadratic Random-Coefficients Analysis of Diastolic Blood Pressure in the Extended Design With Time Scaled in Months

Source	E(MS)
T(quad)G:C	$\dfrac{\sigma^2_{e(y)}}{\sigma^2_{e(t)}(mt-f-1)}+\sigma^2_{t(quad)g:c}$
M:TG:C	$\sigma^2_{e(y)}$

Source	Estimate
T(quad)G:C	$\dfrac{104}{181623(148.4*19.83-95-1)}+0.000372=0.0003722$
M:TG:C	104

181,623 (not shown). Using these values, the mean squares are estimated in Table 7.83.

Given 0.0003722 as the estimate of $MS_{t(quad)g:c}$, the standard error of the intervention effect is computed using Equation 5.26:

$$\hat{\sigma}_\Delta=\sqrt{2\left(\frac{\hat{MS}_{t(quad)g:c}}{g}\right)}=\sqrt{2\left(\frac{0.0003722}{3}\right)}=0.01575$$

Table 7.84 presents the regression coefficients for selected fixed effects in the model. The standard error for the IMONTH2 term was given as 0.01574, which is in good agreement with the value estimated from the variance components.

Table 7.84. Fixed-Effect Regression Coefficients From the Quadratic Random-Coefficients Analysis of Diastolic Blood Pressure in the Extended Design With Time Scaled in Months

Parameter	Estimate	SE	DDF	T	Pr>|T|
INTERCEPT	71.56128043	3.83696397	18E3	18.65	0.0001
COND I	-0.96330938	1.33754238	4	-0.72	0.5112
COND C	0.00000000	.	.	.	.
MONTH	-0.03048808	0.01205179	4	-2.53	0.0647
IMONTH	0.01462564	0.01578692	4	0.93	0.4067
MONTH2	0.00014672	0.01112891	4	0.01	0.9901
IMONTH2	-0.00010756	0.01573844	4	-0.01	0.9949

Table 7.85. Model-Fitting Information From the Quadratic Random-Coefficients Analysis and From the Quadratic Trend Analysis of Diastolic Blood Pressure in the Extended Design With Time Scaled in Months

Description	Random Coefficients	Trend Analysis
− 2 REML Log Likelihood	131856.4	131601.5
Akaike's Information Criterion	− 65935.2	− 65803.7
Schwarz's Bayesian Criterion	− 65962.4	− 65815.4

Neither IMONTH nor IMONTH2 had significant *t*-tests. As a result, there is no basis to reject the null hypothesis of no difference in the mean quadratic patterns between the two conditions over the course of the study.

Having examined the results from the random-coefficients analysis, it is of interest to determine whether the random-coefficients analysis is necessary. The model-fitting information from the random-coefficients analysis and from the trend analysis in the ANCOVA presented previously are shown in Table 7.85.

The ANCOVA analysis has values of the − 2 REML Log Likelihood, AIC, and BIC that were closest to zero. Thus, all three of these criteria point toward the trend analysis in the mixed-model ANCOVA as the better fitting of the two analyses. The three models cannot be distinguished in terms of the number of observations, as both were based on 17,658. However, the ANCOVA involves only 4 covariance parameters, while the random-coefficients analysis requires 8; thus, the principle of parsimony also favors the ANCOVA analysis.[31]

Given this result, the investigator may choose to report the results of the trend analysis in the mixed-model ANCOVA, as there is good evidence that the ANCOVA model fits the data better than does the quadratic random-coefficients model. However, where the evidence favors the random-coefficients analysis, the investigator should report the results of that analysis.

Summary

This chapter has presented examples of many of the analyses appropriate for group-randomized trials that employ a nested cross-sectional design. Several general points can be made in summary of the material in this chapter.

Even though they were not all presented, every analysis shown in this chapter for diastolic blood pressure was also run for smoking status. In each case, the results from the analysis performed using software based on the General Linear Mixed Model closely approximated those from the analysis performed using software based on the Generalized Linear Mixed Model. This pattern is consistent with the recent report by Hannan and Murray (1996) that analyses based on the two models gave equivalent Type I and II error rates in simulations involving a variety of conditions common to group-randomized trials. The Central Limit Theorem provides the basis for this result, as it gives expectation for means to be distributed Gaussian even for decidedly non-Gaussian data as long as there is a moderate number of observations per mean. Because analyses based on the General Linear Mixed Model are easier to perform and interpret, and because they are generally faster, they are preferred for analysis of data from most group-randomized trials, even when the outcome is dichotomous.

For most analyses involving variance components fixed at zero by default using REML estimation, reanalysis using the nobound option resulted in negative estimates and smaller p-values for the effects of interest. This finding is consistent with the recent report by Murray et al. (1996) that the non-negativity constraint common to programs based on ML and REML estimation dramatically deflated the Type I error rate and power for a group-randomized trial when the true *ICC* was small and estimated with limited degrees of freedom. This pattern also has important practical implications given the other challenges facing investigators involved in group-randomized trials. Analysts will not want to artificially reduce the power of their analysis through the acceptance of seemingly appropriate but harmful defaults in their software.

There was considerable variation in size of standard errors, even for the same data. That should come as no surprise to the analytically-inclined reader, as the relative efficiency of the underlying methods has been known for some time. Even so, the considerable variation among the standard errors should provoke investigators and analysts to consider the implications of their designs and analyses for their power to detect effects of interest. That issue is explored further in Chapter 9.

Many of the common analysis strategies used to improve the precision of the analysis operate somewhat differently in the context of mixed-model regression than in the more familiar context of fixed-effects regression. In particular, regression adjustment for covariates does not affect all components of variance in the same way. In each of the analyses presented in this chapter, the residual error was reduced following the regression adjustment for covariates, but other components of variance often increased. Investigators and analysts should be aware of this possibility and take care to use such procedures thoughtfully. This issue is addressed further in Chapter 9.

The analyses presented for Extended Designs included trend analysis in the mixed-model ANOVA/ANCOVA and random coefficients analyses, both linear and quadratic. Analyses for Extended Designs are less developed than those for the simpler Pretest-Posttest Control Group Design, and readers should keep that in mind as they study that material. There is much room for additional research to further develop those methods as well as to develop new methods.

The advent of modern mixed-model regression software allows tremendous flexibility in the analysis of data from a nested cross-sectional design. Though all the analyses presented in this chapter were conducted using SAS PROC MIXED and the GLIMMIX macro, that should not be viewed as an endorsement of those programs over their alternatives. There are now many programs available that are suitable for data from group-randomized trials. Most of the points made in this chapter apply regardless of the software employed. Every program has its own peculiarities and problems, and the user should guard against misuse and misinterpretation. There is no substitute for careful scrutiny of the results and thoughtful study of the defaults and assumptions.

Endnotes

1. The GLIMMIX macro is part of the sample library included with the SAS software. It is an experimental macro and so is not as well tested as other software provided by SAS. In addition, because of its experimental nature, the macro is still evolving, and the changes from version to version have been substantial. All GLIMMIX analyses reported in this book are based on the 06-APR-96 version of the macro. Previous versions have substantially different requirements in terms, of the code and provide substantially different output. The 06-APR-96 version is more flexible and provides output that is more like MIXED than did previous versions. It is available from the Technical Services Division at SAS. It is also available electronically. To obtain GLIMMIX via the World Wide Web, connect to http://www.sas.com/techsup/download/stat/. Select glimmix.sas and glimmixe.sas. The first file is the macro and includes documentation at the beginning of the file. The second file contains examples.

2. MIXED in SAS 6.11 offers four methods to estimate *ddf* (ddfm=residual, ddfm=contain, ddfm=betwithin, ddfm=satterth). The first three methods alternate as the default depending on the analysis specified by the user. Each of the defaults is accurate for the simplest of the designs for which it is the default, but each can give an erroneous result for more complex designs. The fourth method directs MIXED to use a Satterthwaite approximation to compute the *ddf* for the tests of fixed effects (Satterthwaite, 1946). This option provides a reasonable estimate of the *ddf* across a variety of designs, though at the cost of some additional computing time. However, experience has shown that even the Satterthwaite approximation does not always give a correct result. This is why the analyst is encouraged to compute the proper *ddf* whenever possible and to specify the proper *ddf* for each fixed effect in the ddf= option in the model statement.

3. The reduction in processing time accrues because the default method for computing *ddf* is invoked even if all fixed effects are included as effects in the ddf= option. The ddfm=res method is usually the fastest, and that is why it is suggested as a routine option even when all the fixed effects of interest are included as effects in the ddf= option.

4. If there are more than two levels of condition, multiple *t*-tests for pairwise differences will result in an inflated Type I error rate. For this situation, MIXED provides an ad-

just= option for the lsmeans statement, with support for the familiar Bonferroni, Scheffe, Dunnett, and Tukey multiple comparison procedures, among others. Additional details on the adjust= option are available in the SAS documentation (SAS Institute, Inc., 1996; Littell et al., 1996).

5. MIXED overparameterizes the model and so creates a term in the random- or fixed-effects design matrix for every level of each variable in the class statement.

6. There are several options that can be used to speed convergence, though the analyst must be cautious in their application. For example, the default criterion for the sweep operator is E-8; experience has shown that convergence can be improved by adding a singular = 0.000001 option in the model statement without appreciably affecting the parameter estimates. Similarly, the default Hessian criterion for convergence is E-8; experience has shown that convergence can be improved by adding a convh = 0.000001 option to the model statement without appreciably affecting the parameter estimates. Further easing of those criteria may result in poorly estimated parameters. Increasing the maximum number of iterations allowed, via the maxiter= option in the model statement, is not recommended for the same reason.

7. Note that this test is valid only for hierarchical models that differ only in their random effects or in the structure of those random effects. Where the investigator is interested in comparing hierarchical models that differ in their fixed effects, method=ml should be added to the proc mixed statement so that ML estimation is used instead of the default REML.

8. It is important to distinguish the two penalties identified by Cornfield (1978). The first penalty is attached to the variance inflation due to the within-group correlation. The degree of variance inflation is reflected in the magnitude of the *VIF*. When the *VIF* is small, the variance inflation penalty will be small. However, the second penalty may still exact a measurable price for the nested design, as it is attached to the *df* available to estimate the within-group correlation. Where those *df* are limited, there may be an appreciable penalty from the limited *df*, even if the *VIF* is small.

9. Depending on the computer system, the filename may also need to include the location of the GLIMMIX macro file.

10. As for MIXED, the singular= option in the model statement can be used to ease the sweep criterion. The convh= option in the procopt statement can be used to ease the Hessian criterion for convergence within a single call to MIXED. In addition, the converge= statement in the GLIMMIX code can be used to ease the convergence criterion across calls to MIXED. However, if these criteria are eased too much, the parameters may be poorly estimated. Increasing the number of iterations via the maxiter= option in the procopt= statement is not recommended for the same reason.

11. Because it is always faster than the REML or ML, MIVQUE(0) estimation is recommended as a first step whenever the data set is large or the model for the analysis is complex. If the residual error accounts for >90% of the variance, the analyst can use the results from the MIVQUE(0) analysis. If not, little has been lost, and the analyst can either proceed with REML or ML estimation, or perhaps modify the analysis based on the results from the MIVQUE(0) analysis.

12. As documented by Kish (1965), point estimates such as means are unaffected by intraclass correlation, whether positive or negative.

13. Deviance and scaled deviance statistics are not helpful as goodness-of-fit statistics when the number of cells in the multidimensional matrix defined by the terms in the model is large relative to the number of observations per cell. This is often the case in analyses applied to member-level data in large data sets and is true of most of the analyses reported

in this book. This is simply another reason for caution in the interpretation of the deviance and scaled deviance statistics provided by the GLIMMIX macro in the analyses reported here.

14. The same problem exists for the related `estimate` and `contrast` statements, discussed later in this chapter.

15. Readers should understand that the equivalence of the MIXED and GLIMMIX results is due to the Central Limit Theorem as it operates in group-randomized trials. The two approaches may not give equivalent results for other study designs; in those cases, GLIMMIX is preferred over MIXED.

16. The dependent variable used in these analyses, `dbp`, was adjusted for seasonal trend and cuff size in a preliminary data step. As a result, all analyses of `dbp` are adjusted for seasonal trend and cuff size, including those described as unadjusted.

17. The order of the *ddf* specified in the `ddf=` option must be the same as the order of the fixed effects in the `model` statement. If not, the *ddf* will not be assigned correctly.

18. For example, if another variable in the `class` statement is nested within the levels of the offending variable in the `class` statement, the offending variable can't be removed from the `class` statement, and there is no way to compute adjusted means based on the observed marginal distribution.

19. In spite of the considerable progress represented by the `om` option, there are some problems with its implementation in SAS 6.11. For example, if least-squares means are requested for a variable that is involved in an interaction, use of the `om` option will result in a message that those adjusted means are not estimable, when in fact they are.

20. To demonstrate the effect of the `om` option, the adjusted analysis was rerun without that option. The least-squares means and differences of least-squares means computed without the `om` option are shown below:

LEAST-SQUARES MEANS

Level	LSMEAN	SE
COND I	77.50827	2.71387
COND C	76.84008	2.71828

DIFFERENCES OF LEAST-SQUARES MEANS

Level 1	Level 2	Diff	SE
COND I	COND C	0.66818	1.53040

As expected, the least-squares means computed on the assumption of balanced data are different from those computed based on the observed marginal distribution of the fixed effects listed in the `class` statement but not involved in the `lsmeans` effect. The absolute differences in this case are not great, though the standard errors for the means are much larger with the imposed balance. The estimate of the intervention effect is unaffected, as is its standard error.

21. The increased intervention effect reflects confounding due to the covariates included in the adjusted analysis. Confounding is assessed by comparing the adjusted and unadjusted parameter estimates for the term of interest. The investigator must use judgment rather than a statistical test to determine if the difference is large enough to be evidence of confounding. Given a difference of 10%–15%, most investigators conclude that the unadjusted estimate is confounded and report the adjusted estimate. In this case, the unadjusted estimate

of the intervention effect is $+0.434$. The adjusted estimate reported in this section is $+0.668$. The relative difference between those two estimates is:

$$\frac{(+0.668)-(+0.434)}{(+0.434)}\times 100 = +53.9\%$$

Given the magnitude of this relative difference, the adjusted estimate should be reported.

22. The efficiency occurs because the `subject=` option specifies a block-diagonal structure for the between-member random-effects covariance matrix with identical blocks for each level of the effect in the `subject=` option. That reduces the processing time, because the program only estimates the parameters in the blocks and assigns zeros to the positions in the matrix outside those blocks; it also saves memory, as there is less information to store. In fact, for very large problems, the analysis may fail with the original specification due to insufficient memory.

23. Type III F-tests are somewhat controversial (Nelder, 1994) and often misinterpreted, particularly tests for main effects in the presence of interactions (Rodriguez et al., 1995). The meaning of such Type III main-effect F-tests is best explicated by delineating their null hypotheses. The F-test for COND tests the null hypothesis that there is no effect due to condition at the average level of time. Similarly, the F-test for TIME tests the null hypothesis that there is no effect due to time at the average level of condition. SAS has for some time reported Type III F-tests for main effects in the presence of an interaction, arguing that if the interaction is not significant, the F-tests for the main effects provide approximate tests for the main effects. They are approximate because the inclusion of the nonsignificant interaction term will reduce the *ddf* and inflate the standard errors for the tests of the main effects involved in that interaction. If the interaction is nonsignificant, it is best to delete the interaction from the model and rerun the analysis rather than to report the approximate Type III main-effect tests.

24. In SAS 6.11, the tests reported in the tests of effect slices tables are interpretable as tests of simple main effects only when the effect specified in the `lsmeans` statement is a two-way interaction. If the `slice=` option is used for a three-way or higher-order interaction, the test is an omnibus test of the slice effect across all the combinations of levels of the other effects involved in the interaction. As such, they are not tests of simple interactions as defined, for example, in Winer et al. (1991). Analysts should be careful when interpreting tests based on the `slice=` option when they involve three-way or higher-order interactions.

25. The grouping of observations by year as presented here is slightly different from the scheme used by the MHHP investigators and reported, for example, in Luepker et al. (1994). This scheme groups observations based on the actual time of the survey, whereas the MHHP investigators grouped observations based on the intended time of the survey. Because some participants were seen early and others quite late, this difference in definitions causes some observations to be grouped into different years than was the case in the original analysis.

26. In this example $f=95$. There are 95 fixed-effect parameters in the model in addition to the intercept: `cond`, `month`, `month2`, `imonth`, `imonth2`, `age`, `sex`, `educlvl` (7), `bpobsrvr` (79) and `bplocatn` (2).

27. In this example $f=93$. There are 93 fixed-effect parameters in the model in addition to the intercept: `cond`, `month`, `imonth`, `age`, `sex`, `educlvl` (7), `bpobsrvr` (79), and `bplocatn` (2).

28. The careful reader will note that the slope in the intervention condition was less

negative than that observed in the control condition, which is opposite the pattern seen in the trend analysis. That apparent reversal is entirely due to the substantial regression coefficient estimated for COND: -1.047. Because the regression coefficient for IMONTH ignores the difference in intercepts, a plot of the corrected slopes would place the intervention condition slope above that for the control condition. At the same time, a plot of the uncorrected slopes would place the intervention condition slope below that for the control condition. This illustrates the sometimes substantial effect that the difference in y-intercepts can have on the estimated difference between the two conditions at some point in time. The null hypothesis does not involve y-intercepts, and the proper test is provided in the test of the difference in slopes, given as the test for IMONTH.

29. In fact, most of the difference in the -2 LL is due to the covariance, not the slope component of variance. However, it makes little sense to fit slopes and intercepts in a group without letting them covary, and so the test of interest is the test of both vs. neither.

30. It is inappropriate to compare the ANCOVA and the random-coefficients models using a LR chi-square test, as the two are not hierarchical. Indeed, the -2LL for the more complex random-coefficients analysis with 5 covariance parameters is 96352.53, while the -2 LL for the simpler ANCOVA with 4 covariance parameters is 96230.66. The LR chi-square would be 96230.66–96352.53–96686.73 $= -121.87$.

31. Again, it is not appropriate to compare these two models using the LR chi-square, as they are not hierarchical.

8

Applications of Analyses for Nested Cohort Designs

The analyses appropriate for data from a nested cohort design are illustrated in this chapter with data from the cohort survey of the Minnesota Heart Health Program (MHHP). The MHHP design supports most of the analyses presented in Chapter 6.

MHHP had an unusual cohort survey design (Jacobs et al., 1986). Respondents who participated in the 2–4 baseline cross-sectional surveys in each community were selected at random to be cohort participants. As a result, the baseline data were collected over a period of 2–4 years, though no one person was seen more than once during that period. To minimize the effect of repeated testing, the follow-up surveys were structured so that roughly half the cohort was sought after two years of intervention, while the other half was sought after four years of intervention; all cohort participants were sought after seven years of intervention.[1] This plan resulted in the staggered series of cohort surveys in each community shown in Figure 7.1. The cohort data set includes observations on more than 7000 individuals.

Posttest-Only Control Group Design

The primary differences between the cohort and cross-sectional versions of the Posttest-Only Control Group Design are the eligibility criteria used to select members for the posttest survey. In the cross-sectional version, all current members are eligible for the posttest survey. In the cohort version, only members who were present at the beginning of the study are eligible for the posttest survey. Even with this difference in eligibility criteria, the analysis of the data is identical in the two versions of the design. Those methods are illustrated in Chapter 7 and are not repeated here.

Pretest-Posttest Control Group Design

The MHHP cohort design can be reduced to a Pretest-Posttest Control Group Design with two changes in the structure of the data. First, all baseline data are treated as though they were collected at the same time. Second, all data collected 2 years and 4 years after the onset of the intervention are treated as though they had been collected 3 years after the onset of the intervention. With these changes, MHHP provides $c = 2$ conditions, $g = 3$ communities per condition, $t = 2$ time intervals for each community, and observations on several hundred members per community per time interval.

Unadjusted Time × Condition Analysis

Implementation for Gaussian Data

There are several different ways to implement this analysis for diastolic blood pressure using SAS PROC MIXED. The most flexible is based on the repeated statement, which presumes that each member is assigned a unique identification number. Using that approach, the code shown in Table 8.1 is appropriate.

In the analyses for the nested cross-sectional design, member was never included explicitly in the code. This was because member was always the residual error and the residual error is never specified in the MIXED code. The situation is different in a nested cohort design because the residual error is now time*member(group). As a result, member must be added to the class statement so that member can be included in the analysis. To avoid listing all the member identification numbers in the output, the noclprint option is included in the proc mixed statement.

The model statement is identical to that employed in the corresponding

Table 8.1. SAS PROC MIXED Code for the Unadjusted Time × Condition Analysis of Diastolic Blood Pressure in the Pretest-Posttest Control Group Design

```
proc mixed info order=internal noclprint;
  class cond group member time;
  model dbp=cond time cond*time/ddf=4,4,4 ddfm=res;
  repeated time/type=cs subject=member(group*cond)
    r=1 to 3 rcorr=1 to 3;
  random int time/subject=group(cond);
  lsmeans cond*time/slice=cond slice=time cl e;
  estimate '(I3-I0)-(C3-C0)' cond*time 1 -1 -1 1/cl e;
run;
```

analysis in Chapter 7. `Time` is included both as a main effect and as an interaction with `cond`. The table of expected mean squares presented in Chapter 6 (Table 6.1) shows that the *ddf* for the first fixed effect are $c(g-1)=4$ and for the second and third fixed effects are $(t-1)c(g-1)=4$.

The `random` statement is also identical to that employed in the corresponding analysis in Chapter 7. As noted there, the `random` statement is used to model random variation between members. Because there are repeat observations on each `group(cond)`, that term is used as the effect in the `subject=` option. Because the other random effects are crossed with `group(cond)`, they are included in the same `random` statement, following the factorization method described in Chapter 7. The benefits in terms of efficiency that were described in Chapter 7 also accrue here.

Because the `type=` option is not used in the `random` statement, the structure for the between-member random-effects covariance matrix is presumed to be variance components. Because the `group=` option is not used, that structure is presumed to be homogeneous across all between-member grouping factors.

In Chapter 7, the `random` statement was all that was required to model the random variation in the data, since all the examples were based on nested cross-sectional designs. However, in a cohort design, the analyst must be concerned with random variation within members as well as between members. In MIXED, the `repeated` statement is used to model random variation within members. The only effect in the `repeated` statement is `time`, as it is the variable that defines the spacing in time of the repeated observations.[2]

The `subject=` option in the `repeated` statement is functionally equivalent to the `subject=` option in the `random` statement.[3] The effect of the `subject=` option is the effect upon which repeated measures are taken. In the terminology of this book, that is the member. The `subject=` option is required in an analysis based on the `repeated` statement, as that is the only way to allow for within-member correlation over time.[4]

The `type=` option in the `repeated` statement is used to define the structure for the identical blocks of the within-member random-effects covariance matrix. In this example, that structure is defined as compound symmetry via `type=cs`. As noted in Chapter 6, under compound symmetry both the member and member $\times$ time components of variance are assumed constant over all time intervals; that is equivalent to an assumption of constant correlation over time. Given only two time intervals in the Pretest-Posttest Control Group Design, that assumption is easily justified.

The `r` and `rcorr` options in the `repeated` statement add the block of the within-member random-effects covariance and correlation matrices for the first members to the output. Because no `group=` option is used in the `repeated` statement, the within-member random-effects covariance structure is presumed to be homogeneous across the levels of all within-member grouping factors.

The `lsmeans` statement is identical to that used in the corresponding analysis in Chapter 7. It requests the interaction means rather than the main-effect means. The `slice = time` option provides tests of condition at each level of time. The `slice = cond` option provides tests of the time trend in each condition.

Table 8.2 summarizes the structure of the model. It confirms that the between-member random-effects covariance matrix has a variance-components structure and that the within-member random-effects covariance matrix has a compound-symmetry structure. Two subject effects are identified, GROUP(COND) from the `random` statement and MEMBER(COND*GROUP) from the `repeated` statement. The residual method is listed as the degrees-of-freedom method because of the `ddfm = res` option in the `model` statement.[5]

Table 8.3 reflects the four covariance parameters in the model, adding member(group*cond) to the three that were present in the corresponding analysis in Chapter 7. The columns for the fixed- and random-effects design matrices are the same as those in the nested cross-sectional version of the design, though the labeling of the columns in Z is slightly different. The 9 columns in the fixed-effects design matrix are for the intercept (1), `cond` (2), `time` (2), and `cond*time` (4). The 3 columns in the random-effects design matrix for each group(cond) are int(1) and `time` (2). The subjects reported refer to the number of groups, which is the effect in the `subject =` option in the `random` statement, not the number of members, which is the effect in the `subject =` option in the `repeated` statement. The total observations re-

Table 8.2. Model Information From the Unadjusted Time × Condition Analysis of Diastolic Blood Pressure in the Pretest-Posttest Control Group Design

Description	Value
Data Set	WORK.COHORT
Dependent Variable	DBP
Covariance Structures	Variance Components and Compound Symmetry
Subject Effects	GROUP(COND) and MEMBER(COND*GROUP)
Residual Variance Method	Profile
Fixed Effects SE Method	Model-Based
Degrees of Freedom Method	Residual
Estimation Method	REML

Table 8.3. Dimensions of the Unadjusted Time × Condition Analysis of Diastolic Blood Pressure in the Pretest-Posttest Control Group Design

Description	Value
Covariance Parameters	4
Columns in X	9
Max Cols in Z Per Subject	3
Subjects	6
Max Obs Per Subject	2199
Observations Used	10729
Observations Not Used	0
Total Observations	10729

ported refers to the total number of member × time-interval observations, in this case 10,729.

Table 8.4 presents the covariance-parameter estimates. The comments from Chapter 7 concerning the appropriateness of the asymptotic z-tests apply equally here. The LR chi-square test described by Self and Liang (1987) is recommended instead.

The names of the first two covariance parameters stem from the use of the subject= option in the random statement, in which group(cond) was represented as int and time*group(cond) was represented as time. Thus, the component of variance for group(cond) is estimated as 0.449 and the component of variance for time*group(cond) is estimated as 1.70.

The third covariance parameter is labeled as TIME CS. This label suggests that the estimate in that row is the diagonal element of the within-member random-effects covariance matrix, which under compound symmetry is the sum of two variance components, residual error and member (group*cond). In fact, this estimate is the off-diagonal element of that

Table 8.4. Covariance-Parameter Estimates (REML) From the Unadjusted Time × Condition Analysis of Diastolic Blood Pressure in the Pretest-Posttest Control Group Design

Cov Parm	Estimate
INTERCEPT	0.44894
TIME	1.69858
TIME CS	61.85343
Residual	48.99720

matrix, and so it is simply the component of variance for member (group*cond).

That is confirmed in the R matrix presented in Table 8.5. That matrix is generated by the r option in the repeated statement and consists of the first block from the block-diagonal within-member random-effects covariance matrix. Since all blocks are identical, unless a member is missing an observation, one usually need print only a few blocks in order to see a full block, and in this case one block was sufficient.

The diagonal elements in the R matrix are the same in all blocks, as dictated by the type = cs option, and represent the sum of the TIME CS and RESIDUAL components of variance. In this case, that is the sum of the member and residual components of variance. The off-diagonal elements are also the same in all blocks and represent the TIME CS or member component of variance.

The TIME CS estimate as a fraction of the total within-member variation in the data is an estimate of the within-member correlation over time, written as $r_{yy(m)}$. In this case, that estimate is:

$$\hat{r}_{yy(m)} = \frac{\hat{\sigma}^2_{m:g:c}}{\hat{\sigma}^2_e + \hat{\sigma}^2_{mt:g:c} + \hat{\sigma}^2_{m:g:c}} = \frac{61.85}{49.0 + 61.85} = 0.558$$

This correlation is also available via the rcorr = option in the model statement. Table 8.5 presents the correlation matrix.

The off-diagonal elements in the correlation matrix are the same for all members due to the type = cs option and equal the within-member correlation over time. Recall that the baseline data were collected over a period of four years and that the posttest data were collected after two years or four years of intervention. As a result, the average time lag between the two obser-

Table 8.5. R Matrix and R Correlation Matrix from the Unadjusted Time × Condition Analysis of Diastolic Blood Pressure in the Pretest-Posttest Control Group Design

R MATRIX		
Row	COL1	COL2
1	110.85064	61.85343
2	61.85343	110.85064
R CORRELATION MATRIX		
Row	COL1	COL2
1	1.00000	0.55798
2	0.55798	1.00000

vations on a member was five years. Given this time lag, the correlation is about what one might expect for diastolic blood pressure.

The residual variance is estimated as 49.0. Recall from the corresponding analysis in Chapter 7 that the residual variance in the nested cross-sectional version of this design was 112.4. Since neither analysis reflects any covariate adjustments, the dramatic reduction in residual variance is attributable to the within-member correlation over time, reflecting one of the major benefits of a cohort analysis. Given an estimate of the within-member correlation over time of 0.558, one would expect the residual variation to be reduced by a factor of about $(1 - r_{yy(m)}) = (1 - 0.558) = 0.442$, even if no other factors were operative. This would reduce the residual variation from 112.4 to $112.4*0.442 = 49.8$, quite close to the observed value.

The covariance-parameter estimates can be used to estimate the mean squares for the random effects in the model, drawing on the table of expected mean squares given in Chapter 6. Given 10,729 observations and $g = 3$ groups in each of $c = 2$ conditions observed at each of $t = 2$ time intervals, the average $m = 894$. Using these values, the mean squares are estimated in Table 8.6.

Given 1569 as the estimate for $MS_{tg:c}$, the standard error for the intervention effect is estimated using Equation 6.3:

$$\hat{\sigma}_\Delta = \sqrt{2*2\left(\frac{\hat{MS}_{tg:c}}{mg}\right)} = \sqrt{2*2\left(\frac{1569}{894*3}\right)} = 1.53$$

The ICC of interest in this analysis is different from the ICC of interest in the cross-sectional version of this analysis, because there are repeat observations on each member. The ICC of interest is $ICC_{mt:g:c}$ and is estimated as:

$$I\hat{C}C_{mt:g:c} = \frac{\hat{\sigma}^2_{tg:c}}{\hat{\sigma}^2_e + \hat{\sigma}^2_{mt:g:c} + \hat{\sigma}^2_{tg:c}} = \frac{1.70}{49.0 + 1.70} = 0.0335$$

Because the ICC is different in this design, so too is the VIF. The $VIF_{mt:g:c}$ is estimated as:

$$V\hat{I}F_{mt:g:c} = \left(1 + (m-1)I\hat{C}C_{mt:g:c}\right) = \left(1 + (894 - 1)0.0335\right) = 30.9$$

Table 8.6. Selected Mean-Square Estimates for the Unadjusted Time × Condition Analysis of Diastolic Blood Pressure in the Pretest-Posttest Control Group Design

Source	E(MS)	Estimate
TG:C	$\sigma^2_e + \sigma^2_{mt:g:c} + m\sigma^2_{tg:c}$	$49.0 + 894*1.70 = 1569$
Member:TG:C	$\sigma^2_e + \sigma^2_{mt:g:c}$	49.0

Table 8.7. Tests of Fixed Effects From the Unadjusted Time ×
Condition Analysis of Diastolic Blood Pressure in the Pretest-Posttest
Control Group Design

Source	NDF	DDF	Type III F	Pr > F
COND	1	4	1.31	0.3163
TIME	1	4	0.18	0.6935
COND*TIME	1	4	0.05	0.8312

Even though the $ICC_{mt:g:c}$ is modest, the *VIF* is quite large. It indicates that the variance of the intervention effect is 30.9 times as large as it would have been with random assignment of individual members to study conditions.

Table 8.7 presents the tests of fixed effects for the two main effects of COND and TIME, and for the interaction COND*TIME. The test of interest is the test for COND*TIME, as it is the test of the intervention effect. Indeed, the tests listed for COND and TIME are generally of little interest in this analysis.[6] In this case, the *F*-test for COND*TIME is 0.05 and is clearly not significant.

Table 8.8 presents the least-squares means from this analysis. The label COND*TIME I 0 refers to the intervention condition at Time 0 (the pretest). The label COND*TIME C 1 refers to the control condition at Time 1 (the posttest). The other labels follow the same general pattern. The means suggest a decline of about 0.15 mm Hg in the intervention condition and a decline of about 0.50 in the control condition. The results of the slice= options (not shown) can be helpful for interpreting intervention effects when they are pres-

Table 8.8. Least-Squares Means From the Unadjusted Time × Condition
Analysis of Diastolic Blood Pressure in the Pretest-Posttest Control Group
Design

Level	LSMEAN	SE	DDF	T	Pr > |T|
COND*TIME I 0	74.78435	0.87014	4	85.95	0.0001
COND*TIME I 3	74.63424	0.87075	4	85.71	0.0001
COND*TIME C 0	76.06211	0.87022	4	87.41	0.0001
COND*TIME C 3	75.56385	0.87068	4	86.79	0.0001
Level			Alpha	Lower	Upper
COND*TIME I 0			0.05	72.3685	77.2002
COND*TIME I 3			0.05	72.2166	77.0518
COND*TIME C 0			0.05	73.6460	78.4782
COND*TIME C 3			0.05	73.1465	77.9813

Table 8.9. Estimate for (I3-I0)-(C3-C0) From the Unadjusted Time $\times$ Condition Analysis of Diastolic Blood Pressure in the Pretest-Posttest Control Group Design

Parameter	Estimate	SE	DDF	T
(I3-I0)-(C3-C0)	0.34815	1.53010	4	0.23
	Pr>|T|	Alpha	Lower	Upper
	0.8312	0.05	−3.9001	4.5964

ent and supported by the omnibus F-test. In the absence of a significant F-test, they should be interpreted cautiously.

Table 8.9 presents the results from the estimate statement. The t-test that accompanies the estimate is the square root of the F-test for the COND*TIME interaction presented above, and the p-values for the two tests will be the same. Note that the standard error for the intervention effect is exactly as computed above from the components of variance. The positive value of the estimate reflects the fact that the decline in diastolic blood pressure over the time interval represented was greater in the control condition than in the intervention condition.

Implementation for Dichotomous Data

To implement the analysis for smoking status in SAS PROC MIXED, the code shown in the upper panel of Table 8.10 is appropriate. To implement the analysis for smoking status in the GLIMMIX macro, the code shown in the lower panel of Table 8.10 is appropriate.

The MIXED code is identical to that used for diastolic blood pressure, except that the name of the endpoint is now smkstat. The GLIMMIX code reflects the requirements of the macro. The data file must be named explicitly in the data = cohort statement. The lsmeans and estimate statements are omitted from the GLIMMIX analysis, as they can give misleading results; instead, the solution option is added to the model statement to provide the parameter estimates from the mixed-model logistic regression analysis.

Table 8.11 presents the dimensions of the analysis from GLIMMIX and confirms the number of covariance parameters and the size of the fixed- and random-effects design matrices. It also provides information on the number of observations included in the analysis. As noted above, the number of subjects refers to the number of levels of the effect in the subject = option in the random statement. The table from MIXED is identical except for minor differences in the column headings.

Table 8.10 SAS PROC MIXED and GLIMMIX Code for the Unadjusted Time × Condition Analysis of Smoking Status in the Pretest-Posttest Control Group Design

MIXED CODE
```
proc mixed info order=internal noclprint;
  class cond group member time;
  model smkstat=cond time cond*time/ddf=4,4,4 ddfm=res;
  repeated time/type=cs subject=member(group*cond)
    rcorr=1 to 3;
  random int time/subject=group(cond);
  lsmeans cond*time/slice=cond slice=time cl e;
  estimate '(I3-I0)-(C3-C0)' cond*time -1 1 1 -1/cl e;
run;
```

GLIMMIX CODE
```
%include 'glimmix.sas';
%glimmix(
  procopt=info order=internal noclprint,
  data=cohort,
  stmts=%str(
    class cond group member time;
    model smkstat=cond time cond*time
      /ddf=4,4,4 ddfm=res solution;
    repeated time/type=cs subject=member(group*cond)
      rcorr=1 to 3;
    random int time/subject=group(cond);
    ),
  error=binomial,
  link=logit);
run;
```

Table 8.11. Dimensions of the Unadjusted Time × Condition Analysis of Smoking Status in the Pretest-Posttest Control Group Design

Description	Value
Covariance Parameters	4
Columns in X	9
Max Cols in Z Per Subject	3
Subjects	6
Max Obs Per Subject	2224
Observations Used	10883
Observations Not Used	0
Total Observations	10883

Table 8.12 presents the covariance-parameter estimates included in the default GLIMMIX output in the upper panel and the estimates from the default MIXED output in the lower panel. The names of the first two covariance parameters are taken from the code used in the `random` statement and represent `group(cond)` and `time*group(cond)`.

As noted in Chapter 7, the variance components included in the GLIMMIX output are scaled in terms of the variance function:

$$\sigma^2_{\text{scaled}} \cong \frac{\sigma^2_{\text{unscaled}}}{(\text{variance function})^2} \tag{8.1}$$

In this example, where the variance function is binomial, the `group(cond)` variance component as presented is related to the `group(cond)` variance in the original scale approximately as:

$$\sigma^2_{\text{scaled}} \cong \frac{\sigma^2_{\text{unscaled}}}{(\bar{p}(1-\bar{p}))^2}, \tag{8.2}$$

where $\bar{p}$ is the average prevalence rate for smoking in the sample. Here, that value is obtained in a separate analysis as 0.285, so that the factor $\bar{p}(1-\bar{p})$ is 0.2038. To return the scaled estimate to the original scale,

$$\sigma^2_{\text{unscaled}} \cong \sigma^2_{\text{scaled}}(\bar{p}(1-\bar{p}))^2 \tag{8.3}$$

Table 8.12 MIXED and GLIMMIX Covariance-Parameter Estimates (REML) From the Unadjusted Time × Condition Analysis of Smoking Status in the Pretest-Posttest Control Group Design

MIXED COVARIANCE PARAMETER ESTIMATES	
Cov Parm	*Estimate*
INTERCEPT	0.00014905
TIME	0.00005081
TIME CS	0.16062658
Residual	0.04270357

GLIMMIX COVARIANCE PARAMETER ESTIMATES	
Cov Parm	*Estimate*
INTERCEPT	0.00355365
TIME	0.00121029
TIME CS	0.78954949

For example, for the INTERCEPT term,

$$\hat{\sigma}^2_{\text{unscaled}} \cong 0.00355 * \left((0.285 * (1-0.285))\right)^2 = 0.000147$$

For the TIME term,

$$\hat{\sigma}^2_{\text{unscaled}} \cong 0.00121 * \left(0.285 * (1-0.285)\right)^2 = 0.0000502$$

Both unscaled estimates agree closely with the estimates provided by MIXED that are in the original scale.

The TIME CS estimate is the component of variance for member(group* cond). Because it is at the individual level, its scaling factor is different:

$$\sigma^2_{\text{unscaled}} \cong \frac{\sigma^2_{\text{scaled}}}{(\text{variance function})} \tag{8.4}$$

For individual-level variance components, the rescaling factor is the variance function, here $\bar{p}(1-\bar{p})$, not the square of the variance function. As a result, the TIME CS estimate is related to the member(group*cond) variance in the original scale approximately as:

$$\sigma^2_{\text{scaled}} \cong \frac{\sigma^2_{\text{unscaled}}}{\bar{p}(1-\bar{p})} \tag{8.5}$$

To return the scaled estimate to the original scale, $\hat{\sigma}^2_{\text{unscaled}} \cong \hat{\sigma}^2_{\text{scaled}} (\bar{p}(1-\bar{p})$ $= 0.7895 * (0.285 * (1-0.285)) = 0.161$. Again, the result agrees closely with the estimate provided by MIXED in the original scale.

The factor $\bar{p}(1-\bar{p})$ is also the theoretical residual variance under the binomial distribution. GLIMMIX reports an extra-dispersion scale *(EDS)* as 0.2085. This value represents the ratio of the observed residual variance to the variance function. As such, the observed residual variance may be estimated as:

$$\sigma^2_{\text{residual}} \cong EDS \times \sigma^2_{\text{theoretical}} = EDS \times \bar{p}(1-\bar{p}) \tag{8.6}$$

In this case, the residual variance is computed as:

$$\hat{\sigma}^2_{\text{residual}} = 0.2085 * \left(0.285 * (1-0.285)\right) = 0.0425$$

The MIXED estimate of the residual variance is 0.0427; again, the agreement is quite good.

This residual variance is considerably smaller than the theoretical variance because of the high within-member correlation over time. The subject component of variance, as a fraction of the total within-member variance, represents the within-member correlation over time and so is estimated as:

$$\hat{r}_{yy(m)} = \frac{\hat{\sigma}^2_{m:g:c}}{\hat{\sigma}^2_e + \hat{\sigma}^2_{mt:g:c} + \hat{\sigma}^2_{m:g:c}} = \frac{0.161}{0.0425 + 0.161} = 0.791$$

It is appreciably higher than the correlation obtained for diastolic blood pressure, but is about what one would expect given the stability of smoking among adults, even over a five-year average lag period.

Table 8.13 presents the correlation as found in the correlation matrix available in GLIMMIX via the `rcorr` option in the `repeated` statement combined with the `options = mixprintlast` statement or in MIXED via the `rcorr` option alone.[7]

The theoretical residual error is much reduced from the observed residual error, by the factor of $EDS = 0.2085$. That value is approximately the one's complement of the within-member correlation over time, $(1 - 0.791) = 0.209$ and reflects the reduction in the residual error due to repeated measures on the same subjects.

Given 10,883 observations and $g = 3$ groups in each of $c = 2$ conditions observed at each of $t = 2$ time intervals, the average $m = 907$. Using the unscaled values from GLIMMIX, the mean squares are estimated in Table 8.14.

Given 0.0880 as the estimate for $MS_{tg:c}$, the standard error for the intervention effect is estimated using Equation 6.3:

$$\hat{\sigma}_\Delta = \sqrt{2 * 2\left(\frac{\hat{MS}_{tg:c}}{mg}\right)} = \sqrt{2 * \left(\frac{0.0880}{907 * 3}\right)} = 0.0114$$

Table 8.13. R Correlation Matrix From the Unadjusted Time × Condition Analysis of Smoking Status in the Pretest-Posttest Control Group Design as Estimated in GLIMMIX and MIXED

GLIMMIX Row	COL1	COL2
1	1.00000	0.79108
2	0.79108	1.00000
MIXED Row	COL1	COL2
1	1.00000	0.78997
2	0.78997	1.00000

Table 8.14. Selected Mean-Square Estimates for the Unadjusted Time × Condition Analysis of Smoking Status in the Pretest-Posttest Control Group Design

Source	E(MS)	Estimate
TG:C	$\sigma_e^2 + \sigma_{mt:g:c}^2 + m\sigma_{tg:c}^2$	$0.0425 + 907*0.0000502 = 0.0880$
M:TG:C	$\sigma_e^2 + \sigma_{mt:g:c}^2$	0.0425

The standard error computed from the MIXED results is 0.0115.

The $ICC_{mt:g:c}$ is estimated as:

$$I\hat{C}C_{mt:g:c} = \frac{\hat{\sigma}_{tg:c}^2}{\hat{\sigma}_e^2 + \hat{\sigma}_{mt:g:c}^2 + \hat{\sigma}_{tg:c}^2} = \frac{0.0000502}{0.0425 + 0.0000502} = 0.00118$$

The $VIF_{mt:g:c}$ is estimated as:

$$V\hat{I}F_{mt:g:c} = \left(1 + (m-1)I\hat{C}C_{mt:g:c}\right) = \left(1 + (907-1)0.00118\right) = 2.07$$

Table 8.15 presents the tests of fixed effects and provides no evidence of an intervention effect. Note again the very close agreement between the GLIMMIX and MIXED analyses.

Table 8.16 presents the least-squares means from MIXED. They suggest a decline of about 5.9% is smoking prevalence in the intervention condition and a decline of about 5.8% in the control condition.

Table 8.15. GLIMMIX and MIXED Tests of Fixed Effects From the Unadjusted Time × Condition Analysis of Smoking Status in the Pretest-Posttest Control Group Design

GLIMMIX Source	NDF	DDF	Type III F	Pr > F
COND	1	4	0.04	0.8542
TIME	1	4	101.88	0.0005
COND*TIME	1	4	0.03	0.8693
MIXED Source	NDF	DDF	Type III F	Pr > F
COND	1	4	0.04	0.8475
TIME	1	4	101.15	0.0005
COND*TIME	1	4	0.04	0.8486

Table 8.16. MIXED Least-Squares Means From the Unadjusted Time × Condition Analysis of Smoking Status in the Pretest-Posttest Control Group Design

Level	LSMEAN	SE	DDF	T	Pr>|T|
COND*TIME I 0	0.31782	0.01184	4	26.84	0.0001
COND*TIME I 3	0.25874	0.01190	4	21.74	0.0001
COND*TIME C 0	0.31341	0.01187	4	26.40	0.0001
COND*TIME C 3	0.25668	0.01190	4	21.56	0.0001
Level			Alpha	Lower	Upper
COND*TIME I 0			0.05	0.2849	0.3507
COND*TIME I 3			0.05	0.2257	0.2918
COND*TIME C 0			0.05	0.2805	0.3464
COND*TIME C 3			0.05	0.2236	0.2897

The preferred point estimate from the GLIMMIX output is the parameter estimate. When `error = binomial` and `link = logit`, as they are in this example, the parameter estimates are mixed-model logistic regression coefficients. These parameter estimates can be combined to compute log odds for the four cells in this Pretest-Posttest Control Group Design. The log odds can then be converted to probabilities using the inverse link function for the logit link:

$$\text{probability} = \text{invlink}(\ln(\text{odds})) = \frac{\exp(\ln(\text{odds}))}{1 + \exp(\ln(\text{odds}))}$$

Table 8.17 presents the parameter estimates from GLIMMIX. The estimate for the INTERCEPT is the log odds of smoking among persons at the reference levels of condition and time. Those persons are in the control condition at posttest, as shown by the 0.0000 for the EST for COND C and for TIME 3. Exponentiating -1.0642 gives 0.345 as the odds. Applying the inverse link function to this result gives 0.2565 as the probability of smoking in that cell.

Table 8.18 mirrors the design under consideration here. Each cell computes the ln(odds) and the probability of smoking, based on the parameter estimates in the GLIMMIX output. The computed probabilities agree quite closely with the means generated by MIXED in this instance, but that is only because the log odds are calculated as unweighted sums of parameter estimates.

Table 8.19 presents the intervention-effect estimate given by MIXED. It indicates that smoking declined over time more in the intervention condition than in the control condition, but not by much: -0.234%. Note the close

Table 8.17. GLIMMIX Parameter Estimates From the Unadjusted Time $\times$ Condition Analysis of Smoking Status in the Pretest-Posttest Control Group Design

Parameter	Estimate	SE	DDF	T	$Pr > \|T\|$
INTERCEPT	−1.0642	0.0594	10879	−17.93	0.0001
COND I	0.0102	0.0839	4	0.12	0.9090
COND C	0.0000	.	.	.	.
TIME 0	0.2800	0.0399	4	7.02	0.0022
TIME 3	0.0000	.	.	.	.
COND*TIME I 0	0.0099	0.0565	4	0.18	0.8693
COND*TIME I 3	0.0000	.	.	.	.
COND*TIME C 0	0.0000	.	.	.	.
COND*TIME C 3	0.0000	.	.	.	.

agreement between the standard error estimated from the variance components and the value given by MIXED.

Table 8.20 presents the intervention-effect estimate from GLIMMIX. It is in the form of a log odds ratio for the COND*TIME I 0 interaction. The t-statistics and p-values are quite similar for the two analyses because both test the same null hypothesis. However, the point estimate provided by GLIMMIX is not very useful apart from the role it plays in the calculations in Table 8.18.

The results of GLIMMIX and MIXED applied to the same dichotomous endpoint agree quite closely in many respects, just as they did in their application to data from a nested cross-sectional design in Chapter 7. Given the close

Table 8.18. Application of the Parameter Estimates From GLIMMIX to Compute the Probability of Smoking in Each Cell in the Design

Condition	Pretest	Posttest
Intervention	ln(odds) = −1.0642 +0.0102 +0.2800 +0.0099 = −0.7641 probability = 0.3178	ln(odds) = −1.0642 +0.0102 = −1.0540 probability = 0.2585
Control	ln(odds) = −1.0642 +0.2800 = −0.7743 probability = 0.3134	ln(odds) = −1.0642 probability = 0.2565

Table 8.19. MIXED Estimate for (I3-I0)-(C3-C0) From the Unadjusted
Time × Condition Analysis of Smoking Status in the Pretest-Posttest Control
Group Design

Parameter	Estimate	SE	DDF	T
(I3-I0)-(C3-C0)	−0.00234	0.01151	4	−0.20
	$Pr > \lvert T \rvert$	Alpha	Lower	Upper
	0.8486	0.05	−0.0343	0.0296

agreement between MIXED and GLIMMIX when used properly in the analysis of data from group-randomized trials, and the potential for misinterpretation of the GLIMMIX results, MIXED is preferred over GLIMMIX for the
analysis of data from most group-randomized trials.[8] As a result, though all
subsequent analyses of dichotomous endpoints in this chapter were run in both
GLIMMIX and MIXED, only the MIXED results are presented as long as the
two approaches gave equivalent results.

Adjusted Time × Condition Analysis

Implementation for Gaussian Data

The covariates chosen for the adjusted analysis of diastolic blood pressure are
educational attainment, location of the blood pressure measurement, and blood
pressure observer. All three covariates are likely to change in value over time,
though not necessarily for all members. Table 8.21 presents the MIXED code
for the adjusted analysis.

There are several changes in this code compared to that for the unadjusted
analysis. First, the covariates are added to the `class` and `model` statements,
as appropriate. Second, the `om` option in the `lsmeans` statement ensures that
the adjusted means are computed based on the marginal distribution of the
covariates. Third, the `convh=0.000001` option is added to the `proc
mixed` statement to ease the convergence criteria. Fourth, the `singu-`

Table 8.20. GLIMMIX Effect Estimate From the Unadjusted Time × Condition
Analysis of Smoking Status in the Pretest-Posttest Control Group Design

Parameter	Estimate	SE	DDF	T	$Pr > \lvert T \rvert$
COND*TIME I 0	0.0099	0.0565	4	0.18	0.8693

Table 8.21. SAS PROC MIXED Code for the Adjusted Time × Condition Analysis of Diastolic Blood Pressure in the Pretest-Posttest Control Group Design

```
proc mixed info order=internal noclprint convh=0.000001;
  class cond group member time educlvl bpobsrvr
    bplocatn;
  model dpb=cond time cond*time educlvl bpobsrvr bplocatn
    /ddfm=res ddf=4,4,4 singular=0.000001;
  random int time/subject=group(cond);
  repeated time/type=cs subject=member (group*cond)
    r=1 to 3 rcorr=1 to 3;
  lsmeans cond*time/om slice=cond slice=time cl e;
  estimate '(I3-I0)-(C3-C0)' cond*time -1 1 1 -1/cl e;
run;
```

`lar=0.000001` option is added to the `model` statement to ease the sweep criterion. Experience has shown that easing these criteria to 0.000001 can improve the running time without measurably affecting the parameter estimates or their standard errors.

The addition of the covariates reduced the residual-error variance only slightly in these data (Table 8.22), in sharp contrast to the experience in the cross-sectional data. This indicates that the covariates were simply not well related to diastolic blood pressure after adjustment for the other terms in the model. Of course, one of those "other terms in the model" was the member. That the covariates were not well related to the diastolic blood pressure after adjustment for the member is in large part a function of the high within-member correlation over time in diastolic blood pressure.

The TIME CS estimate as a fraction of the total within-member variation in the data is an estimate of the within-member correlation over time, $r_{yy(m)}$. In this case, that correlation is little affected by the regression adjustment for the covariates. It is estimated as:

Table 8.22. Covariance-Parameter Estimates (REML) From the Adjusted Time × Condition Analysis of Diastolic Blood Pressure in the Pretest-Posttest Control Group Design

Cov Parm	Estimate
INTERCEPT	0.30595
TIME	1.48078
TIME CS	61.68925
Residual	47.18577

$$\hat{r}_{yy(m)} = \frac{\hat{\sigma}^2_{m:g:c}}{\hat{\sigma}^2_e + \hat{\sigma}^2_{mt:g:c} + \hat{\sigma}^2_{m:g:c}} = \frac{61.7}{47.2 + 61.7} = 0.567$$

Given 10,729 observations and $g = 3$ groups in each of $c = 2$ conditions at each of $t = 2$ time intervals, the average $m = 894$. Using these values, the mean squares are estimated in Table 8.23.

The standard error for the intervention effect is estimated using Equation 6.6:

$$\hat{\sigma}_\Delta = \sqrt{2 * 2 \left(\frac{\hat{MS}_{tg:c}}{mg} \right)} = \sqrt{2 * 2 \left(\frac{1370}{894 * 3} \right)} = 1.43$$

The adjusted $ICC_{mt:g:c}$ is estimated as:

$$\hat{ICC}_{mt:g:c} = \frac{\hat{\sigma}^2_{tg:c}}{\hat{\sigma}^2_e + \hat{\sigma}^2_{mt:g:c} + \hat{\sigma}^2_{tg:c}} = \frac{1.48}{47.2 + 1.48} = 0.0303$$

The ICC was reduced only slightly. This indicates that the covariates included in the analysis did little to account for the correlation among observations taken during the same the time $\times$ group survey.

The $VIF_{mt:g:c}$ is estimated as:

$$\hat{VIF}_{mt:g:c} = \left(1 + (m - 1) \hat{ICC}_{mt:g:c} \right) = \left(1 + (894 - 1) 0.0303 \right) = 28.1$$

This indicates that the variance of the intervention effect in this group-randomized trial was 28.1 times larger than it would have been had individuals been randomized to study conditions.

Neither the F-tests (not shown), the adjusted means (not shown), nor the simple main-effects tests (not shown) provided any indication of an intervention effect. The adjusted means were not much different from the crude means.

The positive intervention-effect estimate generated by the estimate statement (Table 8.24) suggests that the decline in blood pressure was slightly more favorable in the control condition than in the intervention condition. That find-

Table 8.23. Selected Mean-Square Estimates for the Adjusted Time $\times$ Condition Analysis of Diastolic Blood Pressure in the Pretest-Posttest Control Group Design

Source	E(MS)	Estimate
TG:C	$\sigma^2_e + \sigma^2_{mt:g:c} + m\sigma^2_{tg:c}$	$47.2 + 894 * 1.48 = 1370$
Member:TG:C	$\sigma^2_e + \sigma^2_{mt:g:c}$	47.2

Table 8.24. Estimate for (I3-I0)-(C3-C0) From the Adjusted Time × Condition Analysis of Diastolic Blood Pressure in the Pretest-Posttest Control Group Design

Parameter	Estimate	SE	DDF	T
(I3-I0)-(C3-C0)	0.11575	1.43712	4	0.08
	$Pr>\|T\|$	Alpha	Lower	Upper
	0.9397	0.05	−3.8743	4.1059

ing is certainly not significant given the magnitude of the estimate relative to its standard error.

Analysis of Posttest Data With Regression Adjustment for Baseline Values

Implementation for Gaussian Data

To implement this analysis in SAS PROC MIXED, the data set must be reformatted into what is sometimes called a *multivariate* file. Previous analyses required that the data from each time interval for each member appear on separate records. This analysis requires that all the data for a single member appear on the same record. In addition, variable names must be revised so as to distinguish between pretest and posttest values of the same variable. Given this new file structure, the code shown in Table 8.25 is appropriate.

This code is quite similar to that presented in Chapter 7 for the adjusted analysis of data in the Posttest-Only Control Group Design. The major difference is that most of the variables now carry an extra character to distinguish between those measured at pretest (e.g., dbp1) and those measured at posttest (e.g., dbp2). If a potential covariate cannot change values over time (e.g.,

Table 8.25. SAS PROC MIXED Code for the Analysis of Diastolic Blood Pressure With Regression Adjustment for Baseline Values in the Pretest-Posttest Control Group Design

```
proc mixed info order=internal;
  class cond group sex educ1 bpobs2 bploc2;
  model dbp2=cond dbp1 age2 sex educ1 bpobs2 pbloc2
    /ddf=4 ddfm=res;
  random group(cond);
  lsmeans cond/om cl e;
  estimate 'I-C' cond -1 1/cl e;
run;
```

sex), either its pretest or posttest value may be used, as they are identical. If a potential covariate can change values over time but cannot be influenced by the intervention, its posttest value is often used to maximize the correlation between that covariate and the outcome (e.g., bploc2). If a potential covariate can change values over time and can be influenced by the intervention, then its pretest value should be used to avoid adjusting out some of the intervention effect, thereby artificially reducing the estimate of the intervention effect.[9]

Note that this analysis includes one covariate that was omitted from the analysis in the previous section. Sex was left out of the adjusted time $\times$ condition analysis because its value did not change over time. As such, it was a fixed covariate and could not affect the within-member tests, including the test for the time $\times$ condition interaction. In this analysis, sex is included as a covariate because it can affect the test for condition.

Note as well that this code does not include the convh = 0.000001 or singular = 0.000001 options that were included for the adjusted time $\times$ condition analysis. The analysis presented in this section will run much faster than the time $\times$ condition analysis, because it models only the between-member random-effects covariance matrix, not both the between-member and within-member random-effects covariance matrices.

Table 8.26 summarizes the size of the design matrices as well as the number of observations included in the analysis. Note that there are 5167 observations included. This value is somewhat smaller than $11,052/2 = 5526$ because 325 persons in the data set are missing either their pretest or posttest observation. Those cases were included in the analyses reported in the previous two sections because SAS PROC MIXED employs REML estimation and avoids the listwise deletion feature common to software that employs OLS estimation.

Table 8.26. Dimensions of the Analysis of Diastolic Blood Pressure With Regression Adjustment for Baseline Values in the Pretest-Posttest Control Group Design

Description	Value
Covariance Parameters	2
Columns in X	62
Columns in Z	6
Subjects	1
Max Obs Per Subject	5167
Observations Used	5167
Observations Not Used	0
Total Observations	5167

Table 8.27. Covariance-Parameter Estimates (REML) From the Analysis of Diastolic Blood Pressure With Regression Adjustment for Baseline Values in the Pretest-Posttest Control Group Design

Cov Parm	Estimate
GROUP(COND)	1.77109
Residual	69.65692

However, those cases are omitted from the analysis reported in this section, as they are effectively missing either the dependent variable (posttest) or one of the covariates (pretest). This is one of the disadvantages of this approach, as it cannot use partial information as readily as the repeated-measures approach.

The total variance for diastolic blood pressure at posttest for this sample is 106.31 (analysis not shown). The random-effects variance components in this analysis sum to 71.43 (Table 8.27). Thus, the seven fixed effects account for about 33% of the variation in diastolic blood pressure at posttest.

Given 5167 observations and $g = 3$ groups in each of $c = 2$ conditions, the average $m = 861$. Using these values, the mean squares are estimated in Table 8.28.

Given 1594 as the estimate for $MS_{g:c}$, the standard error for the intervention effect is estimated using Equation 6.9:

$$\hat{\sigma}_\Delta = \sqrt{2\left(\frac{\hat{MS}_{g:c}}{mg}\right)} = \sqrt{2\left(\frac{1594}{861*3}\right)} = 1.11$$

This standard error is about 70% smaller than the standard error for either the unadjusted or adjusted time $\times$ condition analyses presented in the previous two sections. This reduction demonstrates the precision advantage that this analysis often has over its repeated-measures alternatives.

The adjusted $ICC_{m:g:c}$ is estimated as:

Table 8.28. Selected Mean-Square Estimates From the Analysis of Diastolic Blood Pressure With Regression Adjustment for Baseline Values in the Pretest-Posttest Control Group Design

Source	E(MS)	Estimate
Group:C	$\sigma_e^2 + m\sigma_{g:c}^2$	$69.7 + 861*1.77 = 1594$
Member:G:C	σ_e^2	69.7

$$I\hat{C}C_{m:g:c} = \frac{\hat{\sigma}^2_{g:c}}{\hat{\sigma}^2_e + \hat{\sigma}^2_{g:c}} = \frac{1.77}{69.7 + 1.77} = 0.0242$$

The $VIF_{m:g:c}$ is estimated as:

$$V\hat{I}F = \left(1 + (m-1)I\hat{C}C_{m:g:c}\right) = (1 + (861-1)0.0242) = 21.8$$

Even with the reduction in the standard error, the estimated *VIF* is still very large.

The tests of fixed effects (not shown) provide no indication that the two conditions differ significantly in average diastolic blood pressure at posttest after adjustment for baseline values on diastolic blood pressure and the other covariates. Table 8.29 presents the estimate of the intervention effect, here the difference between the adjusted means. Note the agreement between the standard error for the estimate and the value calculated above from the variance components.

Implementation for Dichotomous Data

To implement this analysis for smoking status in SAS PROC MIXED, the code shown in the upper panel of Table 8.30 is appropriate. To implement this analysis for smoking status in the GLIMMIX macro, the code shown in the lower panel of Table 8.30 is appropriate.

The lsmeans and estimate statements are usually omitted from the GLIMMIX analysis but are retained here as a demonstration. In addition, the solution option is added to the model statement to provide the parameter estimates from the mixed-model logistic regression analysis.

As in the analysis for diastolic blood pressure, covariates are selected from both the baseline and the follow-up data. Baseline values are used for covariates that might be affected by the intervention (dbp1, educ1, and marit1) and follow-up values are used otherwise, since correlations are expected to be higher for more proximal measures.

Table 8.29. Estimate for (I-C) From the Analysis of Diastolic Blood Pressure With Regression Adjustment for Baseline Values in the Pretest-Posttest Control Group Design

Parameter	Estimate	SE	DDF	T
I-C	-0.36732	1.11459	4	-0.33
	Pr>|T|	Alpha	Lower	Upper
	0.7587	0.05	-3.4619	2.7273

Table 8.30. SAS PROC MIXED and GLIMMIX Code for the Analysis of Smoking Status With Regression Adjustment for Baseline Values in the Pretest-Posttest Control Group Design

```
MIXED
proc mixed info order=internal;
  class cond group sex educ1 marit1;
  model smk2=cond smk1 age2 sex educ1 marit1
    /ddf=4 ddfm=res;
  random group(cond);
  lsmeans cond/om c1 e;
  estimate 'I-C' cond 1 -1/c1 e;
run;

GLIMMIX
%include 'glimmix.sas';
%glimmix(
  procopt=info order=internal,
  data=coh_mult,
  stmts=%str(
    class cond group sex educ1 marit1;
    model smk2=cond smk1 age2 sex educ1 marit1
      /ddf=4 ddfm=res solution;
    random group(cond);
    lsmeans cond/om c1 e;
    estimate 'I-C' cond 1 -1/c1 e;
    ),
  error=binomial,
  link=logit);
run;
```

The results from the MIXED and GLIMMIX analyses were quite similar except for the least-squares means and the estimates of the intervention effect. Table 8.31 presents the least-squares means from the MIXED analysis. Those results suggest that after adjustment for baseline, the smoking prevalence rates at posttest were 25.5% and 25.4%, respectively, in the intervention and control conditions.

Table 8.31 also presents the least squares means from the GLIMMIX analysis. Recall that those means are computed by weighting the parameter estimates as directed by the om option and summing the weighted estimates. Under the identity link, this would provide an adjusted mean rate. However, under the logit link, quite different results obtain. The order of the MU is correct, but the absolute values are clearly not. The correct means can be obtained from the parameter estimates, but only with separate calculations. The inverse link applied to the sum of the weighted log odds is simply not the same as the sum of the weighted odds, which is what is wanted. Unfortunately

Table 8.31. MIXED and GLIMMIX Least-Squares Means From the Analysis of Smoking Status With Regression Adjustment for Baseline Values in the Pretest-Posttest Control Group Design

MIXED Level	LSMEAN	SE	DDF	T	$Pr>\|T\|$
COND I	0.25497	0.00669	4	38.10	0.0001
COND C	0.25401	0.00667	4	38.06	0.0001
Level			Alpha	Lower	Upper
COND I			0.05	0.2364	0.2736
COND C			0.05	0.2355	0.2725

GLIMMIX Level	LSMEAN	SE	DDF	T	$Pr>\|T\|$
COND I	-2.2324	0.1149	4	-19.43	0.0001
COND C	-2.2567	0.1152	4	-19.60	0.0001
Alpha	Lower	Upper	MU	Lower MU	Upper MU
0.05	-2.5514	-1.9134	0.0969	0.0723	0.1286
0.05	-2.5764	-1.9369	0.0948	0.0707	0.1260

for the user, it is difficult to program the latter, and that is why most logistic regression programs do not do it.

Table 8.32 presents the estimate of the intervention effect from the MIXED and GLIMMIX analyses. The estimate from MIXED is scaled as the difference in adjusted smoking rates between the two conditions and so is readily interpretable. The estimate from GLIMMIX is scaled as a log odds ratio; the MU are uninformative and potentially misleading. As before, the *t*-tests and *p*-values for the two estimates agree closely, as both test the same null hypothesis.

Stratification or Matching in the Analysis

A Priori Stratification

SAS PROC MIXED and the GLIMMIX macro can be used to implement a stratified analysis for a design based on *a priori* stratification, following the presentation in Chapter 6. However, the MHHP did not employ *a priori* stratification and so the MHHP data cannot be used to illustrate that analysis. In-

Table 8.32. MIXED and GLIMMIX Estimates for (I-C) From the Analysis of
Smoking Status With Regression Adjustment for Baseline Values in the
Pretest-Posttest Control Group Design

MIXED					
Parameter	Estimate	SE	DDF	T	Pr>|T|
I-C	0.0009586	0.009485	4	0.10	0.9244
Alpha	Lower	Upper			
0.05	−0.0254	0.0273			
GLIMMIX					
Parameter	Estimate	SE	DDF	T	Pr>|T|
I-C	0.0242	0.1403	4	0.17	0.8712
Alpha	Lower	Upper	MU	Lower MU	Upper MU
0.05	−0.3653	0.4137	0.5061	0.4097	0.6020

deed, *a priori* stratification was not possible for MHHP, given only three communities in each condition.

Post Hoc Stratification in the Adjusted Time × Condition Analysis

SAS PROC MIXED and the GLIMMIX macro can also be used to implement a *post hoc* stratified time × condition analysis, again following the presentation in Chapter 6. The MHHP investigators employed *post hoc* stratification on age, sex, and educational attainment as a part of their primary analysis (Luepker et al., 1994).

Implementation for Gaussian Data

To implement an analysis for diastolic blood pressure that is stratified on sex, the code shown in Table 8.33 is appropriate.

The `noclprint` option is added to the `proc mixed` statement to prevent printing all the member ID numbers. The `convh=0.000001` option is added in an effort to speed the analysis without measurably affecting the parameter estimates. The `class` statement must include `sex` so that sex can be used as a stratification factor.

To stratify on sex, three fixed-effect interactions involving `sex` are included in the `model` statement, along with the main effect of `sex`. These are sex-

Table 8.33. SAS PROC MIXED Code for the Adjusted Analysis of Diastolic Blood Pressure in the Pretest-Posttest Control Group Design With *Post Hoc* Stratification

```
proc mixed info order=internal noclprint convh=0.000001;
  class cond group member time sex educlvl bpobsrvr
    bplocatn;
  model dbp=cond sex cond*sex time cond*time time*sex
    cond*time*sex age educlvl bpobsrvr bplocatn
    /ddfm=res ddf=4,4,4,4,4,4,4 singular=0.000001;
  random int sex time sex*time/subject=group(cond);
  repeated time/type=cs subject=member(group*cond*sex);
  lsmeans cond*time*sex/om cl e;
  estimate '(I3-I0)-(C3-C0) (m-w)'
    cond*sex*time 1 -1 -1 1 -1 1 1 -1/cl e;
run;
```

*cond, sex*time, and cond*time*sex. The three-way interaction is the term of interest in the stratified analysis.

The *ddf* for the first seven fixed effects are all 4 because there are only two strata and two time points. With additional strata or time points, these *ddf* vary among the fixed effects according to the formulae provided in the table of expected mean squares in Chapter 6 (Table 6.5).

The test of the null hypothesis is the test of the TCS interaction. There is little interest in the six other fixed effects involving condition, time, or strata, and interpretation of those terms is complicated by the presence of the TCS interaction in the model. Even so, the ddf= option ensures that those tests are assessed with the correct *ddf.*

The lsmeans effect is cond*sex*time and provides the cell means that define the null hypothesis in the stratified analysis. To ensure that the least-squares means are computed based on the marginal distribution of the data, the om option is included in the lsmeans statement.

This analysis indicated that several of the variance components had been fixed at zero. The adverse effect of this non-negativity constraint was discussed in Chapter 4. The solution to this problem in the context of nested cross-sectional data is to rerun the analysis using the nobound and method=mivque0 options. The former overrides the non-negativity constraint for estimation of the variance components. The latter specifies a non-iterative estimation method that is much faster than REML or ML and valid as long as the residual error represents at least 90% of the variation in the data (Swallow and Monahan, 1984). While the nobound option is equally applicable in cohort data, the method=mivque0 option often is not, especially in a repeated-measures analysis such as this. Here, the member component of variance represents a very large fraction of the total variation, violating the requirement that the residual error represent at least 90% of the variation in the data. As a result, the analysis was rerun using the nobound option alone. Unfortunately, the nobound analysis failed. Experience has shown that this kind of problem is more likely to happen in SAS PROC MIXED for complex analyses such as this than in the simpler analyses presented earlier in this chapter. At the same time, it leaves the analyst in the less-than-satisfactory position of having only the results from the initial analysis that fixed several of the variance components at zero. There is no good solution for this kind of problem in SAS PROC MIXED, and the analyst must either choose other software, report the available results, abandon the stratified analysis, or switch to post hoc stratification in the context of the analysis of posttest data with regression adjustment for baseline values, presented in the next section.

Post Hoc Stratification in the Analysis of Posttest Data With Regression Adjustment for Baseline Values

Implementation for Gaussian Data

To implement this analysis for diastolic blood pressure, the code shown in Table 8.34 is appropriate.

The code is based on that shown for the unstratified version of this analysis. Sex was already in the class and model statements, but cond*sex was not. Because the cond*sex interaction is now included in the model, sex as a main effect is tested against sex*group(cond) and no longer against the residual error; this is shown in the table of expected mean squares in Chapter 6 (Table 6.6). As a result, the ddf= option is extended to designate 4 ddf for both sex and cond*sex.

The lsmeans requested are for the cond*sex cells, since those adjusted means define the intervention effect, and the slice= option is used to help guide interpretation of the results should the cond*sex interaction prove significant. Finally, the estimate statement generates a net difference in-

Table 8.34. SAS PROC MIXED Code for the Analysis of Diastolic Blood Pressure With Regression Adjustment for Baseline Values in the Pretest-Posttest Control Group Design With *Post Hoc* Stratification

```
proc mixed info order=internal;
  class cond group sex educ1 bpobs2 bploc2;
  model dbp2 =cond sex cond*sex dbp1 age2 educ1 bpobs2 bploc2
    /ddf=4,4,4 ddfm=res;
  random int sex/subject=group(cond);
  lsmeans cond*sex/om slice=sex cl e;
  estimate 'M(I-C)-F(I-C)' cond*sex -1 1 1 -1/cl e;
run;
```

Table 8.35. Covariance-Parameter Estimates (REML) From the Analysis of Diastolic Blood Pressure With Regression Adjustment for Baseline Values in the Pretest-Posttest Control Group Design With *Post Hoc* Stratification

Cov Parm	Estimate
INTERCEPT	1.76918
SEX	0.02534
Residual	69.65275

volving the four adjusted sex × condition means; that net difference is the estimate of the intervention effect in this analysis.

Table 8.35 presents the covariance-parameter estimates. Given 5167 observations and $g = 3$ groups in each of $c = 2$ conditions and crossed with $s = 2$ strata, the average $m = 431$. Using these values, the mean squares are estimated in Table 8.36.

The $MS_{gs:c}$ is dramatically smaller than the $MS_{g:c}$ in the unstratified analysis. However, in the calculation of the standard error, it is combined with a larger multiplier and divided by a smaller denominator, as shown in Equation 6.17:

$$\hat{\sigma}_\Delta = \sqrt{2*2\left(\frac{\hat{MS}_{gs:c}}{mg}\right)} = \sqrt{2*2\left(\frac{80.6}{431*3}\right)} = 0.499$$

This standard error is about 55% smaller than the standard error for the unstratified analysis. This reduction demonstrates the precision advantage that *post hoc* stratification can have.

The adjusted $ICC_{m:gs:c}$ is estimated as:

$$\hat{ICC}_{m:gs:c} = \frac{\hat{\sigma}^2_{gs:c}}{\hat{\sigma}^2_e + \hat{\sigma}^2_{gs:c}} = \frac{0.0253}{69.7 + 0.0253} = 0.000363$$

the $VIF_{m:gs:c}$ is estimated as:

Table 8.36. Selected Mean-Square Estimates From the Analysis of Diastolic Blood Pressure With Regression Adjustment for Baseline Values in the Pretest-Posttest Control Group Design with *Post Hoc* Stratification

Source	E(MS)	Estimate
GS:C	$\sigma^2_e + m\sigma^2_{gs:c}$	$69.7 + 431*0.0253 = 80.6$
Member:GS:C	σ^2_e	69.7

$$V\hat{I}F_{m:gs:c} = \left(1 + (m-1)I\hat{C}C_{m:gs:c}\right) = \left(1 + (431-1)0.000363\right) = 1.16$$

Recall that the unstratified VIF was 21.8; again, this dramatic reduction reflects the advantage that *post hoc* stratification can have.

In spite of the reduction in the VIF, there was no evidence of an intervention effect based on the F-test for the COND*SEX interaction (not shown). Improvements in precision will help to detect effects that are of reasonable size; however, if the effect is small, improvements in precision will still yield a nonsignificant finding.

Table 8.37 presents the intervention-effect estimate generated by the estimate statement; that estimate is the adjusted net difference between the two sex-specific differences. The positive value indicates that there was a somewhat more favorable intervention effect among women than among men. That interpretation is confirmed in the pattern of the least-squares means (not shown). Consistent with the F-test for the condition × sex interaction, this estimate is not significantly different from zero.

Matching in the Analysis

The communities in the MHHP were matched on size, type, and distance from Minneapolis–St. Paul. One city from each of the three pairs was assigned to the intervention condition and the other to the control condition. The primary analysis did not reflect the matching (Luepker et al., 1994), but a matched analysis is possible, following the presentation in Chapter 6.

Implementation for Gaussian Data

To implement the matched analysis for diastolic blood pressure, the code shown in Table 8.38 is appropriate.

In the matched analysis, group is left out of the class and random statements because it is completely confounded with condition × strata.

Table 8.37. Estimate for M(I-C)-F(I-C) From the Analysis of Diastolic Blood Pressure With Regression Adjustment for Baseline Values in the Pretest-Posttest Control Group Design With *Post Hoc* Stratification

Parameter	Estimate	SE	DDF	T
M(I-C)-F(I-C)	0.40194	0.50439	4	0.80
	Pr>|T|	Alpha	Lower	Upper
	0.4701	0.05	−0.9985	1.8024

Table 8.38. SAS PROC MIXED Code for the Analysis of Diastolic
Blood Pressure With Regression Adjustment for Baseline Values in
the Pretest-Posttest Control Group Design With *A Priori* Matching

```
proc mixed info order=internal;
  class cond strata sex educ1 bpobs2 bploc2;
  model dbp2=cond dbp1 age2 sex educ1 bpobs2 bploc2
    /ddf=2 ddfm=res;
  random int cond/subject=strata;
  lsmeans cond/om cl e;
  estimate 'I-C' cond 1 -1/cl e;
run;
```

Strata and its interaction are placed in the random statement. There is no
nesting explicitly shown in the MIXED code, as none of the effects shown is
a nested effect. The member is of course nested within the cells of the CS
interaction, but since that term is the residual error, it is not written explicitly
into the code.

One of the effects of the matching is clearly shown in the ddf= option,
which now specifies *ddf* only for the first fixed effect in the model statement.
Because the adjusted analysis is now based on the number of pairs ($s = 3$), the
ddf are half what they are in an unpaired analysis. The *ddf* for the first fixed
effect are computed as $(c-1)(s-1)=2$, as shown in the table of expected
mean squares in Chapter 6 (Table 6.8). Matching always reduces the *ddf* for
the test of interest by half, absent group-level covariates, and exacts a large
power penalty when the number of matched sets is small.

Table 8.39 presents the covariance-parameter estimates for the matched
analysis. Given 5167 observations and $s = 3$ pairs and $c = 2$ conditions, the
average $m = 861$. Using these values, the mean squares are estimated in Table
8.40.

Given 624 as the estimate for MS_{cs}, the standard error for the intervention
effect is estimated using Equation 6.20:

$$\hat{\sigma}_\Delta = \sqrt{2\left(\frac{\hat{MS}_{cs}}{ms}\right)} = \sqrt{2\left(\frac{624}{861*3}\right)} = 0.695$$

This standard error is about 40% smaller than the standard error from the
unmatched analysis.

The adjusted $ICC_{m:cs}$ is estimated as:

$$I\hat{C}C_{m:cs} = \frac{\hat{\sigma}^2_{cs}}{\hat{\sigma}^2_e + \hat{\sigma}^2_{cs}} = \frac{0.644}{69.7 + 0.644} = 0.00916$$

The $VIF_{m:cs}$ is estimated as:

Table 8.39. Covariance-Parameter Estimates (REML) From
the Analysis of Diastolic Blood Pressure With Regression
Adjustment for Baseline Values in the Pretest-Posttest
Control Group Design With A Priori Matching

Cov Parm	Estimate
INTERCEPT	1.14758
COND	0.64352
Residual	69.65655

$$\hat{VIF}_{m:cs} = \left(1 + (m-1)\hat{ICC}_{m:cs}\right) = \left(1 + (861-1)0.00916\right) = 8.88$$

Even with the reduction in the standard error, the VIF is still very large.

The results for the tests of fixed effects (not shown) were quite similar to those in the unmatched analysis with no evidence of an intervention effect. The adjusted means (not shown) were almost identical to those in the unmatched analysis. The intervention effect is shown in Table 8.41 and is also quite similar to that reported for the unmatched version of this analysis, though the standard error is smaller by almost 40%.

Additional Baseline or Follow-up Intervals

Thus far, the MHHP design has been reduced to two observations per member so as to illustrate analyses appropriate for the Pretest-Posttest Control Group Design, with or without regression adjustment for covariates, stratification, or matching. In fact, the full MHHP cohort design involved up to three observations on each member. The analyses considered thus far involved approximately two-thirds of the full MHHP cohort data set, or about 5000 persons. In fact, the full MHHP cohort data set includes more than 15,000 observations on more than 7,000 persons.

Table 8.40. Selected Mean-Square Estimates From the
Analysis of Diastolic Blood Pressure With Regression
Adjustment for Baseline Values in the Pretest-Posttest
Control Group Design With A Priori Matching

Source	E(MS)	Estimate
CS	$\sigma_e^2 + m\sigma_{cs}^2$	$69.7 + 861*0.644 = 624$
Subject:CS	σ_e^2	69.7

Table 8.41. Estimate for (I-C) From the Analysis of Diastolic Blood Pressure With Regression Adjustment for Baseline Values in the Pretest-Posttest Control Group Design With *A Priori* Matching

Parameter	Estimate	SE	DDF	T
I-C	−0.37390	0.70037	2	−0.53
	Pr > |T|	Alpha	Lower	Upper
	0.6468	0.05	3.3874	2.6396

This section illustrates analyses appropriate for nested cohort designs involving more than two observations on each member. These analyses allow consideration of the entire cohort data set for the MHHP. The analyses for Extended Designs include trend analysis in the mixed-model ANOVA/ ANCOVA and random-coefficients analyses. Analyses for Extended Designs are less developed than for the simpler Pretest-Posttest Control Group Design, and readers must keep that in mind as they study the material in this section.

The Traditional Mixed-Model ANOVA/ANCOVA

Chapter 6 noted three weaknesses in the traditional mixed-model ANOVA/ ANCOVA as applied to the Extended Design. First, when more than two time intervals are included in the design, the assumption that each group in a given condition shares a common slope may be inappropriate. Second, as soon as there are additional time intervals in the design, attention must be paid to the structure of the within-member random-effects covariance matrix. Third, this analysis often has less power for a predictable intervention effect than its alternatives because it casts a very broad net in its estimation of the intervention effect.

This section develops the traditional mixed-model ANOVA/ANCOVA for the full MHHP cohort data set, but only in a limited fashion. In particular, this section illustrates the definition of time, the computation of *ddf* for fixed effects, and the MIXED code for the analysis, but does not present any examples.

Defining Time

The MHHP design provides a good example of a complex nested cohort design. As shown in Figure 7.1, there were 2–4 annual baseline surveys in each community. Persons who participated in the baseline surveys were randomly selected for recruitment to follow-up surveys at either $+2$ years or $+4$ years after the introduction of the intervention in the intervention communities; all participants in the baseline surveys were recruited to a follow-up survey at $+6$ or $+7$ years.[10]

As discussed in Chapter 7, the survey date was recorded for each participant. As a result, it is possible to calculate for each cohort member the time between each survey date and the intervention start-up date for their community pair. Those measures can be computed in days, with negative values for baseline surveys and positive values for intervention surveys. Persons surveyed on the day the intervention began in a given pair are assigned a zero.

Categorization of this time variable provides new variables scaled in terms of years (11 levels, -2 to $+8$), months (56 levels, -34 to $+87$), and weeks (183 levels, -148 to $+375$) from the intervention start-up date. Given 15,630 observations in the cohort data set, most of these levels have many observations, though there are some cells that are empty for some communities or that have only one observation, especially when time is scaled in weeks.[11]

ddf for Fixed Effects

Chapter 7 illustrates the determination of ddf for fixed effects in a complex nested cross-sectional design. Those same methods are used for a nested cohort design. To illustrate, consider the cross-tabulation for year $\times$ community as shown in Table 8.42.

Table 8.42. Cross-tabulation of Survey Year and Community in the Minnesota Heart Health Program Cohort Data

	Community						
Year	M	W	F/M	SF	B	R	Total
-2	0	0	208	404	432	406	1450
-1	0	0	317	254	211	221	1003
0	682	334	257	227	251	228	1979
1	136	412	33	0	231	260	1072
2	314	0	273	418	147	0	1152
3	146	433	122	5	379	535	1620
4	408	0	265	425	2	0	1100
5	72	456	134	1	538	559	1760
7	519	0	438	717	953	954	3581
8	138	574	201	0	0	0	913
Total	2415	2209	2248	2451	3144	3163	15630

Table 8.43. Partition of the *df* for the Traditional Mixed-Model
ANOVA/ANCOVA When Time is Scaled in Years, Months, and Weeks

Source	df	Year	Month	Week
Intercept	1	1	1	1
Condition	$c-1$	1	1	1
Group:C	$c(g-1)-x_{gf}-x_{gv}$	4	4	4
Time	$t-1$	10	55	182
TC	$(t-1)(c-1)$	10	—	—
TG:C	$(t-1)c(g\text{-}1)-x_{gv}$	24	—	—
Total	tgc	50	95	255

The computed variable year has 11 levels, ranging from -2 to 8. Given six communities, the upper limit on the total *df* at the group level is $11*6 = 66$. However, 14 of the cells have 1 or fewer observations, reducing the total *df* to 52; two other cells have 5 or fewer observations and so really can't contribute to the analysis, leaving 50.

Table 8.43 presents the partition of the *df* for the traditional mixed-model ANOVA/ANCOVA when time is scaled in years. This partition is similar to that shown in Table 7.59 for the nested cross-sectional version of this design. One *df* is allocated for the intercept and another for condition $(c-1=1)$. Four are allocated for group(condition). Ten each are allocated for time and condition $\times$ time. Those *df* sum to 26; assuming that there are no group-level covariates, there are 24 *df* available for *TG:C*, the residual error at the group level. Note that the formula for $df_{tg:c} = (t-1)c(g-1) = 32$, which is larger than 24. This can and does happen, and the analyst has no choice but to work with the smaller number.

A parallel analysis of the data when time was scaled as months gave a total *df* of 95 and for time scaled as weeks gave a total *df* of 255. As is the case in Chapter 7, there are so many levels of time available when time is scaled in months or weeks that a categorical representation of time exhausts the total *df* at the group level, leaving no *df* for the group-level error term. As a result, the traditional mixed-model ANOVA/ANCOVA cannot be conducted at the level of the month or week if time is treated as a categorical variable.

Implementation for Gaussian Data

The SAS PROC MIXED code for this analysis is presented in Table 8.44. The code is similar to that presented for the time $\times$ condition analysis in the Pretest-Posttest Control Group Design (cf. Table 8.21). It substitutes `year` for the more generic `time`. It specifies *ddf* for the first three fixed effects based

Table 8.44. SAS PROC MIXED Code for the Traditional Mixed-Model ANCOVA of Diastolic Blood Pressure in the Extended Design

```
proc mixed info order=internal noclprint convh=0.000001;
  class cond group member year educlvl bpobsrvr
    bplocatn;
  model dbp=cond year cond*year educlvl bpobsrvr bplocatn
    /ddfm=res ddf=4,24,24 singular=0.000001;
  random int year/subject=group(cond);
  repeated year/type=cs subject=member(group*cond)
    r=1 to 3 rcorr=1 to 3;
run;
```

on the partition of the 50 total df available at the group level, as shown in Table 8.44. In particular, the ddf for cond are computed as $c(g-1) = 2(3-1) = 4$. The ddf for year and cond*year are the residual df available at the group level, 24.

Note that the code does not include either an lsmeans statement or an estimate statement. Given 11 time intervals and 2 conditions, there are 22 least-squares means. They can be requested using the familiar lsmeans statement, but will be difficult to interpret due to their number. An estimate statement can help considerably here, as it will direct the program to compute an estimate of a specific-intervention effect and a standard error for that effect. This often is a more profitable course than simply requesting all possible least squares means.

Trend Analysis in the Mixed-Model ANOVA/ANCOVA

Coding Time as a Continuous Variable

Having defined time in terms of years, months, and weeks from the introduction of the intervention program, those variables may be used to treat time as a continuous variable. All three measures are scaled in real time and each has an appropriate zero point.

Specifying an Intervention Pattern

The fixed-effects portion of the analysis in this example will be adapted from the trend analysis presented in Chapter 7 for the corresponding analysis in the cross-sectional data. Time will be represented with both linear and quadratic terms, as will the intervention effect; in addition, the intervention effect will be constrained to zero during the baseline period.

Partitioning the Degrees of Freedom

As noted earlier, the total df at the group level for these three levels of time are 50, 95, and 255. The partitioning of the df for these levels of time is shown in Table 8.45.

Because the total df at the group level depends on the number of time intervals, the total df increases dramatically as the number of time intervals increases. Because the representation of the first seven effects is identical in each of the three analyses, their df are identical, and so the df available for the $TG:C$ term benefits directly from the increased number of time intervals.

Implementation for Gaussian Data

SAS PROC MIXED can be used to examine alternate structures for the within-member random-effects covariance matrix using the `type=` option in the `repeated` statement. Several structures are considered here for the MHHP diastolic blood pressure data; to simplify the examples, all models are unadjusted.

There are many different structures that may be specified for the within-member random-effects covariance matrix in SAS PROC MIXED. Wolfinger (1993, 1996) and several pieces of the SAS documentation provide details on the many structures available (SAS, Inc., 1992, 1996). In addition, the recent text on the SAS System for Mixed Models (Littell et al., 1996) provides several examples, though none in the context of a group-randomized trial.

Only a few of these structures are of interest in most group-randomized trials. As described in Chapter 6, those are compound symmetry, first-order autoregressive, and Toeplitz. Those structures presume, respectively, constant

Table 8.45. Partition of the df for the Trend Analysis in the Mixed-Model ANCOVA When Time is Scaled in Years, Months, and Weeks

Source	Generic	Year	Month	Week
Intercept	1	1	1	1
Condition	$c-1$	1	1	1
Group:C	$c(g-1)-x_{gf}-x_{gv}$	4	4	4
Time	1	1	1	1
Time × Time	1	1	1	1
Time × C	$c-1$	1	1	1
Time × Time × C	$c-1$	1	1	1
$TG:C$	res_{tgc}	40	85	245
Total	tgc	50	95	255

correlation over time, correlation that is declining exponentially over time, and correlation that is declining monotonically over time. A fourth structure that can be helpful in the selection of one of these patterns is the unstructured matrix, which allows each correlation to be unique.

As shown previously, to fit a compound-symmetry structure in SAS PROC MIXED, a `type = cs` option is included in the `repeated` statement. To fit one of the other structures, the analyst need only change the effect of the `type=` option. To fit a first-order autoregressive structure, that effect is specified as `ar(1)`. To fit a Toeplitz structure, that effect is specified as `toep`. To fit an unstructured matrix, that effect is specified simply as `un`.

Prior to the MIXED analysis, a data step must be used to define the intervention effect and other variables required in this analysis. For example, the code for the analysis with time scaled in years is shown in Table 8.46.

This code is identical to that employed in the analysis of the cross-sectional data in Chapter 7, though the name of the data file in the data step is different. The `if/else` statement creates a new variable, `iyear`, set equal to time for observations in the intervention condition after the baseline period. As such, that term can be considered a variant on the time × condition interaction, constrained to zero during the baseline period. The `yearcat` variable is set equal to `year` and will be used to reflect time as a categorical variable. This is particularly important in a repeated-measures analysis, as it defines the length of the time intervals between measurements on the same subject and allows the program to properly align the observations in the computation of the within-member random-effects covariance matrix.

The SAS PROC MIXED code for the unadjusted analysis by year with the unstructured within-member random-effects covariance matrix is shown in Table 8.47.

The `title` statement provides documentation in the output and is useful when several alternative models are considered at one time. `Year` is defined as a continuous variable by leaving it out of the `class` statement. `Yearcat` is defined as a categorical variable by putting it into the `class` statement. The combination of `year` and `year2` in the `model` statement defines a com-

Table 8.46. SAS Code to Define the Intervention Effect and Other Variables for the Trend Analysis in the Extended Design

```
data cohort;
  yearcat = year;
  year2 = year*year;
  if year>0 and cond=0 then iyear=year;
  else iyear=0;
  iyear2 = iyear*iyear;
run;
```

Table 8.47. SAS PROC MIXED Code for the Trend Analysis in the Extended Design

```
proc mixed info order = internal noclprint convh = 0.000001;
  title3 'YEAR: UN';
  class cond group member yearcat;
  model dbp = cond year year2 iyear iyear2
    /ddf = 4,40,40,40,40 ddfm = res solution
    singular = 0.000001;
  repeated yearcat/type = un subject = member(group*cond);
  random int yearcat/subject = group(cond);
run;
```

mon secular trend, with linear and quadratic components, to be estimated from all the data except observations taken in the intervention condition after the baseline period. Separate intercepts are allowed for the two conditions by putting cond into the model statement. Iyear and its quadratic form, iyear2, represent the deviation observed in the intervention condition from the common secular trend after the baseline period. Note that the lsmeans and estimate statements are omitted, as the intervention effect is no longer defined as a pattern of means. Instead, the intervention effect is reflected in the coefficients for iyear and iyear2, obtained through the solution option in the model statement.

The ddf = option specifies the *ddf* for the tests of fixed effects. The error term for cond is group(cond), with 4 *df*. The error term for year, year2, iyear, and iyear2 is yearcat*group(cond), with 40 *df*.

The repeated statement is used as in previous sections in this chapter. The only effect listed in the repeated statement is yearcat, as that is the term that provides information for the alignment of the time intervals. Effects listed in the repeated statement must be class variables, and year would not serve this purpose; however, yearcat does. The unstructured within-member covariance matrix is specified via the type = un option. The repeated-measures factor is identified with the subject = option as member(cond*group).

Note that yearcat is used in the random statement; this variable was set equal to year in the data step. The use of the categorical representation of time in the random statement ensures that the *tgc* time × group surveys are represented as distinct entities so that the group-level residual-error term is based on the variation among the time × group means. It is also necessary in order for the within-member covariance matrix to be created properly.

The dimensions of the analysis are summarized in Table 8.48. The 57 covariance parameters reflect the unstructured within-member random-effects covar-

Table 8.48. Dimensions of the Trend Analysis of Diastolic Blood Pressure in the Extended Design With Time Scaled in Years and an Unstructured Within-Member Random-Effects Covariance Matrix

Description	Value
Covariance Parameters	57
Columns in X	7
Max Cols in Z Per Subject	11
Subjects	6
Max Obs Per Subject	3153
Observations Used	15532
Observations Not Used	0
Total Observations	15532

iance matrix. In an unstructured matrix, each element is estimated as a separate parameter. There are 15,532 observations in the full cohort data set.

Given 57 covariance parameters, the list of covariance parameters is quite long, as seen in Table 8.49. The INTERCEPT term has its usual meaning and represents the component of variance for group(cond). The YEARCAT term represents the component of variance for yearcat*group(cond). The next 55 entries in the table provide the elements of the within-member random-effects covariance matrix, indexed by their position in the matrix. For example, UN(1,1) is the variance for yearcat = 1, while UN(10,10) is the variance for yearcat = 10. UN(5,1) is the covariance between yearcat = 5 and yearcat = 1. The residual term should be ignored in the context of an unstructured within-member random-effects covariance matrix.

It is very difficult to see any pattern in such a list. It is much easier to see a pattern after transforming the list into a 10 × 10 matrix, shown in Table 8.50. The row and column headings refer to the value of yearcat.

Several features stand out in this matrix. First, several of the covariances are zero, especially in the early years. Second, there is a tendency for the covariances to decrease as they move farther away from the main diagonal. Third, the variances on the main diagonal decline somewhat over time.

The first pattern is easily explained by the unusual cohort design employed in the MHHP. Recall that persons who participated in the cross-sectional survey during the first four years were recruited to participate as cohort members in later years. As a result, no one person was seen more than once during the first four years. For that reason, there can be no covariances involving years 1, 2, 3, or 4.

The second pattern is consistent with the expectation that blood pressure

Table 8.49. Covariance-Parameter Estimates (REML) From the Trend Analysis of Diastolic Blood Pressure in the Extended Design With Time Scaled in Years and an Unstructured Within-Member Random-Effects Covariance Matrix

Parameter		Estimate	Parameter	Estimate	Parameter	Estimate
INTERCEPT		0.409				
YEARCAT		3.535				
YEARCAT	UN(1,1)	111.156	UN(6,5)	0.000	UN(9,3)	50.192
	UN(2,1)	0.000	UN(6,6)	101.792	UN(9,4)	60.029
	UN(2,2)	138.679	UN(7,1)	51.613	UN(9,5)	62.475
	UN(3,1)	0.000	UN(7,2)	61.325	UN(9,6)	52.870
	UN(3,2)	0.000	UN(7,3)	52.863	UN(9,7)	52.591
	UN(3,3)	103.710	UN(7,4)	58.806	UN(9,8)	61.089
	UN(4,1)	0.000	UN(7,5)	44.550	UN(9,9)	100.446
	UN(4,2)	0.000	UN(7,6)	63.788	UN(10,1)	38.498
	UN(4,3)	0.000	UN(7,7)	101.788	UN(10,2)	49.915
	UN(4,4)	116.287	UN(8,1)	62.265	UN(10,3)	46.841
	UN(5,1)	67.840	UN(8,2)	58.029	UN(10,4)	52.225
	UN(5,2)	77.070	UN(8,3)	57.289	UN(10,5)	43.408
	UN(5,3)	65.914	UN(8,4)	65.768	UN(10,6)	41.507
	UN(5,4)	67.894	UN(8,5)	85.900	UN(10,7)	55.194
	UN(5,5)	109.860	UN(8,6)	63.754	UN(10,8)	54.914
	UN(6,1)	60.615	UN(8,7)	0.000	UN(10,9)	0.000
	UN(6,2)	56.924	UN(8,8)	108.104	UN(10,10)	99.605
	UN(6,3)	59.743	UN(9,1)	48.472		
	UN(6,4)	70.827	UN(9,2)	52.048	Residual	1.001

measurements taken close together will be more highly correlated than measurements taken far apart.

The third pattern is weaker than the other two. It may be due in part to attrition over time, as fewer members of the cohort were measured in later years. To the extent that those who remained were more homogeneous than the full cohort, one would expect smaller variances over time.

To make it easier to see the correlation pattern, the variances and covariances can be used to compute the correlations, using the formula:

$$\text{corr}(1,2) = \frac{\text{cov}(1,2)}{\sqrt{\text{var}(1) * \text{var}(2)}} \tag{8.7}$$

The resulting correlation matrix is shown in Table 8.51. In that matrix, it is easy to see the pattern of the correlations over time. Though there is some

Table 8.50. Covariance-Parameter Estimates (REML) From the Trend Analysis of Diastolic Blood Pressure in the Extended Design With Time Scaled in Years and an Unstructured Within-Member Random-Effects Covariance Matrix, Rearranged Into a 10 × 10 Matrix

Year	1	2	3	4	5	6	7	8	9	10
1	110.6									
2	0.0	135.0								
3	0.0	0.0	103.4							
4	0.0	0.0	0.0	115.5						
5	70.9	80.5	65.9	67.5	109.8					
6	60.3	55.9	59.4	70.5	0.0	101.5				
7	63.5	59.7	53.3	59.5	44.2	68.6	97.8			
8	61.9	57.5	57.0	65.2	88.0	63.5	0.0	107.8		
9	48.2	51.5	50.1	59.7	62.7	52.6	53.9	60.9	100.3	
10	30.3	43.0	48.1	54.6	43.7	42.5	56.7	56.1	0.0	97.7

variation, there is clearly a pattern of declining correlation with increasing lag between measurements. However, that pattern does not follow the exponential pattern anticipated in the first-order autoregressive structure and may be better fit by the Toeplitz structure. It is also possible, given the variations in the pattern, that the compound-symmetry structure will suffice.

To compare the four structures, the analysis must be run four times, changing the structure through the type= option in the repeated statement. Information concerning the model fit from those four analyses is summarized in Table 8.52.

Recall that the REML Log-Likelihood, Akaike's Information Criterion, and Schwarz's Bayesian Criterion may be used to compare models. Of these, Schwarz's Bayesian Criterion is the most stringent but also the most broadly applicable (Kass and Raftery, 1995). The model with the value closest to zero is deemed to fit the data better than the other models. In this case, that is the model with the Toeplitz structure, though the model with the compound-symmetry structure has a very similar value for the Schwarz criterion. The Akaike criterion is not as stringent and favors the unstructured matrix, while the model with the Toeplitz structure ranks second on that index. The same pattern holds for the −2 REML Log Likelihood. The matrix with the first-order autoregressive structure ranks last on all indicators.

Parsimony is also a consideration in selecting models (Wolfinger, 1996) and the four structures vary considerably in the number of parameters. The unstructured matrix has 57 covariance parameters, the Toeplitz matrix has 12,

Table 8.51. Over-Time Correlations from the Trend Analysis of Diastolic Blood Pressure in the Extended Design with Time Scaled in Years and an Unstructured Within-Member Random-Effects Covariance Matrix, Rearranged Into a 10 × 10 Matrix

Year	1	2	3	4	5	6	7	8	9	10
1	1.000									
2	0.000	1.000								
3	0.000	0.000	1.000							
4	0.000	0.000	0.000	1.000						
5	0.644	0.661	0.618	0.599	1.000					
6	0.569	0.478	0.580	0.651	0.000	1.000				
7	0.610	0.520	0.530	0.560	0.427	0.688	1.000			
8	0.567	0.477	0.540	0.584	0.808	0.607	0.000	1.000		
9	0.457	0.443	0.492	0.555	0.598	0.522	0.544	0.586	1.000	
10	0.292	0.375	0.478	0.515	0.422	0.426	0.580	0.547	0.000	1.000

while both the compound-symmetry and the first-order autoregressive matrix have only 4 parameters.

Taking all factors into consideration, the Toeplitz structure appears to be a good choice for the analysis in which time is scaled in years. It has the most favorable Schwarz criterion and it allows the gradual decline over time observed among the correlations estimated using the unstructured matrix. At the same time, it requires considerably fewer parameters than the unstructured matrix. In addition, while a number of the cells in the matrix were zero by design, it is quite reasonable to assume that the correlations in those cells, were they estimable, would follow the pattern estimated from the Toeplitz matrix, shown in Table 8.53.

Because the Toeplitz and compound-symmetry structures had quite similar Schwarz criteria for the analysis when time was scaled in years, both structures were used in parallel analyses for time scaled in months and weeks (not

Table 8.52. Model-fitting Information From the Trend Analysis of Diastolic Blood Pressure in the Extended Design With Four Alternative Structures for the Within-Member Random-Effects Covariance Matrix

Model Fitting Criteria	UN	CS	Toeplitz	AR(1)
−2 REML Log Likelihood	112696.2	112928.4	112843.8	113769.2
Akaike's Criterion	−56405.1	−56468.2	−56433.9	−56888.6
Schwarz's Criterion	−56623.1	−56483.5	−56479.8	−56903.9

Table 8.53. Over-Time Correlations From the Trend Analysis of Diastolic Blood Pressure in the Extended Design With Time Scaled in Years and a Toeplitz Within-Member Random-Effects Covariance Matrix, Rearranged Into a 10 × 10 Matrix

Year	1	2	3	4	5	6	7	8	9	10
1	1.000									
2	0.595	1.000								
3	0.577	0.595	1.000							
4	0.564	0.577	0.595	1.000						
5	0.536	0.564	0.577	0.595	1.000					
6	0.535	0.536	0.564	0.577	0.595	1.000				
7	0.493	0.535	0.536	0.564	0.577	0.595	1.000			
8	0.475	0.493	0.535	0.536	0.564	0.577	0.595	1.000		
9	0.446	0.475	0.493	0.535	0.536	0.564	0.577	0.595	1.000	
10	0.351	0.446	0.475	0.493	0.535	0.536	0.564	0.577	0.595	1.000

shown). In both cases, the compound-symmetry structure yielded the better Schwarz criterion value and easily was the more parsimonious of the two structures. This finding is not surprising, as the number of covariance parameters is quite large with the Toeplitz structure when time is scaled in months or weeks. In contrast, the compound-symmetry structure remains at 4 parameters whether time is scaled in years, months, or weeks. Thus, while the Toeplitz structure offered some advantage over compound symmetry for the analysis in which time was scaled in years, the compound-symmetry structure was satisfactory for the analyses in which time was scaled in months or weeks.

The next step is to compare the models that have the best fit in terms of the within-member random-effects covariance matrix for their time scale so as to select a final model for the random effects. Table 8.54 presents key lines from the analysis with time scaled by year using the Toeplitz structure and from the analyses with time scaled by month and week using the compound-symmetry structure. The Schwarz criterion can be used to compare these models. It sug-

Table 8.54. Model-Fitting Information From the Trend Analysis in the Extended Design

Model-Fitting Information	Year (Toeplitz)	Month (CS)	Week (CS)
−2 REML Log Likelihood	112843.8	112905.4	112932.4
Akaike's Information Criterion	−56433.9	−56456.7	−56470.2
Schwarz's Bayesian Criterion	−56479.8	−56472.0	−56485.5

Table 8.55. Covariance-Parameter Estimates (REML) From the Trend Analysis of Diastolic Blood Pressure in the Extended Design With Time Scaled in Months and a Compound-Symmetry Within-Member Random-Effects Covariance Matrix

Cov Parm	Estimate
INTERCEPT	0.28981
MONCAT	3.82111
MONCAT CS	56.58029
Residual	49.87532

gests that the model using the compound-symmetry structure with time scaled in months is the best fitting of the three. As a result, the balance of the presentation for diastolic blood pressure is based on that model.

Table 8.55 presents the covariance-parameter estimates for this analysis. The MONCAT CS estimate as a fraction of the total within-member variation in the data is an estimate of the within-member correlation over time, $r_{yy(m)}$. In this case, that estimate is:

$$\hat{r}_{yy(m)} = \frac{\hat{\sigma}^2_{m:g:c}}{\hat{\sigma}^2_{mt:g:c} + \hat{\sigma}^2_{m:g:c}} = \frac{56.6}{49.9 + 56.6} = 0.531$$

With the compound-symmetry structure, this result is assumed appropriate for all possible over-time correlations within subjects. As seen in the previous section, some of those correlations were zero by design. Others will be higher or lower than 0.531. Even so, the model comparisons presented in the previous section indicate that the assumption of a constant correlation of 0.531 is acceptable in these data.

Table 8.56 presents the tests of fixed effects for this analysis. The tests

Table 8.56. Tests of Fixed Effects From the Trend Analysis of Diastolic Blood Pressure in the Extended Design With Time Scaled in Months and a Compound-Symmetry Within-Member Random-Effects Covariance Matrix

Source	NDF	DDF	Type III F	Pr > F
COND	1	4	1.00	0.3734
MONTH	1	85	2.76	0.1003
MONTH2	1	85	2.11	0.1501
IMONTH	1	85	0.35	0.5542
IMONTH2	1	85	0.61	0.4375

for the terms of interest, imonth and imonth2, provide no evidence of an intervention effect. Normally, the quadratic term would be deleted from the model if it were found to be nonsignificant. However, the Type III F-test for imonth is also not close to statistical significance, so there is little chance the result would change even with the slight improvement in precision that would be afforded by dropping the quadratic term. That finding is consistent with the original report on these data (Luepker et al., 1994).

The Random-Coefficients Analysis

The random-coefficients model presented in Chapter 6 is the simplest model of that type that focuses on linear time trends in the context of an Extended Design. The assumed structure of the condition mean slopes in that model is that they are strictly linear, though they can vary among the conditions. The assumed structure of the member- and group-specific slopes is that they are also strictly linear, though they can vary among the members and groups.

Such a model is plausible for a nested cohort design with a single baseline observation on each member. Given such a design, separate condition slopes allow, for example, an intervention effect in the form of linear slopes diverging from a common initial level. Such a model also is appropriate for the MHHP data, because each member was observed only once during the baseline period.

In other designs, this linear random-coefficients model may not be sufficient, especially where the investigators suspect some curvature in the member-specific trends. In that case, quadratic components could be added to the model, both for the fixed and random effects, adapting the example given in Chapter 7 for the nested cohort design. However, to do so requires three or more measurements on each member. As a result, the example given in this section follows the model presented in Chapter 6.

Implementation for Gaussian Data

To implement the linear random-coefficients analysis presented in Chapter 6 for diastolic blood pressure, the code shown in Table 8.57 is appropriate.

The method=mivque0 option is not included in the proc mixed statement in anticipation that the residual error will account for less than 90% of the total variation in the data.[12] The ddf= option sets the *ddf* for the three fixed effects at 4, consistent with the formulae in the table of expected mean squares for this model that is presented in Chapter 6 (Table 6.12). Those formulae give $c(g-1)$ as the *ddf* for the tests of cond, time and cond*time. In this example, the generic time is replaced by month and the generic cond *time is replaced by imonth. No covariates are included in this example.

Table 8.57. SAS PROC MIXED Code for the Linear Random-Coefficients Analysis of Diastolic Blood Pressure in the Extended Design

```
proc mixed info order=internal noclprint convh=0.000001;
  title3 'Random Coefficients Linear';
  class cond group member;
  model dbp=cond month imonth
    /ddf=4,4,4 ddfm=res solution singular=0.000001;
  random int month/subject=group(cond) type=un;
  random int month/subject=member(group*cond) type=un;
run;
```

In the fixed effects, the intercept estimates the *y*-intercept in the control condition and the cond term estimates the difference between the *y*-intercepts for the two conditions. The month term estimates the time trend in the control condition. In this analysis, imonth is set equal to month for all observations in the intervention condition and to zero for all observations in the control condition. As a result, the imonth term estimates any difference between the time trend in the intervention and control conditions.

This code includes two random statements. The first structures the random coefficients for the groups. The second structures the random coefficients for the members. Both statements allow for random intercepts and random linear slopes. Both also allow the intercepts and slopes to covary via the type=un option.[13]

The dimensions of this analysis are summarized in Table 8.58. The code specifies seven covariance parameters: group(cond), month*group-(cond), the covariance between those two parameters, member-(group*cond), month*member(group*cond), the covariance be-

Table 8.58. Dimensions for the Linear Random-Coefficients Analysis of Diastolic Blood Pressure in the Extended Design

Description	Value
Covariance Parameters	7
Columns in X	5
Max Cols in Z Per Subject	2268
Subjects	6
Max Obs Per Subject	3153
Observations Used	15532
Observations Not Used	0
Total Observations	15532

tween those two parameters, and residual error. The full data set with 15,332 observations is available for the analysis.

The most striking result in Table 8.58 is the value for the maximum number of columns in the Z matrix per subject. Recall that this is the number of columns in the random-effects design matrix, in this case for each group. In this analysis, that value is 2268, which is very large. This job required 46 hours of CPU time, and most of that was probably spent inverting a matrix of size 2268×2268.[14] Indeed, the iteration history indicated that the model converged in only a single iteration, also pointing to the matrix inversion as the probable culprit in terms of the long processing time.

Table 8.59 presents the covariance-parameter estimates from this analysis. The first three covariance parameters represent the parameters defined in the first random statement. So the first (1.989) is the component of variance for the group intercepts. The third (0.001356) is the component of variance for the group slopes. The second is the covariance between the group intercepts and slopes. The second three covariance parameters represent the parameters defined in the second random statement. The fourth parameter (66.58) is the component of variance for the member intercepts. The sixth (0.002888) is the component of variance for the member slopes. The fifth is the covariance between those member components. As expected, the covariance parameters other than residual error are small, except for the component of variance for the member intercepts. Residual error accounts for less than half of the variation in the data; based on Swallow and Monahan's report (1984), MIVQUE(0) estimation would be inappropriate.

The covariance-parameter estimates can be used to construct the mean squares for the random effects in the model, drawing on the table of expected mean squares given in Chapter 6 (Table 6.12). Given 15,532 observations in $tgc = 95$ group $\times$ time surveys, the average $m = 163.5$ while $g = 3$ and the

Table 8.59. Covariance-Parameter Estimates (REML) From the Linear Random-Coefficients Analysis of Diastolic Blood Pressure in the Extended Design With Time Scaled in Months

Cov Parm		Estimate
INTERCEPT	UN(1,1)	1.98932118
	UN(2,1)	−0.04857265
	UN(2,2)	0.00135566
INTERCEPT	UN(1,1)	66.57865061
	UN(2,1)	−0.17206911
	UN(2,2)	0.00288813
Residual		45.35013457

Table 8.60. Selected Mean-Square Estimates for the Linear Random-Coefficients Analysis of Diastolic Blood Pressure in the Extended Design With Time Scaled in Months

Source	E(MS)
$T(\text{lin}):G:C$	$\dfrac{\sigma^2_{e(y)}}{\sigma^2_{e(t)}(t-f-1)}+\sigma^2_{mt(\text{lin}):g:c}+m\sigma^2_{t(\text{lin})g:c}$

Source	Estimate
$T(\text{lin}):G:C$	$\dfrac{45.35}{373.9(15.83-3-1)}+0.002888+163.5*0.001356$
	$=0.2348$

average $t=15.83$. From a separate analysis the remaining parameter, $\sigma^2_{e(t)}$, is estimated as 373.85. Using these values, the mean squares are estimated in Table 8.60.

Given 0.2348 as the estimate of $MS_{t(\text{lin})g:c}$, the standard error of the intervention effect is computed using Equation 6.26:[15]

$$\hat{\sigma}_\Delta = \sqrt{2\left(\frac{\hat{MS}_{t(\text{lin})g:c}}{mg}\right)} = \sqrt{2\left(\frac{0.2348}{163.5*3}\right)} = 0.0309$$

The solution option provides the solution coefficients for each of the terms in the model, including the intervention effect. Those coefficients are presented in Table 8.61. The coefficient for month indicates a change per month of -0.00677 mm Hg in the control condition from the last baseline survey until

Table 8.61. Fixed-Effect Regression Coefficients From the Linear Random-Coefficients Analysis of Diastolic Blood Pressure in the Extended Design With Time Scaled in Months

Parameter	Estimate	SE	DDF	T	Pr>|T|
INTERCEPT	76.02708	0.83571	16E3	90.97	0.0001
COND I	-1.32688	1.18174	4	-1.12	0.3243
COND C	0.00000	.	.	.	.
MONTH	-0.00677	0.02138	4	-0.32	0.7673
IMONTH	0.01687	0.03024	4	0.56	0.6066

Table 8.62. Tests of Fixed Effects From the Linear Random-Coefficients Analysis of Diastolic Blood Pressure in the Extended Design With Time Scaled in Months

Source	NDF	DDF	Type III F	Pr > F
COND	1	4	1.26	0.3243
MONTH	1	4	0.10	0.7673
IMONTH	1	4	0.31	0.6066

the end of the study. The coefficient for IMONTH indicates that the change per month in the intervention condition was $(-0.00677 + 0.0169) = +0.0101$ mm Hg. Note that the standard error for the IMONTH term is given as 0.0302, which is in good agreement with the value estimated from the variance components as 0.0309.

Table 8.62 presents the tests of fixed effects. The F-test for imonth is the square of the t-test for imonth given in Table 8.61. Neither provides any basis to reject the null hypothesis of no difference in the mean linear slopes between the two conditions.

Having examined the results from the random-coefficients analysis, it is of interest to determine whether the random-coefficients analysis is necessary. If not, the simpler ANOVA/ANCOVA models are valid (Murray et al., in press).

Table 8.63 presents the model-fitting information from the random-coefficients analysis and from the trend analysis in the ANCOVA presented earlier in this chapter.

The ANCOVA analysis provides the -2 REML Log Likelihood, AIC and BIC values closest to zero. In general, a model with -2 REML Log Likelihood, AIC, and BIC values closest to zero is considered a better fit to the data. Thus, all three of these criteria point toward the ANCOVA as the better fitting of the two analyses. The models cannot be distinguished in terms of the number of observations, as both are based on 15,532 observations. However, the

Table 8.63. Model-Fitting Information from the Linear Random-Coefficients Analysis and From the Quadratic Trend Analysis of Diastolic Blood Pressure in the Extended Design with Time Scaled in Months

Description	Random Coefficients	Trend Analysis
-2 REML Log Likelihood	113006.4	112905.4
Akaike's Information Criterion	-56510.2	-56456.7
Schwarz's Bayesian Criterion	-56537.0	-56472.0

ANCOVA involves only 4 covariance parameters, while the random-coefficients analysis requires 7; thus, the principle of parsimony also favors the ANCOVA analysis.[16]

Given this result, the investigator may choose to report the results of the trend analysis in the mixed-model ANCOVA, as there is good evidence that the ANCOVA model fits the data better than the random-coefficients model. However, where the evidence favors the random-coefficients model, the investigator should report the results of that analysis.

Summary

This chapter presented examples of many of the analyses appropriate for group-randomized trials that employ a nested cohort design. Several of the summary points made at the end of Chapter 7 are equally appropriate here:

- For analyses involving a dichotomous outcome, the results from the analyses performed using software based on the General Linear Mixed Model closely approximated those from the analyses performed using software based on the Generalized Linear Mixed Model.
- For most analyses involving variance components fixed at zero by default using REML estimation, the nobound option was helpful in avoiding artificial depression of the Type I error rate.
- Across the analyses considered, there was considerable variation in size of standard errors, even for the same data.
- Many of the common analysis strategies used to improve the precision of the analysis operate somewhat differently in the context of mixed-model regression than in the more familiar context of fixed-effects regression.

In addition to these points, there were a number of methods illustrated that are unique to cohort data. For example, demonstrated in this chapter were the use of several alternative structures for the within-member covariance matrix, including unstructured, compound symmetry, first-order autoregressive, and Toeplitz. Traditional methods require the use of the compound-symmetry structure, accompanied as it must be with assumptions that are often difficult to justify. The alternative structures offer greater flexibility. More important, they should allow a much closer match between the assumed and the observed structure for the within-member random-effects covariance matrix.

The analyses presented for Extended Designs included trend analysis in the mixed-model ANOVA/ANCOVA and random-coefficients analyses. Analyses for Extended Designs are less developed than for the simpler Pretest-Posttest Control Group Design, and readers will want to keep that in mind as they study that material. There is much room for additional research to further develop the methods presented in that section, as well as to develop new methods.

As noted at the end of Chapter 7, modern software often allows rapid fitting of complex models, including models like those illustrated in this chapter. Investigators and analysts alike should take care that they understand the models they are fitting as well as the software they are using, so as to ensure that their results are interpretable. The need to pore over the defaults and details of the output only increases with the complexity of the models.

Endnotes

1. The final cohort surveys in Bloomington and Roseville were conducted after six years of intervention. At that time, funding for the following year was uncertain, and the decision was made to advance the date of the follow-up survey rather than risk losing that survey.

2. Depending on the structure of the data, it may not be necessary to include `time` as an effect in the `repeated` statement. For example, if the number of time intervals is the same for all groups and members and if the spacing of those intervals is constant, it is not necessary to include `time` as an effect. If those conditions don't apply, it is necessary to include `time` in order to define the spacing of the time intervals for proper construction of the within-member random-effects covariance matrix.

3. It specifies a block-diagonal structure for the within-member random-effects covariance matrix with identical blocks for each level of its effect. This improves processing time in the same way that it does in the `random` statement.

4. Note that the `subject=` effect includes both `group` and `cond` within the parentheses; if only the `group` is listed, the savings in processing time otherwise available via the `subject=` option in the `random` statement are not available.

5. In this example, the *ddf* for all the fixed effects in the model are defined in the `ddf=` option in the `model` statement and so the `ddfm=res` option is not necessary. However, because it often improves processing time, it is included routinely for that reason.

6. The interpretation of the Type III *F*-tests for main effects in the presence of an interaction is discussed in Chapter 7, Endnote 23.

7. The `options=mixprintlast` statement was not shown in the GLIMMIX code at the beginning of this section. However, the only way to get the `rcorr=` table in the 06-APR-96 version of GLIMMIX is to include that statement in the GLIMMIX code.

8. Readers should understand that the equivalence of the MIXED and GLIMMIX results is due to the Central Limit Theorem as it operates in group-randomized trials. The two approaches may not give equivalent results for other study designs; in those cases, GLIMMIX is preferred over MIXED.

9. This phenomenon is sometimes called overadjustment or overmatching.

10. The Mankato-Winona pair also had a cross-sectional survey two years after the introduction of the intervention program.

11. The grouping of observations by year as presented here is slightly different from the scheme used by the MHHP investigators and reported, for example, in Luepker et al. (1994). This scheme groups observations based on the actual time of the survey, whereas the MHHP investigators grouped observations based on the intended time of the survey.

Because some participants were seen early and others quite late, this difference in definitions will cause some observations to be grouped into different years than was the case in the original analysis.

12. MIVQUE(0) estimation would be much faster than either REML or ML for this complex analysis on this large data set, but MIVQUE(0) estimators are not valid unless residual error accounts for at least 90% of the variance in the data (Swallow and Monahan, 1984). Anticipating that the default REML analysis would be slow, the code was developed and debugged using `method = mivque0` in a random sample of the total cohort before the code was applied to the full cohort under REML. That work was well worth the effort, as the jobs run on a 10% random sample required only a few minutes of CPU time, while the full job required 46 hours of CPU time.

13. The two `random` statements must be listed in this order. If their order is reversed, the job will not run.

14. Given how long this analysis took on a computer operating at 275 MHz, even with 512 Mb virtual memory available, it is unlikely that most users would even consider it for similar-size problems, at least in SAS PROC MIXED. If software designed especially for hierarchical linear models would be appreciably faster, it would have a clear advantage over the SAS procedure. The run time for the same analysis based on a random sample of only 10%, or about 500 persons with 3 observations each, was only a few minutes' CPU time. Thus the SAS procedure may be a reasonable alternative for smaller problems, but clearly it is slow for large problems.

15. In this example $f = 3$, as there are 3 fixed-effect parameters in the model in addition to the intercept: `cond`, `month`, `imonth`.

16. It is not appropriate to compare the ANCOVA and random-coefficients models using the LR chi-square, as the two models are not hierarchical.

9

Sample Size, Detectable Difference, and Power

> . . . from the point of view of inference on the effects of treatments, the experimental unit must be considered as a whole, and the variation between the observational units within an experimental unit is usually of little value in assessing the errors of estimates of treatment effects.
>
> Kempthorne (1952), p. 163

The power of a group-randomized trial is the power of the test of the intervention effect for the primary endpoint. More precisely, it is the probability that Letan intervention effect of a given size will be statistically significant. If the probability is 80% that a test will detect an intervention effect of one standard deviation in magnitude as statistically significant, the study has 80% power for an effect of that size or larger.

In most textbooks on research design and analysis methods, the methods to estimate sample size, detectable difference, and power are presented in one of the early chapters. That is because these methods are an essential part of the planning process and should be used early in the development of a research proposal. While I fully agree with that proposition, I do not think that those methods should be studied before the methods of data analysis are presented. That is because the methods for estimation of sample size, detectable difference, and power depend substantially on the methods selected for data analysis. Without a clear understanding of those methods, estimation of sample size, detectable difference, or power must be a black-box exercise. In an effort to take those techniques out of the black box, I have postponed their presentation until after the discussion of analysis methods in Chapters 5–8.

From the outset, it is important to note that a power analysis is only as good as the formulae and parameter estimates that are used and the analyst who uses them. Power analysis should be done by someone who understands the formulae and why they are structured as they are. This allows the analyst to tailor the formulae to the particular needs of the study. In addition, investigators should take care that the parameter estimates accurately reflect the expected state of affairs in the population to be studied. Without good estimates, power analysis is only guesswork.

Factors That Determine Power

There are many factors that influence the power of a statistical test. These include the expectations of the investigator, the structure of the design, the structure of the variables, and the structure of the analysis.

The Expectations of the Investigator

The expectations of the investigator play an important role in any power analysis. Those expectations emerge in three different areas.

The first is the expectation for the form and magnitude of the intervention effect. The investigators must determine in advance what form and magnitude of effect is worth detecting in terms of its clinical or public health significance.

That expectation leads directly to a test statistic to evaluate the intervention effect. If the investigator anticipates an intervention effect that is well described as a difference between two means, then the test statistic should be constructed to evaluate such a difference. If the investigator anticipates an intervention effect that is well described as a difference between two slopes, then the test statistic should be constructed to evaluate such a difference. If the investigator anticipates an intervention effect that changes in magnitude over time, reflecting both development and decay, then the test statistic should be constructed to evaluate such a pattern. The pattern expected from the intervention is cast as the alternative hypothesis and the pattern expected in the absence of the intervention effect is cast as the null hypothesis. The test statistic should be chosen to be sensitive to the form and magnitude of the departures from the null hypothesis that define the intervention effect.

The investigators may ask the analyst, "What kind of effect can I get out of this design?" The standard reply should be, "What kind and magnitude of effect is important to detect from a clinical or public health perspective?" If the investigators only stare back blank-faced, the analyst might ask, "What kind and magnitude of effect would be viewed as important by experts in the field?"

The original question put to the analyst by the investigators is an example of approaching the problem from the wrong direction. The form and magnitude of the desired intervention effect should lead the way in planning the study; they should not emerge only at the end, as a finishing touch in the planning process. For example, if the investigators want to examine change, there must be observations taken both before and after the intervention program and the design must be structured to include those observations. If the investigators expect the intervention effect to follow a particular pattern, the design must be structured to include enough observations scheduled at the proper times to be able to detect that pattern. If the investigators expect the intervention to take some time to develop and have its effect, sufficient time must be provided after the introduction of the intervention so that the effect can mature and be captured in full force.

The second area in which the expectations of the investigators emerge is in the form of their decisions concerning the Type I and II error rates for the primary analysis. The Type I error rate is the rate at which the intervention will be reported as effective due to chance alone. In general, investigators try to minimize that rate. The Type II error rate is the rate at which the intervention will be reported as ineffective when it actually achieved the desired result. In general, investigators try to minimize that rate as well. Unfortunately, the forces that govern the Type I and II error rates often act in opposition, so that reducing one error rate serves to increase the other.

The research community has come to look at 5% as an acceptable Type I error rate. Many view 10% or 20% as an acceptable Type II error rate. In fact, the Type I and II error rates should be matched to the study at hand, in consideration of the relative danger of making a Type I or Type II error. If a Type I error would be serious, that rate should be set quite low. If a Type II error would be serious as well, that rate should also be set quite low. On the other hand, if one or both errors would be troublesome but not ruinous, their rates might be set somewhat higher. Setting the rates should be done in full recognition that they have a substantial effect on the size of the study.

The desired Type I and II error rates define the critical values in the distribution against which the observed value of the test statistic is assessed. The actual values depend both on the Type I and II error rates and on the expected distribution of the test statistic under the null hypothesis.

The third area in which the expectations of the investigator influence power is the choice of a one- or two-tailed test. If the investigator expects that the intervention effect will be in a particular direction, and if the investigator doesn't care if the direction is reversed, then a one-tailed test is appropriate. If the investigator is not sure of the direction of the effect, or if the investigator cares if the effect is in the unexpected direction, a two-tailed test should be used.

Often investigators remember only the first part of each of those two rules. Many think that as long as they have a clear *a priori* expectation that the effect will be in a particular direction, they should use a one-tailed test. In fact, that is only half of the requirement. Because it is far more likely that the investigators will care if the result is in the unexpected direction, two-tailed tests should be standard in group-randomized trials.

The Structure of the Design

By definition, the size of a study increases as the number of conditions, groups, members, time intervals, and strata increase. In general, so does the power of the study. However, the relationship between power and these factors is not linear. There are common circumstances in which the power of a study is reduced as the number of conditions, time intervals, and strata are increased, depending largely on the form and magnitude of the desired intervention effect. If the intervention effect increases in complexity as the study grows larger, power often declines. If the intervention effect remains simply structured, power usually improves.

Under almost any circumstances, as the number of groups per condition and members per group increases, the power of the study increases. Indeed, the single most important factor in the power of a group-randomized trial is usually the number of groups allocated to each condition. Increasing the number of members in each group also improves power. However, the law of diminishing returns is at work both for groups and members, and more so for the latter, such that the improvement in power is smaller with each additional group or member added to the design.

The Structure of the Variables

In general, an analysis of Gaussian data is more powerful than an analysis of non-Gaussian data, other factors constant. Here, power depends entirely on the variance because the mean and variance are independent. For non-Gaussian variables, power often depends on both the mean and the variance, because the two are often related. In both cases, power increases as the variance decreases, through better measurement, adoption of a more precise endpoint, or analytic strategies.

Group-randomized trials stand apart from most clinical trials in the expectation that the data are correlated, not only within persons but also between persons. As discussed in Chapter 1, allocation of identifiable groups to study conditions guarantees some measure of intraclass correlation, usually positive, and any positive intraclass correlation increases the variation among the groups. Because the proper analysis of a group-randomized trial assesses the variation of the conditions against the variation of the groups, such positive intraclass correlation reduces power.

The impact of even modest positive intraclass correlation can be dramatic. For example, compared to an intraclass correlation of zero, an intraclass correlation of 0.01 observed in groups of 100 members doubles the variance of the group mean. An intraclass correlation of 0.05 observed in groups of 100 members increases the variance of the group mean sixfold. Unfortunately, that is the range for intraclass correlations observed in many group-randomized trials (e.g., Hannan et al., 1994; Murray, Rooney et al., 1994; Murray and Short, 1995, 1996, 1997; Siddiqui et al., 1996).

The Structure of the Analysis

Any action that reduces the standard error of the intervention effect will improve power, other factors constant. The size of the standard error of the intervention effect is jointly influenced by the residual error and by one or more additional variance components, with the combination dependent upon the particular analysis applied to the data.

As seen in Chapters 7 and 8, analytic tools such as regression adjustment for covariates, stratification, matching, and repeat observations on groups and members can be applied in a group-randomized trial. Each of these techniques can improve power, though none is guaranteed to do so. It is particularly important to remember that these procedures can affect the variance components that define the standard error of the intervention effect unevenly. Reductions in one component may be more than offset by increases in another so that the net effect is an increase in the standard error. There is no substitute for prior experience with similar data in terms of guiding the analyst's expectations for the study under consideration.

Fundamentals of Power Analysis

Several excellent treatments of power analysis are available. Cohen's (1988) text provides a good background discussion of power analysis, many useful formulae, and, for the computationally reticent, extensive tables of power and sample size for a variety of metrics and analyses. Fleiss (1981) provides a good discussion of power analysis for rates and proportions and also provides tables of sample size as a function of the magnitude of the expected intervention effects and the desired Type I and II error rates. Other familiar texts on clinical trials and observational studies also include material on power analysis (e.g., Kelsey et al., 1996; Meinert, 1986; Schlesselman, 1982). However, none of this material is written for group-randomized trials and none of the tables should be used without adaptation. Unfortunately, the adaptation of this material to the context of group-randomized trials is often quite complicated.

Several papers published in the last 15 years have described the methods appropriate for power analysis in simple group-randomized trials. These include articles by teams at the University of Western Ontario (Donner, 1984b, 1992; Donner et al., 1981), the University of Minnesota (Hannan et al., 1994; Murray and Hannan, 1990; Murray, Rooney et al., 1994; Murray and Short, 1995, 1996, 1997), the University of Washington (Feng and Grizzle, 1992; Koepsell et al., 1991; Martin et al., 1993), the National Institutes of Health (Freedman et al., 1990; Gail et al., 1992; Zucker et al., 1995), and elsewhere (Feldman and McKinlay, 1994; Hsieh, 1988). This presentation draws heavily on those articles. It also includes much new material as it extends the discussion to more complex designs and analyses.

These papers demonstrate that even for a single research question, endpoint, design, and analysis, there are many different approaches to power analysis. Some analysts focus on computing power. Others focus on computing detectable differences. Others focus on computing the number of members or groups required to detect an intervention effect of a given magnitude. Even if two analysts intend to compute the same quantity, they may use different formulae. Add the rich variety in research questions, endpoints, designs, and analyses, and a power analysis for a group-randomized trial can seem very complex.

One of the reasons for the apparent complexity is that there are so many factors that influence power. Any equation that has many parameters can be written in many different ways, with each formulation solving for a different parameter. At first glance, these formulae may appear to be quite different when in fact most of the basic formulae can be manipulated into a common form. Unfortunately, the algebra can get complicated, and for the inexperienced, it is easier to believe that all those formulae are doing different things. But that simply is not so. They use estimates for many different parameters to compute detectable differences, power, sample size, or some other single parameter that is temporarily treated as the dependent variable in a complex expression.

Another reason for the apparent complexity is that there is no standard notation for power analysis. The inexperienced can look at two formulae that are in fact equivalent and believe that they are different simply because they use different notation.

Another reason for the apparent complexity is that not all writers include the same set of parameters in their equations. This is particularly true for parameters like the expected rate of attrition, noncompliance, and others. Formulae that ignore such parameters are effectively assuming that their value is zero. On the other hand, the author may simply plan to deal with those factors at a later time.

Yet another reason for the apparent complexity is that discussions of power analysis are often cast in the context of a particular scale of measurement or a particular analysis plan. Certainly the scale of measurement and analytic plan affect the power analysis, but it also is possible to structure the formulae so that they can accommodate a wide variety of measurement scales and analytic plans.

No single presentation can resolve all these issues. What is possible is to be consistent across the designs and analyses to be considered.

Steps in a Power Analysis

There are seven steps involved in a power analysis. The first step is to specify the form and magnitude of the intervention effect. The second step is to select a test statistic for that effect. The third step is to determine the distribution of that test statistic under the null hypothesis. The fourth step is to select the critical values in that distribution that determine whether or not the investigator will reject the null hypothesis. The fifth step is to develop an expression for the variance of the intervention effect under the null hypothesis in terms of parameters that are easily estimated. The sixth step is to gather estimates of those parameters. The seventh step is to estimate power given the results of the first six steps. This seventh step should include a sensitivity analysis that varies the estimates of the most important parameters. At that point, the power analysis is largely done. The investigator should select the design and analysis that optimizes power and cost for the effect of interest under assumptions that are easily defended.

Power in a Simple Clinical Trial

The simplest clinical trial design is a Posttest-Only Control Group design with m members allocated to each of two conditions. The model for this design is:

$$Y_{i:l} = \mu + C_l + \varepsilon_{i:l} \tag{9.1}$$

The observed value for the ith member in the lth condition is a function of the grand mean and the effect of the lth condition; any difference between the observed value and the predicted value is allocated to the residual error ($\varepsilon_{i:l}$).

Assume that the investigator determines that the intervention effect is well described by a difference between the two conditions in their posttest means. Let $\hat{\Delta} = \hat{\bar{y}}_I - \hat{\bar{y}}_C$ estimate that difference. Let $\hat{\sigma}_{\Delta}^2 = \hat{\sigma}_{\bar{y}_I - \bar{y}_C}^2$ estimate the variance of that difference under the null hypothesis. Assuming the residual error is distributed Gaussian, the intervention effect is evaluated using a t-statistic in combination with the appropriate df. The general form of that t-statistic is:

$$\hat{t} = \frac{\hat{\Delta}}{\hat{\sigma}_\Delta} \tag{9.2}$$

In this case, the t-statistic is estimated as:

$$\hat{t} = \frac{\hat{\bar{y}}_I - \hat{\bar{y}}_C}{\hat{\sigma}^2_{\bar{y}_I - \bar{y}_c}} \tag{9.3}$$

The expected distribution of this t-statistic is determined by its df, here $2(m-1)$, where there are m members in each of the two conditions.

Assume further that the investigator has determined that the desired Type I and II error rates are 5% and 20%, respectively. Assume as well that the investigator expects a positive intervention effect but would be concerned about a negative effect; as a result, the investigator chooses a two-tailed test. These decisions define the critical values that are used to determine whether or not to reject the null hypothesis.

At this point, the investigator is ready to develop an expression for the variance of the intervention effect under the null hypothesis in terms of parameters that are easily estimated. In this case, that variance is the variance of a difference between two condition means, given earlier as $\hat{\sigma}^2_\Delta = \hat{\sigma}^2_{\bar{y}_I - \bar{y}_c}$. That form is not given in terms of parameters that are easily estimated, and some elaboration is required.

Given the random assignment of members to conditions, it is reasonable to assume that the two study conditions are independent. The variance of the difference between two independent conditions means is:

$$\hat{\sigma}^2_{\bar{y}_I - \bar{y}_c} = \hat{\sigma}^2_{\bar{y}_I} + \hat{\sigma}^2_{\bar{y}_c} \tag{9.4}$$

The estimated variance of a single condition mean is the estimated variance of the members, $\hat{\sigma}^2_y$, divided by the number of members contributing to that mean, m:[1]

$$\hat{\sigma}^2_{\bar{y}_c} = \frac{\hat{\sigma}^2_y}{m_c}$$

The variances for the two condition means are then estimated as:

$$\hat{\sigma}^2_{\bar{y}_I} = \frac{\hat{\sigma}^2_{y_I}}{m_I} \text{ and } \hat{\sigma}^2_{\bar{y}_I} = \frac{\hat{\sigma}^2_{y_C}}{m_C}$$

If the number of members observed in each condition is assumed equal, $m_I = m_C = m$, and the variances in the two conditions are assumed equal, $\hat{\sigma}^2_{y_I} = \hat{\sigma}^2_{y_C} = \hat{\sigma}^2_y$, then:

$$\frac{\hat{\sigma}^2_{y_I}}{m_I} = \frac{\hat{\sigma}^2_{y_C}}{m_C} = \frac{\hat{\sigma}^2_y}{m}$$

The estimate of the variance of the difference becomes:

$$\hat{\sigma}^2_\Delta = \frac{2\hat{\sigma}^2_y}{m} \tag{9.5}$$

As a result, the t-statistic is estimated as:

$$\hat{t} = \frac{\hat{\Delta}}{\sqrt{\dfrac{2\hat{\sigma}^2_y}{m}}} \tag{9.6}$$

The advantage of this formulation is that it is written in terms of three simple parameters: the usual population variance, estimated as $\hat{\sigma}^2_y$, the number of members per condition, m, and the difference between the two sample means, estimated as $\hat{\Delta} = \hat{\bar{y}}_I - \hat{\bar{y}}_C$. These parameters are relatively easy to estimate, drawing on data from published reports, from analyses of existing data, or from preliminary studies.

To ensure that the two-tailed Type I error rate is α, $\hat{t}$ is considered statistically significant only if $|\hat{t}| > t_{\text{critical: } \alpha/2}$, where $t_{\text{critical: } \alpha/2}$ defines the $\alpha/2$ percentile of the t-distribution for the available df. Figure 9.1 illustrates the division of the t-distribution into two tails, each containing 2.5% of the distribution. The probability that $|\hat{t}| > t_{\text{critical: } \alpha/2}$ will be the sum of the probabilities in the tails, or 5%. Thus under the null hypothesis (H$_o$), the probability that $|\hat{t}| > t_{\text{critical: } \alpha/2}$ will be α.

The observed $\hat{t}$ also is but one possible value from the sampling distribution under the alternative hypothesis (H$_a$) that the point estimate has some specified nonzero value. If the alternative hypothesis is true, we want to reject the null hypothesis as often as possible. To fail to do so would be a Type II error. To ensure that the Type II error rate is β, the probability that $|\hat{t}| > t_{\text{critical: } \alpha/2}$ must be $1 - \beta$ for the expected value of the point estimate under the alternative

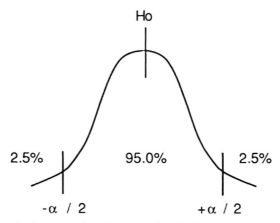

Figure 9.1. By selecting cutpoints for the *t*-distribution to be $+\alpha/2$, the analyst ensures that they Type I error rate will be α.

hypothesis. This happens only when $\hat{t} > t_{\text{critical: } \alpha/2} + t_{\text{critical:}\beta}$, or equivalently, when $\hat{t} > t_{\text{critical: } \alpha/2} - t_{\text{critical: } 1-\beta}$. Here $t_{\text{critical:}\beta}$ and $t_{\text{critical: } 1-\beta}$ define the β and $1 - \beta$ percentiles, respectively, of the sampling distribution under the alternative hypothesis that the point estimate has some specified nonzero value, given the available *df*. Figure 9.2 illustrates the relationship between the distribution of $\hat{t}$ under both the null and alternative hypotheses.

Written quite generally, the power for a single *df* contrast of size $\hat{\Delta}$ and evaluated via the *t*-test given in Equation 9.2 is:

$$\text{power} = \text{prob}(\hat{t} \le \hat{t}_\beta), \text{ where } \hat{t}_\beta = \frac{\hat{\Delta}}{\hat{\sigma}_\Delta} - t_{\text{critical: } \alpha/2} \qquad (9.7)$$

or equivalently as:

$$\text{power} = \text{prob}(\hat{t} \ge \hat{t}_{1-\beta}), \text{ where } \hat{t}_{1-\beta} = t_{\text{critical: } \alpha/2} - \frac{\hat{\Delta}}{\hat{\sigma}_\Delta} \qquad (9.8)$$

Written in terms of m, $\hat{\sigma}_y^2$, and $t_{\text{critical: } \alpha/2}$, the structure of $\hat{\sigma}_\Delta^2$ is made explicit and the power to detect a difference as large as or larger than $\hat{\Delta}$ is estimated as:

$$\text{power} = \text{prob}(\hat{t} \le \hat{t}_\beta), \text{ where } \hat{t}_\beta = \frac{\hat{\Delta}}{\sqrt{\dfrac{2\hat{\sigma}_y^2}{m}}} - t_{\text{critical: } \alpha/2} \qquad (9.9)$$

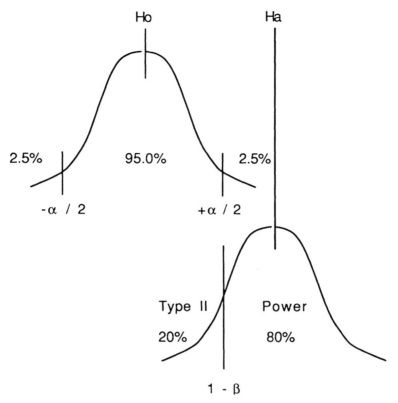

Figure 9.2. The relationship between the distribution of $\hat{t}$ under both the null and alternative hypotheses.

or equivalently as:

$$\text{power} = \text{prob}\left(\hat{t} \geq \hat{t}_{1-\beta}\right), \text{ where } \hat{t}_{1-\beta} = t_{\text{critical: } \alpha/2} - \frac{\hat{\Delta}}{\sqrt{\dfrac{2\hat{\sigma}_y^2}{m}}} \qquad (9.10)$$

To illustrate, consider the example in Table 9.1. The values for the observed $\hat{t}$ and the *a priori* $t_{\text{critical: } \alpha/2}$ are arbitrary. The values for $\hat{t}_{1-\beta}$ and $\hat{t}_{\beta}$ are calculated using Equations 9.7 and 9.8. The probabilities are determined for the computed values of $\hat{t}_{1-\beta}$ and $\hat{t}_{\beta}$ assuming many *df*. When the effect is large enough to generate a value of $\hat{t} = 2.80$, the probability $\text{prob}(\hat{t} \geq \hat{t}_{1-\beta})$ is 80%, as is the probability $\text{prob}(\hat{t} \leq \hat{t}_{\beta})$. That indicates that the power of the test is 80% to find an effect that large or larger to be statistically significant. That result is achieved whether power is calculated based on $\hat{t}_{1-\beta}$ or $\hat{t}_{\beta}$ as long as

Table 9.1. The Relationship Between $\hat{t}$, $\hat{t}_{1-\beta}$, $\hat{t}_\beta$, and Power When the Type I Error Rate is Fixed and df are Many

$\hat{t} = \dfrac{\hat{\Delta}}{\hat{\sigma}_\Delta}$	$t_{\text{critical}:\alpha/2}$	$\hat{t}_{1-\beta}$	$prob(\hat{t} \geq \hat{t}_{1-\beta})$ (%)	$\hat{t}_\beta$	$prob(\hat{t} \leq \hat{t}_\beta)$ (%)
0	1.96	1.96	2.5	−1.96	2.5
1.96	1.96	0.00	50	0.00	50
2.80	1.96	−0.84	80	0.84	80

the proper expression is used.[2] When the effect is large enough to generate a value of $\hat{t} = 1.96$, the test is still large enough to be reported as statistically significant, but the power to detect an effect that large or larger is reduced to only 50%. When the intervention effect is zero, so that $\hat{t} = 0$, the probabilities $prob(\hat{t} \geq \hat{t}_{1-\beta})$ and $prob(\hat{t} \leq \hat{t}_\beta)$ each represent one tail of the two-tailed Type I error rate.

There are several different ways to characterize the power of a study. Investigators may report power for a given $\hat{\Delta}$, or for a range of $\hat{\Delta}$, where the range reflects variations in the assumptions made for the parameters that are used in the calculations. Another way is to report the sample size required for the study; here, too, a range of sample sizes may be reported. Yet another way is to report the detectable intervention effect, often called the detectable difference when the intervention effect is estimated as a difference. Here, too, a range of detectable differences may be reported. These three approaches (detectable difference, sample size, and power) are simply three different ways of arranging the terms that help the investigator determine the size of the study.

Written in terms of $\hat{\sigma}_\Delta^2$, the detectable difference between two independent condition means is estimated as:

$$\hat{\Delta} = \sqrt{\hat{\sigma}_\Delta^2 (t_{\text{critical}:\ \alpha/2} + t_{\text{critical}:\beta})^2} \qquad (9.11)$$

Written in terms of m, $\hat{\sigma}_y^2$, $t_{\text{critical}:\ \alpha/2}$, the structure of $\hat{\sigma}_\Delta^2$ is made explicit and the same detectable difference is estimated as:

$$\hat{\Delta} = \sqrt{\frac{2\hat{\sigma}_y^2 (t_{\text{critical}:\ \alpha/2} + t_{\text{critical}:\beta})^2}{m}} \qquad (9.12)$$

In either form, the values for $t_{\text{critical}:\ \alpha/2}$ and $t_{\text{critical}:\beta}$ depend on the df for the t-test.

Written in terms of $\hat{\sigma}_\Delta^2$, the sample size per condition required for a specified value of $\hat{\Delta}$ is estimated as:

$$m = \frac{m\hat{\sigma}_\Delta^2 (t_{\text{critical: } \alpha/2} + t_{\text{critical:}\beta})^2}{\hat{\Delta}^2} \qquad (9.13)$$

Written in terms of $\hat{\sigma}_y^2$, $t_{\text{critical: } \alpha/2}$, and $t_{\text{critical:}\beta}$, the structure of $\hat{\sigma}_\Delta^2$ is made explicit and the same sample size is estimated as:

$$m = \frac{2\hat{\sigma}_y^2 (t_{\text{critical: } \alpha/2} + t_{\text{critical:}\beta})^2}{\hat{\Delta}^2} \qquad (9.14)$$

The solution of either expression may require two or three iterations. The initial values of $t_{\text{critical: } \alpha/2}$ and of $t_{\text{critical:}\beta}$ often have to be changed given the preliminary result and its effect on the *df*.

Power in a Simple Group-Randomized Trial

The methods for a clinical trial must be adapted for group-randomized trials wherein identifiable groups rather than individuals are allocated to each condition. The Posttest-Only Control Group design presented in Chapter 5 is the group-randomized trial analog to the simple clinical trial. In the unadjusted analysis of posttest data, the model was presented in Equation 5.1 as:

$$Y_{i:k:l} = \mu + C_l + G_{k:l} + \varepsilon_{i:k:l}$$

Assume that the investigator has determined that the intervention effect is well-described by a difference between two posttest condition means. Let $\hat{\Delta}$ estimate that difference. Let $\hat{\sigma}_\Delta^2$ estimate the variance of that difference. Then the *t*-statistic given in Equation 9.2 is used to assess that effect. The distribution of $\hat{t}$ is determined by the available *df*. The critical values in that distribution in turn are determined by decisions on the Type I and II error rates and on whether to conduct a one- or two-tailed test.

The investigator still must develop an expression for the standard error of the difference between two condition means under the null hypothesis. Consider first the variance of the group mean. If that mean were based on m independent observations, the variance of that mean would be estimated as shown in Equation 1.1:

$$\hat{\sigma}_{\bar{y}_g}^2 = \frac{\hat{\sigma}_y^2}{m}$$

However, because the members within an identifiable group almost always show positive intraclass correlation, $ICC_{m:g:c}$, those observations cannot be assumed independent. As shown in Chapter 1, this intraclass correlation reflects an extra component of variance attributable to the groups nested within conditions, $\sigma_{g:c}^2$. As a result, the variance of the group mean in the group-randomized trial is estimated as shown in Equations 1.6 and 1.7 as: [3]

$$\hat{\sigma}_{\bar{y}_g}^2 = \frac{\hat{\sigma}_e^2}{m} + \hat{\sigma}_{g:c}^2 = \frac{\hat{\sigma}_y^2}{m}\left(1 + (m-1)I\hat{C}C_{m:g:c}\right) \qquad (9.15)$$

The condition mean is estimated as the average of g group-specific means. Assuming equality across conditions for the components of variance, the number of members per group, the number of groups per condition, and the intraclass correlation among the members within a group, the estimated variance of the condition mean under the null hypothesis is:

$$\hat{\sigma}_{\bar{y}_c}^2 = \frac{\hat{\sigma}_{\bar{y}_g}^2}{g} = \frac{\hat{\sigma}_y^2\left(1 + (m-1)I\hat{C}C_{m:g:c}\right)}{mg} \qquad (9.16)$$

The estimate of the variance of the difference between two independent condition means is then:

$$\hat{\sigma}_{\Delta}^2 = \frac{2\hat{\sigma}_y^2\left(1 + (m-1)I\hat{C}C_{m:g:c}\right)}{mg} \qquad (9.17)$$

Given a moderate number of members per group and groups per condition, the t-statistic to assess the difference between the two such means is estimated as:

$$\hat{t} = \frac{\hat{\Delta}}{\sqrt{\dfrac{2\hat{\sigma}_y^2(1 + (m-1)I\hat{C}C_{m:g:c})}{mg}}} \qquad (9.18)$$

The df for this t-statistic are $df = 2(g-1)$.

Where the presentation for the clinical trial made the explicit assumption that the data were Gaussian, that assumption is not made here. In a group-randomized trial, the variance of the condition mean is based not on the variance of the member-level data, which may have a decidedly non-Gaussian error distribution, but on the variance of the group mean. Under the Central Limit Theorem, the group means have errors that are distributed approximately Gaussian, even if the member-level errors are non-Gaussian, as long as there is a moderate number of members within each group and groups within each condition. A recent simulation study confirmed that the Central Limit Theorem provides good protection for a dichotomous endpoint in a group-randomized trial with only four groups per condition and 30 members per group (Hannan and Murray, 1996).

The formulae presented for power, detectable difference, and sample size from the clinical trial are easily adapted to accommodate the variance of the condition mean in the group-randomized trial. Written quite generally, power is estimated as shown in Equation 9.7:

$$\text{power} = \text{prob}(\hat{t} \le \hat{t}_\beta), \text{ where } \hat{t}_\beta = \frac{\hat{\Delta}}{\hat{\sigma}_\Delta} - t_{\text{critical: } \alpha/2}$$

or equivalently as shown in Equation 9.8:

$$\text{power} = \text{prob}(\hat{t} \ge \hat{t}_{1-\beta}), \text{ where } \hat{t}_{1-\beta} = t_{\text{critical: } \alpha/2} - \frac{\hat{\Delta}}{\hat{\sigma}_\Delta}$$

In this form, the only difference between the clinical trial and the group-randomized trial is in the structure of $\hat{\sigma}_\Delta^2$.

Written in terms of m, g, $\hat{\sigma}_y^2$, $I\hat{C}C_{m:g:c}$, and $t_{\text{critical: } \alpha/2}$, the structure of $\hat{\sigma}_\Delta^2$ is made explicit and the power to detect a difference as large as or larger than $\hat{\Delta}$ is estimated as:

$$\text{power} = \text{prob}(\hat{t} \le \hat{t}_\beta)$$
$$\text{where } \hat{t}_\beta = \frac{\hat{\Delta}}{\sqrt{\dfrac{2\hat{\sigma}_y^2(1 + (m-1)I\hat{C}C_{m:g:c})}{mg}}} - t_{\text{critical: } \alpha/2} \qquad (9.19)$$

or as:

$$\text{power} = \text{prob}(\hat{t} \ge \hat{t}_{1-\beta})$$
$$\text{where } \hat{t}_{1-\beta} = t_{\text{critical: } \alpha/2} - \frac{\hat{\Delta}}{\sqrt{\dfrac{2\hat{\sigma}_y^2(1 + (m-1)I\hat{C}C_{m:g:c})}{mg}}} \qquad (9.20)$$

Written in terms of $\hat{\sigma}_\Delta^2$, the detectable difference is estimated as shown in Equation 9.11:

$$\hat{\Delta} = \sqrt{\hat{\sigma}_\Delta^2(t_{\text{critical: } \alpha/2} + t_{\text{critical}:\beta})^2}$$

Written in terms of m, g, $\hat{\sigma}_y^2$, $I\hat{C}C_{m:g:c}$, $t_{\text{critical: } \alpha/2}$, and $t_{\text{critical}:\beta}$, the structure of $\hat{\sigma}_\Delta^2$ is made explicit and the same detectable difference is estimated as:

$$\hat{\Delta} = \sqrt{\frac{2\hat{\sigma}_y^2(1+(m-1)I\hat{C}C_{m:g:c})(t_{\text{critical: }\alpha/2}+t_{\text{critical}:\beta})^2}{mg}} \qquad (9.21)$$

In either form, the values selected for $t_{\text{critical: }\alpha/2}$ and $t_{\text{critical}:\beta}$ depend on the *df* for the *t*-test, $df = 2(g\text{-}1)$.

Written in terms of $\hat{\sigma}_\Delta^2$, the sample size of groups per condition required for a specified value of $\hat{\Delta}$ is computed using a modification of Equation 9.13:

$$g = \frac{g\hat{\sigma}_\Delta^2(t_{\text{critical: }\alpha/2}+t_{\text{critical}:\beta})^2}{\hat{\Delta}^2} \qquad (9.22)$$

Written in terms of m, $\hat{\sigma}_y^2$, $I\hat{C}C_{m:g:c}$, $t_{\text{critical: }\alpha/2}$, and $t_{\text{critical}:\beta}$, the structure of $\hat{\sigma}_\Delta^2$ is made explicit and the same sample size is computed as:

$$g = \frac{2\hat{\sigma}_y^2(1+(m-1)I\hat{C}C_{m:g:c})(t_{\text{critical: }\alpha/2}+t_{\text{critical}:\beta})^2}{m\hat{\Delta}^2} \qquad (9.23)$$

Either form may require two or more iterations. The initial values of $t_{\text{critical: }\alpha/2}$ and of $t_{\text{critical}:\beta}$ often have to be changed given the preliminary result for *g*.

Written in terms of $\hat{\sigma}_\Delta^2$, the sample size of members per group required for a specified value of $\hat{\Delta}$ is computed as shown in Equation 9.13:

$$m = \frac{m\hat{\sigma}_\Delta^2(t_{\text{critical: }\alpha/2}+t_{\text{critical}:\beta})^2}{\hat{\Delta}^2}$$

Written in terms of g, $\hat{\sigma}_y^2$, $I\hat{C}C_{m:g:c}$, $t_{\text{critical: }\alpha/2}$, and $t_{\text{critical}:\beta}$, the structure of $\hat{\sigma}_\Delta^2$ is made explicit and the same sample size is computed as:

$$m = \frac{2\hat{\sigma}_y^2(1+(m-1)I\hat{C}C_{m:g:c})(t_{\text{critical: }\alpha/2}+t_{\text{critical}:\beta})^2}{g\hat{\Delta}^2} \qquad (9.24)$$

Either form may require two or more iterations, because the value of $\hat{\sigma}_\Delta$ will change with the value of *m*.

Extension to Other Design and Analysis Plans

The first step in any power analysis is the specification of the form and magnitude of the intervention effect, Δ. The research question should define both the design and the analysis, which in turn define the structure of Δ. If the question is whether two conditions differ in the average level of y, after adjustment for baseline levels, the study is a nested cohort design with pretest and posttest measures and the analysis is built around a comparison of two means after regression adjustment for baseline values. In that case, Δ is defined as shown in Chapter 6. If the question is whether the average group-specific slope in the intervention condition departs from the average group-specific slope in the control condition, the study is an extended nested cross-sectional design and the analysis is a random-coefficients analysis. In that case, Δ is defined as shown in Chapter 5. Other questions may lead to other designs and analyses and to other definitions for Δ.

To simplify the power analysis, the investigator should simplify the structure of Δ as much as possible. For example, if several contrasts among means, slopes, mean slopes, or their differences are of interest, the investigator should pick one as primary and focus the power analysis on that contrast. Similarly, if there are more than two conditions, the investigators should pick the two that define the primary contrast of interest and focus the power analysis on that contrast. All the methods presented in this chapter presume that Δ is defined as a single df contrast among condition-level statistics.

The second step is to select a test for that effect. As long as the intervention effect is defined as a single df contrast among condition-level statistics, and as long as there are a moderate number of members per group and groups per condition, the familiar t-test in Equation 9.2 is appropriate.

The third step is to determine the distribution of that test under the null hypothesis. With the t-test, the distribution is known as soon as the df are known.

The fourth step is to select the critical values in that distribution that determine whether or not the investigator will reject the null hypothesis. The critical values are tied to the investigator's decisions on the Type I and II error rates and the use of a one- or two-tailed test.

The fifth step is to develop an expression for the variance of the intervention effect under the null hypothesis in terms of parameters that are easily estimated from the literature, from available data, or from new data. This is the reason that the formulae presented above were written in terms of parameters like m, g, and σ_y^2. Those parameters are far easier to estimate than parameters such as $\sigma_{\bar{y}_I-\bar{y}_C}^2$.

The sixth step is to gather estimates of those parameters. This is a critical step, as the quality of the power analysis depends substantially on the quality of the estimates of the parameters. Investigators should seek to estimate the parameters from data that are similar to the data likely to be collected in the study. For example, if the study will involve schoolchildren from a predominantly Hispanic neighborhood, estimates drawn from children of a different age or ethnic group may not be valid. It would be far better to gather limited data from the target population and develop the estimates from those data.

Once the estimates are available, the seventh step is the mechanical generation of the detectable differences, sample sizes, or power estimates, usually across a range of levels for several of the parameters. Here computer spreadsheets can be very helpful, as they often have built-in statistical functions and can perform repetitive calculations more accurately than can be done by hand. Of course, care must be taken to ensure that the spreadsheet is created and used properly.

Once the calculations are complete, the investigators should review the results and choose the combination of groups per condition and members per group that provides adequate power at a reasonable cost. There are always many different combinations of groups per condition and members per group that provide adequate power, but those combinations often differ considerably in their cost.

The least familiar step in this sequence often is working out the structure of σ_Δ^2. Earlier sections in this chapter did that for $\hat{\Delta} = \hat{\bar{y}}_I - \hat{\bar{y}}_C$ in the context of a simple Posttest-Only Control Group Design, both for the clinical trial and for the group-randomized trial. This section will offer guidelines for other designs and analyses.

Variance of the Intervention Effect and the Expected Mean Squares

In Equation 9.17, the variance of the difference between two condition means from the Posttest-Only Control Group nested cross-sectional design was defined as:

$$\sigma_\Delta^2 = \frac{2\sigma_y^2(1 + (m-1)ICC_{m:g:c})}{mg}$$

This form of the variance is familiar to those who have followed the literature on sample size and power analysis for group-randomized trials over the last 15 years (cf. Donner et al., 1981; Feldman and McKinlay, 1994; Hsieh, 1988; Koepsell et al., 1991; Murray and Hannan, 1990).

In Equation 5.3, the variance of the intervention effect for the same design and analysis was given in a different form:

$$\sigma_\Delta^2 = 2\left(\frac{MS_{g:c}}{mg}\right)$$

· The first form is written in terms of easily estimated parameters. That form is quite helpful for anyone who wants to conduct a power analysis. The second form is written in terms of the results from the mixed-model regression analysis. It can be helpful to anyone who wants to compute the variance of the intervention effect from the results of the analysis.

In fact, these two formulations are equivalent. To see this, recall from Chapter 1 that the endpoint variance is the sum of two components:

$$\sigma_y^2 = \sigma_e^2 + \sigma_{g:c}^2$$

The correlation among observations taken in the same group was defined in Equation 1.5 as an intraclass correlation:

$$ICC_{m:g:c} = \frac{\sigma_{g:c}^2}{\sigma_e^2 + \sigma_{g:c}^2}$$

As a result, the expected mean squares for groups and members can be written in two different forms, shown in Table 9.2. The first form is as given in Table 5.1. The second form is as given in Snedecor and Cochran (1989, p. 242). A little algebra will show that for each row, the two forms of the $E(MS)$ are equivalent.

By elaborating the alternative forms of the $MS_{g:c}$, the meaning of the variance of the intervention effect becomes increasingly clear:

$$\sigma_\Delta^2 = 2\left(\frac{MS_{g:c}}{mg}\right) = 2\left(\frac{\sigma_e^2 + m\sigma_{g:c}^2}{mg}\right) = 2\left(\frac{\sigma_y^2(1 + (m-1)ICC_{m:g:c})}{mg}\right) \quad (9.25)$$

The first expression is from Equation 5.3. The third expression is from Equation 9.17. The second expression reflects the underlying variance components that define the $MS_{g:c}$, σ_y^2 and $ICC_{m:g:c}$, as shown in Table 5.1.

For this simplest case, σ_e^2 and $\sigma_{g:c}^2$ capture all of the variation attributable to the members and groups. However, in more complex designs, that variation is shared among several components of variance. In anticipation of those more

Table 9.2. Two Equivalent Forms of the Expected Mean Squares for the Posttest-Only Comparison Group Design Presented in Chapter 5

Source	E(MS)	E(MS)
Group:C	$\sigma_e^2 + m\sigma_{g:c}^2$	$\sigma_y^2(1 + (m-1)ICC_{m:g:c})$
Member:G:C	σ_e^2	$\sigma_y^2(1 - ICC_{m:g:c})$

complex designs, let the total member variance be designated as σ_m^2 and the total group variance be designated as σ_g^2. Then the most general form for the variance of the intervention effect in the nested cross-sectional version of the Posttest-Only Control Group Design involving two conditions is an adaptation of the second expression:

$$\sigma_{\Delta}^2 = 2\left(\frac{\sigma_m^2 + m\sigma_g^2}{mg}\right) \tag{9.26}$$

This more general form is elaborated in the next several sections to accommodate more complex designs and analyses.

Repeat Observations on Groups

In a group-randomized trial, the simplest kind of repeat observations occurs in the cross-sectional version of the Pretest-Posttest Control Group Design where there are repeat observations on the same groups. The model for that analysis was presented in Equation 5.7:

$$Y_{i:jk:l} = \mu + C_l + T_j + TC_{jl} + G_{k:l} + TG_{jk:l} + \varepsilon_{i:jk:l}$$

Based on this model, there are two sources of variation among the groups:

$$\sigma_g^2 = \sigma_{g:c}^2 + \sigma_{tg:c}^2 \tag{9.27}$$

Those two components are related through the over-time correlation within groups, $r_{yy(g)}$, as:

$$\sigma_{g:c}^2 = \sigma_g^2(r_{yy(g)}) \text{ and } \sigma_{tg:c}^2 = \sigma_g^2(1 - r_{yy(g)}) \tag{9.28}$$

where

$$r_{yy(g)} = \frac{\sigma_{g:c}^2}{\sigma_{g:c}^2 + \sigma_{tg:c}^2} \tag{9.29}$$

As a result, the variance of the intervention effect in this analysis can be written in terms of the original σ_m^2 and σ_g^2 as:

$$\sigma_{\Delta}^2 = 2*2\left(\frac{MS_{tg:c}}{mg}\right) = 2*2\left(\frac{\sigma_e^2 + m\sigma_{tg:c}^2}{mg}\right) = 2*2\left(\frac{\sigma_m^2 + m\sigma_g^2(1 - r_{yy(g)})}{mg}\right) \tag{9.30}$$

Any of these expressions for σ_{Δ}^2 can be used in the power analysis and the choice will usually depend on which estimates are available.

To illustrate the estimation of the over-time correlation within groups and its use in the development of standard error estimates, consider the example from the corresponding section in Chapter 7. Table 9.3 reproduces the covariance-parameter estimates from that example (from Table 7.39). The three estimates represent $\hat{\sigma}_{g:c}^2$, $\hat{\sigma}_{tg:c}^2$ and $\hat{\sigma}_e^2$, respectively. The total variation attributable to group is estimated as:

$$\hat{\sigma}_g^2 = \hat{\sigma}_{g:c}^2 + \hat{\sigma}_{tg:c}^2 = 3.61 + 2.78 = 6.39$$

The over-time correlation within groups, $r_{yy(g)}$, is estimated as:

$$\hat{r}_{yy(g)} = \frac{\hat{\sigma}_{g:c}^2}{\hat{\sigma}_{g:c}^2 + \sigma_{tg:c}^2} = \frac{3.61}{3.61 + 2.78} = 0.565$$

This is a large correlation and suggests that the level of blood pressure observed in one of the MHHP communities at baseline is well related to the level observed a year later.

Cast in terms of the $MS_{tg:c}$, the standard error of the intervention effect was estimated in Chapter 7 as:

$$\hat{\sigma}_{\Delta} = \sqrt{2*2\left(\frac{\hat{MS}_{tg:c}}{mg}\right)} = \sqrt{2*2\left(\frac{1024}{328*3}\right)} = 2.04$$

Cast in terms of σ_m^2 and σ_g^2 and $r_{yy(g)}$, the standard error of the intervention effect is estimated as:

$$\hat{\sigma}_{\Delta} = \sqrt{2*2\left(\frac{\hat{\sigma}_m^2 + m\hat{\sigma}_g^2(1 - \hat{r}_{yy(g)})}{mg}\right)} = \sqrt{2*2\left(\frac{112 + 328*6.39(1 - 0.565)}{328*3}\right)} = 2.04$$

Table 9.3. Covariance-Parameter Estimates From the Time × Condition Analysis of Diastolic Blood Pressure From the Pretest-Posttest Control Group Design Example in Chapter 7

Cov Parm	Estimate
INTERCEPT	3.61318
TIME	2.77915
Residual	112.41756

Repeat Observations on Members

The simplest form of over-time correlation within members occurs in the cohort version of the Pretest-Posttest Control Group Design. The model for that analysis was presented in Equation 6.1:

$$Y_{ij:k:l} = \mu + C_l + T_j + TC_{jl} + G_{k:l} + M_{i:k:l} + TG_{jk:l} + MT_{ij:k:l} + \varepsilon_{ij:k:l}$$

Based on this model, there are two sources of variation among the groups, as defined in Equation 9.27. In addition, there are three sources of variation among the members:

$$\sigma_m^2 = \sigma_{m:g:c}^2 + \sigma_{mt:g:c}^2 + \sigma_e^2 \tag{9.31}$$

The three components of the member variance are related through the over-time correlation within members, $r_{yy(m)}$, as:

$$\sigma_{m:g:c}^2 = \sigma_m^2(r_{yy(m)}) \text{ and } \sigma_{mt:g:c}^2 + \sigma_e^2 = \sigma_m^2(1 - r_{yy(m)}) \tag{9.32}$$

where

$$r_{yy(m)} = \frac{\sigma_{m:g:c}^2}{\sigma_{m:g:c}^2 + \sigma_{mt:g:c}^2 + \sigma_e^2} \tag{9.33}$$

The variance of the intervention effect can be written in terms of the original σ_m^2 and σ_g^2 and the two over-time correlations as:

$$\begin{aligned}
\sigma_\Delta^2 &= 2*2\left(\frac{MS_{tg:c}}{mg}\right) \\
&= 2*2\left(\frac{\sigma_e^2 + \sigma_{mt:g:c}^2 + m\sigma_{tg:c}^2}{mg}\right) \\
&= 2*2\left(\frac{\sigma_m^2(1 - r_{yy(m)}) + m\sigma_g^2(1 - r_{yy(g)})}{mg}\right)
\end{aligned} \tag{9.34}$$

Any of these expressions for σ_Δ^2 can be used in the power analysis and the choice will usually depend on which estimates are available.

To illustrate the estimation of the over-time correlation within members and groups and their use in the development of standard-error estimates, consider the example from the corresponding section in Chapter 8. Table 9.4 reproduces the covariance-parameter estimates from that example (from Table 8.4).

Table 9.4. Covariance-Parameter Estimates From the Time $\times$ Condition Analysis of Diastolic Blood Pressure From the Pretest-Posttest Control Group Design Example in Chapter 8

Cov Parm	Estimate
INTERCEPT	0.44894
TIME	1.69858
TIME CS	61.85343
Residual	48.99720

The four estimates represent $\hat{\sigma}^2_{g:c}$, $\hat{\sigma}^2_{tg:c}$, $\hat{\sigma}^2_{m:g:c}$, and $\hat{\sigma}^2_{mt:g:c} + \hat{\sigma}^2_e$. The total variation attributable to groups is estimated as:

$$\hat{\sigma}^2_g = \hat{\sigma}^2_{g:c} + \hat{\sigma}^2_{tg:c} = 0.449 + 1.70 = 2.15$$

The over-time correlation within group, $r_{yy(g)}$, is estimated as:

$$\hat{r}_{yy(g)} = \frac{\hat{\sigma}^2_{g:c}}{\hat{\sigma}^2_{g:c} + \hat{\sigma}^2_{tg:c}} = \frac{0.449}{0.449 + 1.70} = 0.209$$

This correlation suggests that the level of blood pressure observed in an MHHP community at baseline is only modestly related to the level observed a year later, after adjustment for repeat measures on the same individuals.

The total variation attributable to members is estimated as:

$$\hat{\sigma}^2_m = \hat{\sigma}^2_{m:g:c} + \hat{\sigma}^2_{mt:g:c} + \hat{\sigma}^2_e = 61.85 + 49.0 = 111$$

The over-time correlation within member, $r_{yy(m)}$, is estimated as:

$$\hat{r}_{yy(m)} = \frac{\hat{\sigma}^2_{m:g:c}}{\hat{\sigma}^2_e + \hat{\sigma}^2_{mt:g:c} + \hat{\sigma}^2_{m:g:c}} = \frac{61.85}{49.0 + 61.85} = 0.558$$

This correlation suggests that the level of blood pressure observed for a person at baseline is well related to the level observed a year later, even after adjustment for repeat measures on the same communities.

Cast in terms of the $MS_{tg:c}$, the standard error of the intervention effect was estimated in Chapter 8 as shown in the upper panel of Table 9.5. Cast in terms of the original variance components σ^2_m and σ^2_g and the two over-time correlations, the standard error of the intervention effect is estimated as shown in the lower panel of Table 9.5.

Table 9.5. Standard Error of the Intervention Effect From the Time ×
Condition Analysis of Diastolic Blood Pressure From the Pretest-Posttest
Control Group Design Example in Chapter 8

AS ESTIMATED IN CHAPTER 8

$$\hat{\sigma}_\Delta = \sqrt{2*2\left(\frac{\hat{MS}_{tg:c}}{mg}\right)}$$

$$= \sqrt{2*2\left(\frac{1569}{894*3}\right)}$$

$$= 1.53$$

AS ESTIMATED IN CHAPTER 9

$$\hat{\sigma}_\Delta = \sqrt{2*2\left(\frac{\hat{\sigma}_m^2(1-\hat{r}_{yy(m)}) + m\hat{\sigma}_g^2(1-\hat{r}_{yy(g)})}{mg}\right)}$$

$$= \sqrt{2*2\left(\frac{111(1-0.558) + 894(2.15(1-0.209))}{894*3}\right)}$$

$$= 1.53$$

Regression Adjustment for Covariates

In the usual fixed-effects analysis, the impact of the regression adjustment for
covariates is quite simple:

$$\sigma_e^2 = \sigma_y^2(1 - R_{yx}^2) \tag{9.35}$$

The single error term in the fixed-effects analysis is the usual variance of the
endpoint reduced by a factor of $(1 - R_{yx}^2)$, where R_{yx}^2 is the squared multiple
correlation coefficient indexing the proportion of variance explained by the
covariates.

The situation is more complex in a group-randomized trial because there
are always multiple random effects. The total variance is still reduced by the
factor $(1 - R_{yx}^2)$, but the reduction is rarely divided proportionally among the
components of variance. The member component of variance always decreases, with the magnitude of the decline dependent on the strength of the
association. However, the group components of variance may decrease or increase. The effect on σ_Δ^2 is very unpredictable in the absence of prior experience with the variables and populations of interest.

Given the unpredictable effect of the regression adjustment on the components of variance, the situation is well summarized as:

$$\sigma_y^2(1 - R_{yx}^2) = \sigma_m^2\theta_m + \sigma_g^2\theta_g \tag{9.36}$$

where

$$\theta_m = \frac{\text{adjusted } \sigma_m^2}{\text{unadjusted } \sigma_m^2} \text{ and } \theta_g = \frac{\text{adjusted } \sigma_g^2}{\text{unadjusted } \sigma_g^2} \tag{9.37}$$

The first application of regression adjustment for covariates occurred in Chapter 5 in the adjusted analysis for the Posttest-Only Control Group design. The model from that analysis was presented in Equation 5.4:

$$Y_{i:k:l} = \mu + C_l + \sum_{o=1}^{x} \beta_o(X_{oi:k:l} - \overline{X}_{o\ldots}) + G_{k:l} + \varepsilon_{i:k:l}$$

The adjusted member variance is $\sigma_m^2\theta_m$ and is captured entirely by σ_e^2. Similarly, the adjusted group variance is $\sigma_g^2\theta_g$ and is captured entirely by $\sigma_{g:c}^2$. As a result, the variance of the intervention effect for this design and analysis can be written in terms of the original σ_m^2 and σ_g^2 as:

$$\sigma_\Delta^2 = 2\left(\frac{MS_{g:c}}{mg}\right) = 2\left(\frac{\sigma_e^2 + m\sigma_{g:c}^2}{mg}\right) = 2\left(\frac{\sigma_m^2\theta_m + m\sigma_g^2\theta_g}{mg}\right) \tag{9.38}$$

Any of these expressions for σ_Δ^2 can be used in the power analysis and the choice will usually depend on which estimates are available.

To illustrate the estimation of the variance reduction due to regression adjustment for covariates and its use in the development of standard-error estimates, consider the corresponding examples from Chapter 7 for the unadjusted and adjusted analyses of the same data from the Posttest-Only Control Group Design. Table 9.6 reproduces the covariance-parameter estimates from the unadjusted analysis (from Table 7.6). The total variation shared between the two random effects in the design is $2.82 + 107.0 = 109.8$. The covariance-parameter estimates from the adjusted analysis are also presented in Table 9.6 (from Table 7.27). The total variation shared between the same random effects is $3.14 + 95.5 = 98.6$.

The residual error decreased by a factor of:

$$\hat{\theta}_m = \frac{95.5}{107} = 0.893$$

However, the group component of variance increased by a factor of:

$$\hat{\theta}_g = \frac{3.14}{2.82} = 1.113$$

Table 9.6. Covariance-Parameter Estimates From the Unadjusted and Adjusted Analyses of Diastolic Blood Pressure From the Posttest-Only Control Group Design Example in Chapter 7

UNADJUSTED ANALYSIS	
Cov Parm	Estimate
GROUP(COND)	2.81897
Residual	106.99941
ADJUSTED ANALYSIS	
Cov Parm	Estimate
GROUP(COND)	3.14000
Residual	95.48340

This result illustrates the point made in Chapter 7 that some variance components may increase with regression adjustment for covariates.

The R_{yx}^2 in the adjusted analysis is estimated as:

$$\hat{R}_{yx}^2 = 1 - \frac{\hat{\sigma}_m^2 \hat{\theta}_m + \hat{\sigma}_g^2 \hat{\theta}_g}{\hat{\sigma}_y^2} = 1 - \frac{107*0.892 + 2.82*1.113}{109.8} = 0.102$$

Cast in terms of the $MS_{g:c}$, the adjusted standard error of the intervention effect was estimated in Chapter 7 as:

$$\hat{\sigma}_\Delta = \sqrt{2\left(\frac{\hat{MS}_{g:c}}{mg}\right)} = \sqrt{2\left(\frac{1000}{288*3}\right)} = 1.52$$

Cast in terms of the underlying variance components, σ_m^2 and σ_g^2, θ_m and θ_g, the adjusted standard error is estimated as:

$$\hat{\sigma}_\Delta = \sqrt{2\left(\frac{\hat{\sigma}_m^2 \hat{\theta}_m + m\hat{\sigma}_g^2 \hat{\theta}_g}{mg}\right)} = \sqrt{2\left(\frac{107(0.892) + 288(2.82)(1.113)}{288*3}\right)} = 1.52$$

Post Hoc Stratification

In the usual fixed-effects model, the effect of *post hoc* stratification is quite simple:

$$\sigma_e^2 = \sigma_y^2(1 - r_{ys}) \qquad (9.39)$$

The single error term is the usual variance of the endpoint reduced by a factor of $(1 - r_{ys})$, where r_{ys} is the correlation between the endpoint and the stratification factor. To the extent that the stratification factor is related to the endpoint, that correlation is large and the residual error is reduced, improving precision.

The situation is more complex in a group-randomized trial, where there are always multiple random effects. The total variance is still reduced by the factor $(1 - r_{ys})$, but the reduction is rarely divided proportionally among σ_m^2 and σ_g^2. Usually σ_m^2 decreases; on the other hand, σ_g^2 may increase or decrease.

More important, the structure of σ_g^2 is expanded and only a subset of the components of σ_g^2 are of interest in the *post hoc* stratified analysis. This situation is well summarized as:

$$\sigma_y^2(1 - r_{ys}) = \sigma_m^2 \phi_m + \sigma_g^2 \phi_g \qquad (9.40)$$

where,

$$\phi_m = \frac{\text{stratified } \sigma_m^2}{\text{unstratified } \sigma_m^2} \text{ and } \phi_g = \frac{\text{stratified group components of interest}}{\text{unstratified } \sigma_g^2}$$

$$(9.41)$$

To illustrate the estimation of the variance reduction due to *post hoc* stratification and its use in the development of standard-error estimates, consider the example from Chapter 7 for the unstratified analysis of data from a Posttest-Only Control Group Design. The model for that analysis was presented in Equation 5.1 as:

$$Y_{i:k:l} = \mu + C_l + G_{k:l} + \varepsilon_{i:k:l}$$

Now consider *post hoc* stratification by gender in this example. The model for the stratified analysis is:

$$Y_{i:kp:l} = \mu + C_l + S_p + CS_{lp} + G_{k:l} + GS_{kp:l} + \varepsilon_{i:kp:l} \qquad (9.42)$$

In the stratified model, σ_g^2 is expanded from one to two components:

$$\sigma_g^2 = \sigma_{g:c}^2 + \sigma_{gs:c}^2 \qquad (9.43)$$

Only one of these two components is of interest in the *post hoc* stratified analysis, as shown in the expected mean squares in Table 9.7. The intervention effect is captured in the condition $\times$ strata interaction and tested against

Table 9.7. Expected Mean Squares for a Stratified Analysis of Data From the Nested Cross-Sectional Version of the Posttest-Only Control Group Design

Source	df	E(MS)	MS
Condition	$c-1$	$\sigma_e^2 + ms\sigma_{g:c}^2 + mgs\sigma_c^2$	MS_c
Group:C	$c(g-1)$	$\sigma_e^2 + ms\sigma_{g:c}^2$	$MS_{g:c}$
Strata	$s-1$	$\sigma_e^2 + m\sigma_{gs:c}^2 + mgc\sigma_s^2$	MS_s
CS	$(c-1)(s-1)$	$\sigma_e^2 + m\sigma_{gs:c}^2 + mg\sigma_{cs}^2$	MS_{cs}
GS:C	$c(g-1)(s-1)$	$\sigma_e^2 + m\sigma_{gs:c}^2$	$MS_{gs:c}$
Member:GS:C	$gsc(m-1)$	σ_e^2	MS_e

$MS_{gs:c}$. Only the second of the two components of σ_g^2 contributes to that mean square. As a result, for this example,

$$\phi_m = \frac{\text{stratified } \sigma_m^2}{\text{unstratified } \sigma_m^2} \text{ and } \phi_g = \frac{\text{stratified } \sigma_{gs:c}^2}{\text{unstratified } \sigma_g^2} \qquad (9.44)$$

Given this model, the adjusted member variance is $\sigma_m^2\phi_m$ and is captured entirely by σ_e^2. Similarly, the adjusted group variance is $\sigma_g^2\phi_g$ and is captured entirely by $\sigma_{gs:c}^2$. The variance of the intervention effect for the stratified analysis involving two conditions and two strata can be written in terms of the original σ_m^2 and σ_g^2, together with ϕ_m and ϕ_g, as:

$$\sigma_\Delta^2 = 2*2\left(\frac{MS_{gs:c}}{mg}\right) = 2*2\left(\frac{\sigma_e^2 + m\sigma_{gs:c}^2}{mg}\right) = 2*\left(\frac{\sigma_m^2\phi_m + m\sigma_g^2\phi_g}{mg}\right) \qquad (9.45)$$

Table 9.8. Covariance-Parameter Estimates From the Unstratified Analysis of Diastolic Blood Pressure From the Posttest-Only Comparison Group Design Example in Chapter 7, as Well as From a Stratified Analysis of Those Data

UNSTRATIFIED ANALYSIS	
Cov Parm	Estimate
GROUP(COND)	2.81897
Residual	106.99941
STRATIFIED ANALYSIS	
Cov Parm	Estimate
GROUP(COND)	4.11604
SEX*GROUP(COND)	2.32531
Residual	100.37609

Any of these expressions for σ_Δ^2 can be used in the power analysis and the choice will usually depend on which estimates are available.

To illustrate the estimation of the variance reduction due to *post hoc* stratification, and its use in the development of standard-error estimates, consider the results from the unstratified and stratified analyses, presented in Table 9.8.

In the stratified analysis,

$$\hat\phi_m = \frac{\text{stratified } \hat\sigma_m^2}{\text{unstratified } \hat\sigma_m^2} = \frac{100.4}{107} = 0.938 \text{ and } \hat\phi_g = \frac{\text{stratified } \hat\sigma_{gs:c}^2}{\text{unstratified } \hat\sigma_g^2} = \frac{2.33}{2.82} = 0.826$$

The r_{ys} in the adjusted analysis is estimated as:

$$\hat{r}_{ys} = \left(1 - \frac{\hat\sigma_m^2\hat\phi_m + \hat\sigma_g^2\hat\phi_g}{\hat\sigma_y^2}\right) = \left(1 - \frac{107*0.938 + 2.82*0.826}{109.8}\right) = 0.0647$$

The reduction in variance due to stratification is modest in this example and fairly evenly divided between the member and group components of variance. That is not always true.

Cast in terms of the $MS_{gs:c}$, the adjusted standard error of the intervention effect is estimated as:

$$\hat\sigma_\Delta = \sqrt{2*2\left(\frac{\hat{MS}_{gs:c}}{mg}\right)} = \sqrt{2*2\left(\frac{771}{288*3}\right)} = 1.89$$

Cast in terms of the underlying variance components, σ_m^2 and σ_g^2, and ϕ_m and ϕ_g, the adjusted standard error of the intervention effect for this example is estimated as:

$$\hat\sigma_\Delta = \sqrt{2*2\left(\frac{\hat\sigma_m^2\hat\phi_m + m\hat\sigma_g^2\hat\phi_g}{mg}\right)} = \sqrt{2*2\left(\frac{107(0.938) + 288(2.82)(0.826)}{288*3}\right)} = 1.89$$

Note that the standard error from the unstratified analysis given in Chapter 7 is 1.46. As can happen, the standard error increased with *post hoc* stratification. In this case, the r_{ys} was quite small and did not compensate for the increase from 2 to 2*2 as the multiplier in the numerator of the standard error. This example illustrates the point made in Chapter 5 that *post hoc* stratification should be reserved for situations in which the investigator has a genuine interest in the differential effect of the intervention across the strata.

Matching

In the clinical trial, the effect of matching is similar to that of *post hoc* stratification. The residual error is reduced by a factor of $(1 - r_{ys})$, where r_{ys} is the correlation between the endpoint and the matching factor. In addition, the *ddf* for the test of interest are reduced by half.

The situation is more complex in a group-randomized trial, where there are multiple random effects; fortunately, the solution follows the pattern established for *post hoc* stratification in the previous section. The total variance is still reduced by the factor $(1 - r_{ys})$, but the reduction is rarely divided proportionally among σ_m^2 and σ_g^2. Usually σ_m^2 declines; on the other hand, σ_g^2 may increase or decrease. As for the clinical trial, the *ddf* are reduced by half.

The structure of σ_g^2 is expanded and only a subset of the components of σ_g^2 is of interest in the matched analysis. As a result, this situation is well summarized as:

$$\sigma_y^2(1 - r_{ys}) = \sigma_m^2 \phi_m + \sigma_g^2 \phi_g \tag{9.46}$$

where

$$\phi_m = \frac{\text{matched } \sigma_m^2}{\text{unmatched } \sigma_m^2} \text{ and } \phi_g = \frac{\text{matched group components of interest}}{\text{unmatched } \sigma_g^2} \tag{9.47}$$

To illustrate the estimation of the variance reduction due to matching and its use in the development of standard-error estimates, consider again the example from Chapter 7 for the unmatched analysis of data from a Posttest-Only Control Group Design. The model from that analysis was presented in Equation 5.1:

$$Y_{i:k:l} = \mu + C_l + G_{k:l} + \varepsilon_{i:k:l}$$

Now consider matching on community type in this example. The model for the matched analysis is:

$$Y_{i:lp} = \mu + C_l + S_p + CS_{lp} + \varepsilon_{i:lp} \tag{9.48}$$

In the matched model, σ_g^2 is expanded from one to two components as shown above in Equation 9.43:

$$\sigma_g^2 = \sigma_s^2 + \sigma_{gs}^2$$

Table 9.9. Expected Mean Squares for a Matched Analysis of Data from a Posttest-Only Control Group Design

Source	df	E(MS)	MS
Condition	$c-1$	$\sigma_e^2 + m\sigma_{cs}^2 + ms\sigma_c^2$	MS_c
Strata	$s-1$	$\sigma_e^2 + mc\sigma_s^2$	MS_s
CS	$(c-1)(s-1)$	$\sigma_e^2 + m\sigma_{cs}^2$	MS_{cs}
Member:CS	$cs(m-1)$	σ_e^2	MS_e

Only one of these two components is of interest in the matched analysis, as shown in the expected mean squares in Table 9.9.

The intervention effect is captured in the condition main effect and tested against MS_{cs}. Only the second of the two components of σ_g^2 contributes to that mean square. As a result, for this example,

$$\phi_m = \frac{\text{matched } \sigma_m^2}{\text{unmatched } \sigma_m^2} \text{ and } \phi_g = \frac{\text{matched } \sigma_{cs}^2}{\text{unmatched } \sigma_g^2} \qquad (9.49)$$

The adjusted member variance is $\sigma_m^2\phi_m$ and is captured entirely by σ_e^2. The adjusted group variance is $\sigma_g^2\phi_g$ and is captured entirely by σ_{cs}^2. The variance of the intervention effect for the matched analysis is written in terms of the original σ_m^2 and σ_g^2, together with ϕ_m and ϕ_g as:

$$\sigma_\Delta^2 = 2\left(\frac{MS_{cs}}{ms}\right) = 2\left(\frac{\sigma_e^2 + m\sigma_{cs}^2}{ms}\right) = 2\left(\frac{\sigma_m^2\phi_m + m\sigma_g^2\phi_g}{ms}\right) \qquad (9.50)$$

Any of these expressions for σ_Δ^2 can be used in the power analysis and the choice will usually depend on which estimates are available.

To illustrate the estimation of the variance reduction due to matching and its use in the development of standard-error estimates, consider the results from the unmatched and matched analyses of the Posttest-Only Control Group example from Chapter 7, shown in Table 9.10.

In the matched analysis,

$$\hat{\phi}_m = \frac{\text{matched } \hat{\sigma}_m^2}{\text{unmatched } \hat{\sigma}_m^2} = \frac{107}{107} = 1.0 \text{ and } \hat{\phi}_g = \frac{\text{matched } \hat{\sigma}_{cs}^2}{\text{unmatched } \hat{\sigma}_g^2} = \frac{0.984}{2.82} = 0.349$$

The r_{ys} in the matched analysis is:

$$\hat{r}_{ys} = \left(1 - \frac{\hat{\sigma}_m^2\hat{\phi}_m + \hat{\sigma}_g^2\hat{\phi}_g}{\hat{\sigma}_y^2}\right) = \left(1 - \frac{107*1.00 + 2.82*0.349}{109.8}\right) = 0.0165$$

Table 9.10. Covariance-Parameter Estimates From the
Unmatched Analysis of Diastolic Blood Pressure From the
Posttest-Only Comparison Group Design Example in Chapter 7,
as Well as From a Matched Analysis of Those Data

UNMATCHED ANALYSIS	
Cov Parm	Estimate
GROUP(COND)	2.81897
Residual	106.99941
MATCHED ANALYSIS	
Cov Parm	Estimate
STRATA	1.84072
COND*STRATA	0.98409
Residual	106.99910

The reduction in total variance due to matching is very modest in this example. However, it is not evenly divided between the member and group components of variance, and the more important consideration for power is that the reduction is large for the group component of variance.

Cast in terms of the MS_{cs}, the matched standard error of the intervention effect is estimated as:

$$\hat{\sigma}_\Delta = \sqrt{2\left(\frac{\hat{MS}_{cs}}{ms}\right)} = \sqrt{2\left(\frac{390}{288*3}\right)} = 0.950$$

Cast in terms of the underlying variance components, σ_m^2 and σ_g^2, and ϕ_m and ϕ_g, the matched standard error is estimated as:

$$\hat{\sigma}_\Delta = \sqrt{2\left(\frac{\hat{\sigma}_m^2\hat{\phi}_m + m\hat{\sigma}_g^2\hat{\phi}_g}{ms}\right)} = \sqrt{2\left(\frac{107(1.0) + 288(2.82)(0.349)}{288*3}\right)} = 0.950$$

Note that the matched standard error is considerably smaller than the unmatched standard error, given in Chapter 7 as 1.48. At the same time, the *ddf* in the matched analysis are $(c-1)(s-1)=2$, compared to $c(g-1)=4$ in the unmatched analysis. The critical value of the *F*-distribution given 1 and 4 *df* is 7.71. Given only 1 and 2 *df*, the critical value soars to 18.5. It is unlikely that the reduction in the standard error observed in this case could make up for such a large increase in the critical value. However, if the original *df* were larger, the matched analysis might well have more power.

Trend Analysis in Mixed-Model ANOVA/ANCOVA

In the trend analysis in the mixed-model ANOVA/ANCOVA, the intervention effect is not defined in terms of condition means. Instead, it is defined in terms of condition-specific time trends fit to the time $\times$ group means. This section presents the derivation of the variance of that intervention effect in the context of the cross-sectional version of the Extended Design. It also illustrates the calculation of that variance using the example from Chapter 7 for the adjusted analysis of data from an Extended Design.

Let $\hat{\beta}_{t(\text{lin})}$ be the linear regression coefficient estimating the change in y per unit change in time:

$$\hat{\beta}_{t(\text{lin})} = \hat{r}_{yt} \frac{\hat{\sigma}_y}{\hat{\sigma}_t} \qquad (9.51)$$

Here $\hat{\sigma}_y$ and $\hat{\sigma}_t$ are the unbiased estimates of the standard deviations of y and time, $\hat{r}_{yt}$ is the estimated correlation between y and time, and the regression is based on mtg independent observations in one condition.

The variance of the estimate of the bivariate linear regression coefficient for time and y is

$$\sigma^2_{\hat{\beta}_{t(\text{lin})}} = \frac{\hat{\sigma}^2_{y-y'}}{\hat{\sigma}^2_t(mtg-1)} \qquad (9.52)$$

where

$$\hat{\sigma}^2_{y-y'} = \hat{\sigma}^2_y(1 - \hat{r}^2_{yt})\left(\frac{mtg-1}{mtg-2}\right)$$

Combining these formulae, the variance of the estimated bivariate linear regression coefficient in one condition is written as:

$$\sigma^2_{\hat{\beta}_{t(\text{lin})}} = \frac{\hat{\sigma}^2_y(1 - \hat{r}^2_{yt})}{\hat{\sigma}^2_t(mtg-1)}\left(\frac{mtg-1}{mtg-2}\right) = \frac{\hat{\sigma}^2_y(1 - \hat{r}^2_{yt})}{\hat{\sigma}^2_t(mtg-2)} \qquad (9.53)$$

For the multivariate case, three adaptations must be made (Cohen and Cohen, 1983). First, one df is lost for each fixed-effect regression coefficient estimated in the analysis. If there are f coefficients for the fixed effects and one for the intercept, a total of $f+1$ coefficients are estimated. As a result, $(mtg-2)$ becomes $(mtg-(f+1)) = (mtg-f-1)$. Second, some of the variation in the endpoint is explained by the other terms in the analysis, in addition to time. As a result, the term $\hat{\sigma}_y^2(1 - \hat{r}_{yt}^2)$ becomes $\hat{\sigma}_y^2(1 - \hat{R}_{y\cdot xt}^2)$, where $\hat{R}_{y\cdot xt}^2$ reflects the proportion of variance in the endpoint explained by the other terms in the analysis, including time. Third, some of the variation in time is explained by the other predictor variables in the analysis. As a result, the term $\hat{\sigma}_t^2$ becomes $\hat{\sigma}_t^2(1 - \hat{R}_{t\cdot x}^2)$, where $\hat{R}_{t\cdot x}^2$ reflects the proportion of variance in time explained by the other predictor variables in the analysis. Given these modifications, the variance of the multivariate linear regression coefficient characterizing the relationship between time and the endpoint in one condition is written as:

$$\sigma_{\hat{\beta}_{t(\text{lin})}}^2 = \frac{\hat{\sigma}_y^2(1 - \hat{R}_{y\cdot xt}^2)}{\hat{\sigma}_t^2(1 - \hat{R}_{t\cdot x}^2)(mtg - f - 1)} \tag{9.54}$$

Given two conditions, the intervention effect in this analysis is defined as the difference between the two condition-specific regression lines, $\hat{\Delta} = (\hat{\beta}_{t(\text{lin})}|c = I) - (\hat{\beta}_{t(\text{lin})}|c = C)$. Assuming equality across the two conditions for the variances for y and time, as well as for the values of m, t, and g, the variance of the difference between the two linear time trends is estimated as:

$$\hat{\sigma}_\Delta^2 = \frac{2\hat{\sigma}_y^2(1 - \hat{R}_{y\cdot xt}^2)}{\hat{\sigma}_t^2(1 - \hat{R}_{t\cdot x}^2)(mtg - f - 1)} \tag{9.55}$$

Thus far, the formula for the variance has been developed as though the regression were conducted on mtg observations in each condition. In fact, each trend is fit to tg time $\times$ group means, where each mean is based on m observations. As a result, the variance of y is replaced by the variance of the time $\times$ group mean:

$$\hat{\sigma}_{\bar{y}_{tg}}^2 = \frac{\hat{\sigma}_y^2}{m} \tag{9.56}$$

In addition, the mtg in the denominator is replaced by tg. These two actions offset each other, so that the variance of the difference between two linear slopes each fit to tg time $\times$ group means is still estimated as shown in Equation 9.55.

Thus far, the intervention effect has been estimated as the difference between two condition-specific linear time trends estimated separately. In fact, those trends are usually estimated together in a single analysis, as illustrated in Chapter 7. With this approach, the regression coefficient for time (linear) will represent the linear trend in one condition and the coefficient for the time (linear) $\times$ condition interaction will represent the difference between the linear trends in the two conditions. As such, the coefficient for the time (linear) $\times$ condition interaction represents the intervention effect directly so that

$\hat{\Delta} = \hat{\beta}_{t(\text{lin})c}$. In a clinical trial, its variance is esimated as:

$$\hat{\sigma}^2_{\hat{\Delta}} = \frac{\hat{\sigma}^2_y(1 - \hat{R}^2_{y \cdot xtc})}{\hat{\sigma}^2_{tc}(1 - \hat{R}^2_{tc \cdot x})(mtgc - f - 1)} \tag{9.57}$$

Equations 9.55 and 9.57 are quite similar in structure but their elements are different. Both include $\hat{\sigma}^2_y$, and the same estimate may be applied in both formulae. However, the terms $\hat{R}^2_{y \cdot xtc}$ and $\hat{R}^2_{y \cdot xt}$ estimate different fractions of $\hat{\sigma}^2_y$. Similarly, $\hat{\sigma}^2_{tc}$ and $\hat{\sigma}^2_t$ estimate different variances. Certainly $\hat{R}^2_{tc \cdot x}$ and $\hat{R}^2_{t \cdot x}$ estimate different squared multiple correlation coefficients. The quantitites $(mtgc - f - 1)$ and $(mtg - f - 1)$ are different. Finally, Equation 9.57 includes no multiplier in its numerator, while Equation 9.55 includes 2 as a multiplier for a comparison of the time trends esimated separately from two conditions. In spite of these many differences, analysts who match their estimates to the proper formula will get the same results with both formulae, as both estimate the variance of the same intervention effect.

Equations 9.55 and 9.57 were developed as though each tg mean were based on m independent observations. That is an appropriate assumption in a clinical trial, but not in a group-randomized trial. In the group-randomized trial, an additional component of variance must be added to the variance of the time × group means to account for the correlation expected among the observations taken on the members in the same time × group survey. That component was defined in Equation 9.28 as $\sigma^2_{tg:c}$, which is the fraction of the total variation due to groups that is not explained by the within-group correlation over time:

$$\sigma^2_{tg:c} = \sigma^2_g(1 - r_{yy(g)})$$

The variance of the time × group mean in the group-randomized trial is then:

$$\hat{\sigma}^2_{\bar{y}_{tg}} = \frac{\hat{\sigma}^2_m}{m} + \sigma^2_g(1 - r_{yy(g)}) \tag{9.58}$$

Another problem with Equations 9.55 and 9.57 is that they assume that the regression adjustment for covariates affects all components of variance in the same way. As shown earlier in this chapter, regression adjustment for the other terms in the model often affects each component of variance in a different way. Similarly, the variance of time is partitioned into components attributable to the members and the groups and each component is reduced as a function of the regression adjustment for the other terms in the model. However, the variation in time attributable to groups plays no role in the variance of the intervention effect in this analysis.

Combining these elements, Equation 9.55 is rewritten for a group-randomized trial as:

$$\hat{\sigma}_{\Delta}^2 = \frac{2\left(\hat{\sigma}_{m(y)}^2 \hat{\theta}_{m(y \cdot xt)} + m\hat{\sigma}_{g(y)}^2 \hat{\theta}_{g(y \cdot xt)}(1 - \hat{r}_{yy(g)})\right)}{\hat{\sigma}_{m(t)}^2 \hat{\theta}_{m(t \cdot x)}(mtg - f - 1)} \tag{9.59}$$

Equation 9.57 is rewritten for a group-randomized trial as:

$$\hat{\sigma}_{\Delta}^2 = \frac{\hat{\sigma}_{m(y)}^2 \hat{\theta}_{m(y \cdot xtc)} + m\hat{\sigma}_{g(y)}^2 \hat{\theta}_{g(y \cdot xtc)}(1 - \hat{r}_{yy(g)})}{\hat{\sigma}_{m(tc)}^2 \hat{\theta}_{m(tc \cdot x)}(mtgc - f - 1)} \tag{9.60}$$

As in the clinical trial, Equations 9.59 and 9.60 will give the same result if the estimates and formulae are used properly.

To illustrate the calculation of the variance of the difference between two condition slopes computed from time × group means, consider the example from Chapter 7 for the adjusted analysis of an extended cross-sectional design. In that example, time was treated as a continuous variable and scaled in months from the onset of the intervention program. The intervention effect was constrained to be zero during the baseline period and modeled as a departure from the pooled secular trend. Both the intervention effect and the secular trend were modeled with linear and quadratic components. Because the analysis included observations from both conditions and estimated the intervention effect directly, Equation 9.60 is used.

Table 9.11 reproduces the covariance-parameter estimates from the adjusted analysis presented in Chapter 7. Table 9.11 also presents the covariance-parameter estimates from a new analysis of the same data with no fixed effects.

Table 9.11. Covariance-Parameter Estimates From the Adjusted Trend Analysis of Diastolic Blood Pressure From the Extended Design Example in Chapter 7, as Well as From an Analysis of Those Data With No Fixed Effects

ADJUSTED ANALYSIS	
Cov Parm	Estimate
INTERCEPT	0.11482
MONCAT	3.30264
Residual	101.57511
NO FIXED EFFECTS	
Cov Parm	Estimate
INTERCEPT	0.28327
MONCAT	3.64899
Residual	110.89942

The value for $\hat{\sigma}^2_{m(y)}$ is taken as the `Residual` estimate from the unadjusted analysis, 110.9. The value for $\hat{\theta}_{m(y \cdot xtc)}$ is taken as the ratio of the two `Residual` estimates:

$$\hat{\theta}_{m(y \cdot xtc)} = \frac{101.6}{110.9} = 0.9161$$

The value for $\hat{\sigma}^2_{g(y)}$ is taken from the unadjusted analysis as the sum of the group and time $\times$ group components of variance from that analysis:

$$\hat{\sigma}^2_{g(y)} = \hat{\sigma}^2_{g:c(y)} + \hat{\sigma}^2_{tg:c(y)} = 0.2833 + 3.649 = 3.932$$

The value for $\hat{\theta}_{g(y \cdot xtc)}$ is taken as the ratio of the $\hat{\sigma}^2_{g(y)}$ from the adjusted and unadjusted analyses:

$$\hat{\theta}_{g(y \cdot xtc)} = \frac{0.1148 + 3.303}{0.2833 + 3.649} = 0.869$$

The over-time correlation within groups is estimated from the adjusted model as:

$$\hat{r}_{yy(g)} = \frac{\hat{\sigma}^2_{g:c(y)}}{\hat{\sigma}^2_{g:c(y)} + \hat{\sigma}^2_{tg:c(y)}} = \frac{0.1148}{0.1148 + 3.303} = 0.0336$$

In this example, the intervention effect is represented by linear and quadratic terms representing the departure in the intervention condition from the common secular trend. Let the quadratic component be the component of interest. Then the expression $\hat{\sigma}^2_{m(tc)}\hat{\theta}_{m(tc \cdot x)}$ in the formula for the variance becomes $\hat{\sigma}^2_{m(t(\text{quad})c)}\hat{\theta}_{m(t(\text{quad})c \cdot x)}$. Required is an estimate of the component of variance in the quadratic term that is attributed to the members, $\hat{\sigma}^2_{m(t(\text{quad})c)}$, and an estimate of the reduction in that component that is due to the inclusion of the other terms in the analysis, $\hat{\theta}_{m(t(\text{quad})c \cdot x)}$. To get those estimates, two additional analyses are required, in parallel with those for diastolic blood pressure.

An adjusted analysis is required in which the quadratic component is the dependent variable and all the other terms in the original analysis of diastolic

Table 9.12. SAS MIXED Code to Estimate the Residual Variation in the Intervention Effect From the Adjusted Trend Analysis of Diastolic Blood Pressure From the Extended Design Example in Chapter 7

```
proc mixed info order = internal method = mivque0;
  class cond group moncat sex educlvl bpobsrvr
    bplocatn;
  model imonth2 = cond month month2 imonth age sex
    educlvl bpobsrvr bplocatn/ddf = 4,109,109,109 ddfm = res;
  random int/subject = group(cond);
run;
```

blood pressure are retained unless they are confounded with the quadratic component. That regression analysis is conducted using the MIXED code shown in Table 9.12. This analysis is identical to that originally conducted for blood pressure, with two exceptions. First, the imonth2 term is substituted for dbp as the dependent variable. In addition, the moncat*group(cond) term is dropped from the random statement because it would be confounded with imonth2. An analysis is also required that includes no fixed effects.

The covariance parameter estimates from the adjusted analysis of imonth2 are presented in Table 9.13. The covariance parameter estimates from an analysis of the same data with no fixed effects are also presented in Table 9.13.

The value for $\hat{\sigma}^2_{m(t(\text{quad})c)}$ is taken as the Residual estimate from the unadjusted analysis, rounded to 2126000. The value for $\hat{\theta}_{m(t(\text{quad})c \cdot x)}$ is taken as the ratio of the two Residual estimates: [4]

$$\hat{\theta}_{m(t(\text{quad})c \cdot x)} = \frac{75599}{2126000} = 0.03556$$

Cast in terms of the $MS_{tg:c}$, the standard error of the intervention effect was estimated in Chapter 7 as shown in the upper panel of Table 9.14. Cast in terms of the underlying variance components and other parameters developed here, the standard error is estimated as shown in the lower panel in Table 9.14.

Random-Coefficients Model: Cross Section

In the random-coefficients model applied to the nested cross-sectional design, the intervention effect is defined in terms of mean slopes, where each mean slope is the average of g group-specific slopes. One slope is computed for

Table 9.13. Covariance-Parameter Estimates for the Intervention Effect From the Adjusted Trend Analysis of Diastolic Blood Pressure From the Extended Design Example in Chapter 7 and From an Analysis of Those Data with no Fixed Effects

ADJUSTED ANALYSIS	
Cov Parm	Estimate
INTERCEPT	2709.26762
Residual	75598.68659
NO FIXED EFFECTS	
Cov Parm	Estimate
INTERCEPT	851139.16625
Residual	2125773.84900

Table 9.14. Standard Error of the Intervention Effect From the Adjusted Trend Analysis of Diastolic Blood Pressure From the Extended Design Example in Chapter 7

AS ESTIMATED IN CHAPTER 7

$$\hat{\sigma}_\Delta = \sqrt{\frac{\hat{MS}_{tg:c}}{\hat{\sigma}^2_{e(tc)}(mtgc - f - 1)}} = \sqrt{\frac{\hat{\sigma}^2_{e(y)} + m\hat{\sigma}^2_{tg:c}}{\hat{\sigma}^2_{e(tc)}(mtgc - f - 1)}}$$

$$= \sqrt{\frac{591.8}{75599(148.4*19.83*3*2 - 95 - 1)}}$$

$$= 0.000668$$

AS ESTIMATED IN CHAPTER 9

$$\hat{\sigma}_\Delta = \sqrt{\frac{(\hat{\sigma}^2_{m(y)}\hat{\theta}_{m(y \cdot xtc)} + m\hat{\sigma}^2_{g(y)}\hat{\theta}_{g(y \cdot xtc)}(1 - \hat{r}_{yy(g)}))}{\hat{\sigma}^2_{m(t(\text{quad})c)}\hat{\theta}_{m(t(\text{quad})c \cdot x)}(mtgc - f - 1)}}$$

$$= \sqrt{\frac{110.9(0.9161) + 148.4(3.932)(0.869)(1 - 0.0336)}{2126000(0.03556)(148.4*19.83*3*2 - 95 - 1)}}$$

$$= 0.000668$$

---

each of the groups nested within its condition. The intervention effect is represented in the model as $T_{(\text{lin})}C_l$. Given only two conditions, the intervention effect is the simple difference between the two condition mean slopes. This section will derive the variance of that intervention effect in the context of the nested cross-sectional version of the Extended Design. It will also illustrate the estimation of that variance using the example from Chapter 7 for the adjusted analysis of data from an Extended Design.

Let $\hat{\beta}_{t(\text{lin})g:c}$ be the linear regression coefficient estimating the change in y per unit change in time, fit to the mt observations in a single group.

$$\hat{\beta}_{t(\text{lin})g:c} = \hat{r}_{yt}\frac{\hat{\sigma}_y}{\hat{\sigma}_t} \tag{9.61}$$

Here $\hat{\sigma}_y$ and $\hat{\sigma}_t$ are the unbiased estimates of the standard deviations of y and time and $\hat{r}_{yt}$ is the estimated correlation between y and time, and the regression is limited to the mt observations in a single group.

Let $\sigma^2_{\hat{\beta}t(\text{lin})g:c}$ be the variance of that coefficient. Following the discussion in the previous section, that variance is estimated as:

$$\sigma^2_{\hat{\beta}t(\text{lin})g:c} = \frac{\hat{\sigma}^2_y(1 - \hat{R}^2_{y \cdot xt})}{\hat{\sigma}^2_t(1 - \hat{R}^2_{t \cdot x})(mt - f - 1)} \tag{9.62}$$

In this design, the variance of a single condition mean slope is based on g group-specific regression coefficients relating time to the endpoint. When those coefficients are homogeneous across conditions, the variance of a single condition mean slope under the null hypothesis is estimated as:

$$\hat{\sigma}^2_{\beta_{t(\text{lin})c}} = \frac{\sigma^2_{\beta_{t(\text{lin})g:c}}}{g} \qquad (9.63)$$

To extend this expression to the mixed model, an additional component of variance is added to the variance of the regression coefficient in Equation 9.62 to allow for heterogeneity in the group-specific slopes. Under this model, that variation is represented as $\hat{\sigma}^2_{t(\text{lin})g:c}$. In addition, that component as well as the member component of variance may be affected by the regression adjustment for covariates. Finally, the variance of time that is attributable to groups plays no role in the variance of the regression coefficient and the remaining variation attributable to members may be affected by the regression adjustment for covariates.

As a result, the variance of the group-specific slope in the context of a group-randomized trial is estimated as:

$$\sigma^2_{\beta_{t(\text{lin})g:c}} = \frac{\hat{\sigma}^2_{m(y)}\hat{\theta}_{m(y \cdot xt)}}{\hat{\sigma}^2_{m(t)}\hat{\theta}_{m(t \cdot x)}(mt - f - 1)} + \hat{\sigma}^2_{t(\text{lin})g:c}\hat{\theta}_{t(\text{lin})g:c \cdot x} \qquad (9.64)$$

Here, $\hat{\sigma}^2_{m(y)}$ and $\hat{\theta}_{m(y \cdot xt)}$ are defined as in the previous section, as are $\hat{\sigma}^2_{m(t)}$ and $\hat{\theta}_{m(t \cdot x)}$. The term $\hat{\sigma}^2_{t(\text{lin})g:c}$ represents the unadjusted component of variance due to heterogeneity among the group-specific mean slopes and the term $\hat{\theta}_{t(\text{lin})g:c \cdot x}$ represents the effect of the regression adjustment on that component.

Substituting this expression for the estimated variance of the condition mean slope (Equation 9.63) under the null hypothesis,

$$\hat{\sigma}^2_{\beta_{t(\text{lin})c}} = \frac{\sigma^2_{\beta_{t(\text{lin})g:c}}}{g} = \frac{1}{g}\left(\frac{\hat{\sigma}^2_{m(y)}\hat{\theta}_{m(y \cdot xt)}}{\hat{\sigma}^2_{m(t)}\hat{\theta}_{m(t \cdot x)}(mt - f - 1)} + \hat{\sigma}^2_{t(\text{lin})g:c}\hat{\theta}_{t(\text{lin})g:c \cdot x}\right) \qquad (9.65)$$

Under the null hypothesis, the variance of the difference between two condition mean slopes each based on g slopes is written as:[5]

$$\begin{aligned}
\hat{\sigma}^2_{\Delta} &= 2\left(\frac{\hat{MS}_{t(\text{lin})g:c}}{g}\right) = \frac{2}{g}\left(\frac{\hat{\sigma}^2_{e(y)}}{\hat{\sigma}^2_{e(t)}(mt - f - 1)} + \hat{\sigma}^2_{t(\text{lin})g:c}\right) \\
&= \frac{2}{g}\left(\frac{\hat{\sigma}^2_{m(y)}\hat{\theta}_{m(y \cdot xt)}}{\hat{\sigma}^2_{m(t)}\hat{\theta}_{m(t \cdot x)}(mt - f - 1)} + \hat{\sigma}^2_{t(\text{lin})g:c}\hat{\theta}_{t(\text{lin})g:c \cdot x}\right) \qquad (9.66)
\end{aligned}$$

This estimated variance is expressed in terms of a single unit change in time. Cast in terms of a period equal to $t-1$ units of time, the variance is $(t-1)^2 \hat{\sigma}_\Delta^2$. Any of these expressions for $\hat{\sigma}_\Delta^2$ can be used in the power analysis and the choice will depend on which estimates are available.

To illustrate the calculation of this variance in the context of a nested cross-sectional design, consider the example from Chapter 7 that presented an adjusted analysis of an Extended Design in which time was treated as a continuous variable and scaled in months from the onset of the intervention program. In that example, the analysis was limited to data collected during and subsequent to the last baseline survey. The intervention effect was modeled as the difference between the two conditions in their mean linear slope where each mean slope was based on three group-specific slopes.

Table 9.15 presents the covariance-parameter estimates from the adjusted analysis presented in Chapter 7 (from Table 7.75). Table 9.15 also presents the covariance-parameter estimates from a new analysis of the same data with no fixed effects.

The value for $\hat{\sigma}_{m(y)}^2$ is taken as the Residual estimate from the unadjusted analysis, 110.4. The value for $\hat{\theta}_{m(y \cdot xt)}$ is taken as the ratio of the two Residual estimates:

$$\hat{\theta}_{m(y \cdot xt)} = \frac{101.9}{110.4} = 0.923$$

Table 9.15. Covariance-Parameter Estimates From the Random-Coefficients Analysis of Diastolic Blood Pressure From the Extended Design Example in Chapter 7, as Well as From an Analysis of Those Data With no Fixed Effects

RANDOM COEFFICIENTS ANALYSIS		
Cov Parm		Estimate
INTERCEPT	UN(1,1)	5.29087938
	UN(2,1)	−0.10226163
	UN(2,2)	0.00198817
Residual		101.87119326
NO FIXED EFFECTS		
Cov Parm		Estimate
INTERCEPT	UN(1,1)	5.07860600
	UN(2,1)	−0.09904259
	UN(2,2)	0.00205205
Residual		110.37794100

The value for $\hat{\sigma}^2_{t(\text{lin})g:c}$ from the adjusted analysis is 0.002025. The value from the unadjusted analysis is 0.001988. The value for $\hat{\theta}_{t(\text{lin})g:c\cdot x}$ is taken as the ratio of the $\hat{\sigma}^2_{t(\text{lin})g:c}$ from the adjusted and unadjusted analyses:

$$\hat{\theta}_{t(\text{lin})g:c\cdot x} = \frac{0.001988}{0.002052} = 0.969$$

In this example, time is represented as a continuous variable scaled in months and the intervention effect is represented as a difference in mean linear slopes. Then the expression $\hat{\sigma}^2_{m(t)}\hat{\theta}_{m(t\cdot x)}$ in Equation 9.66 becomes $\hat{\sigma}^2_{m(t(\text{lin}))}\hat{\theta}_{m(t(\text{lin})\cdot x)}$. Required is an estimate of the component of variance in the linear term that is attributed to the members, $\hat{\sigma}^2_{m(t(\text{lin}))}$, and an estimate of the reduction in that component that is due to the inclusion of the other terms in the analysis, $\hat{\theta}_{m(t(\text{lin})\cdot x)}$. To get those estimates, two additional analyses are required, following the scheme used in the previous section.

Table 9.16 presents the covariance-parameter estimates from the adjusted analysis of imonth. Table 9.16 also presents the covariance-parameter estimates from an analysis of the same data with no fixed effects.

The value for $\hat{\sigma}^2_{m(t(\text{lin}))}$ is taken as the Residual estimate from the unadjusted analysis, 365.6. The value for $\hat{\theta}_{m(t(\text{lin})\cdot x)}$ is taken as the ratio of the two Residual estimates:

$$\hat{\theta}_{m(t(\text{lin})\cdot x)} = \frac{162.0}{365.6} = 0.443$$

Cast in terms of the $MS_{t(\text{lin})g:c}$, the standard error of the intervention effect was estimated in Chapter 7 as shown in the upper panel in Table 9.17. Cast

Table 9.16. Covariance-Parameter Estimates for the Intervention Effect From the Random-Coefficients Analysis of Diastolic Blood Pressure From the Extended Design Example in Chapter 7 and From an Analysis of Those Data With no Fixed Effects

RANDOM COEFFICIENTS ANALYSIS	
Cov Parm	Estimate
GROUP(COND)	1.20138
Residual	161.98263
NO FIXED EFFECTS	
Cov Parm	Estimate
GROUP(COND)	471.79431
Residual	365.61129

in terms of the underlying variance components and other parameters developed here, the standard error is estimated as shown in the lower panel of Table 9.17.

Random-Coefficients Model: Cohort

In the random-coefficients model applied to the nested cohort design, the intervention effect is defined in terms of condition mean slopes where each condition mean slope is the average of g group-specific mean slopes and where each group-specific mean slope is the average of m member-specific slopes. One slope is computed for each of the members nested within its group and condition. The intervention effect is represented in the model as $T_{(\text{lin})}C_l$. Given only two conditions, the intervention effect is the simple difference between the two condition mean slopes. This section presents the derivation of the variance of that intervention effect in the context of the nested cohort version of the Extended Design. It also illustrates the estimation of that variance using the example from Chapter 8 for the adjusted analysis of data from an Extended Design.

Let $\hat{\beta}_{mt(\text{lin}):g:c}$ be the linear regression coefficient estimating the change in y per unit change in time, fit to the t observations from a single member.

Table 9.17. Standard Error of the Intervention Effect From the Random-Coefficients Analysis of Diastolic Blood Pressure From the Extended Design Example in Chapter 7

AS ESTIMATED IN CHAPTER 7

$$\hat{\sigma}_\Delta = \sqrt{2\left(\frac{\hat{MS}_{t(\text{lin}):g:c}}{g}\right)} = \sqrt{2\left(\frac{\dfrac{\hat{\sigma}^2_{e(y)}}{\hat{\sigma}^2_{e(t)}(mt-f-1)} + \hat{\sigma}^2_{t(\text{lin})g:c}}{g}\right)}$$

$$= \sqrt{2\left(\frac{0.00230}{3}\right)}$$

$$= 0.0392$$

AS ESTIMATED IN CHAPTER 9

$$\hat{\sigma}_\Delta = \sqrt{\frac{2}{g}\left(\frac{\hat{\sigma}^2_{m(y)}\hat{\theta}_{m(y\cdot xt)}}{\hat{\sigma}^2_{m(t)}\hat{\theta}_{m(t\cdot x)}(mt-f-1)} + \hat{\sigma}^2_{t(\text{lin})g:c}\hat{\theta}_{t(\text{lin}):g:c\cdot x}\right)}$$

$$= \sqrt{\frac{2}{3}\left(\frac{110.4(0.923)}{365.6(0.443)(150.5*14.33-93-1)} + 0.002052(0.969)\right)}$$

$$= 0.0392$$

$$\hat{\beta}_{mt(\text{lin}):g:c} = \hat{r}_{yt} \frac{\hat{\sigma}_y(1 - \hat{r}_{yy(m)})}{\hat{\sigma}_t} \qquad (9.67)$$

Here $\hat{\sigma}_y$ and $\hat{\sigma}_t$ are the unbiased estimates of the standard deviations of y and time, $\hat{r}_{yt}$ is the estimated correlation between y and time, $\hat{r}_{yy(m)}$ is the average within-member correlation over time, and the regression is limited to the t observations in a single member. The numerator includes the expression $(1 - \hat{r}_{yy(m)})$ to reflect the reduction in the usual variance due to the repeat observations on the same members.

Let $\sigma^2_{\beta mt(\text{lin}):g:c}$ be the variance of that coefficient. Following the discussion in the previous section, that variance is estimated as:

$$\sigma^2_{\hat{\beta}mt(\text{lin}):g:c} = \frac{\hat{\sigma}^2_y(1 - \hat{r}_{yy(m)})(1 - \hat{R}^2_{y \cdot xt})}{\hat{\sigma}^2_t(1 - \hat{R}^2_{t \cdot x})(t - f - 1)} \qquad (9.68)$$

In this design, the variance of a single group mean slope is based on m member-specific regression coefficients relating time to the endpoint. When those coefficients are homogeneous across groups, the variance of the mean slope for a single group is estimated as:

$$\hat{\sigma}^2_{\hat{\beta} t(\text{lin})g:c} = \frac{\sigma^2_{\hat{\beta}mt(\text{lin}):g:c}}{m} \qquad (9.69)$$

When the mean group slopes are homogeneous across conditions, the variance of a mean slope for a single condition is estimated as

$$\hat{\sigma}^2_{\hat{\beta} t(\text{lin})c} = \frac{\sigma^2_{\hat{\beta} t(\text{lin})g:c}}{g} \qquad (9.70)$$

To extend this expression to the mixed model, an additional component of variance is added to the variance of the member-specific slopes to allow for heterogeneity in the those slopes. In this model, that variation is represented as $\hat{\sigma}^2_{mt(\text{lin}):g:c}$. Another component is added to the variance of the group-specific mean slopes to allow for heterogeneity in those mean slopes. In this model, that variation is represented by $\hat{\sigma}^2_{t(\text{lin})g:c}$. In addition, those components as well as the member component of variance will be affected by the regression adjustment for covariates. Finally, the variance of time that is attributable to groups plays no role in the variance of the regression coefficient and the remaining variation attributable to members may be affected by the regression adjustment for covariates.

As a result, the variance of the group-specific mean slope is:

$$\hat{\sigma}^2_{\bar{\beta}t(\text{lin})g:c} = \frac{1}{m}\left(\frac{\hat{\sigma}^2_{m(y)}(1-\hat{r}_{yy(m)})\hat{\theta}_{m(y\cdot xt)}}{\hat{\sigma}^2_{m(t)}\hat{\theta}_{m(t\cdot x)}(t-f-1)} + \hat{\sigma}^2_{mt(\text{lin}):g:c}\hat{\theta}_{mt(\text{lin}):g:c\cdot x} + m\hat{\sigma}^2_{t(\text{lin})g:c}\hat{\theta}_{t(\text{lin})g:c\cdot x}\right)$$

$$(9.71)$$

Here $\hat{\sigma}^2_{m(y)}$ and $\hat{\theta}_{m(y\cdot xt)}$ are defined as in the previous section, as are $\hat{\sigma}^2_{m(t)}$ and $\hat{\theta}_{m(t\cdot x)}$. The term $\hat{\sigma}^2_{mt(\text{lin}):g:c}$ represents the unadjusted component of variance due to heterogeneity among the member-specific slopes and the term $\hat{\theta}_{mt(\text{lin}):g:c\cdot x}$ represents the effect of the regression adjustment on that component. The term $\hat{\sigma}^2_{t(\text{lin})g:c}$ represents the unadjusted component of variance due to heterogeneity among the group-specific mean slopes and the term $\hat{\theta}_{t(\text{lin})g:c\cdot x}$ represents the effect of the regression adjustment on that component.

Substituting this expression for the estimated variance of the group-specific mean slope into the expression for the estimated variance of the condition mean slope,

$$\hat{\sigma}^2_{\bar{\beta}t(\text{lin})c} = \frac{1}{mg}\left(\frac{\hat{\sigma}^2_{m(y)}(1-\hat{r}_{yy(m)})\hat{\theta}_{m(y\cdot xt)}}{\hat{\sigma}^2_{m(t)}\hat{\theta}_{m(t\cdot x)}(t-f-1)} + \hat{\sigma}^2_{mt(\text{lin}):g:c}\hat{\theta}_{mt(\text{lin}):g:c\cdot x} + m\hat{\sigma}^2_{t(\text{lin}):g:c}\hat{\theta}_{t(\text{lin})g:c\cdot x}\right)$$

$$(9.72)$$

Under the null hypothesis, the variance of the difference between two condition mean slopes is then estimated as:[6]

$$\hat{\sigma}^2_{\Delta} = 2\left(\frac{\hat{MS}_{t(\text{lin})g:c}}{mg}\right) = \frac{2}{mg}\left(\frac{\hat{\sigma}^2_{e(y)}}{\hat{\sigma}^2_{e(t)}(t-f-1)} + \hat{\sigma}^2_{mt(\text{lin}):g:c} + m\hat{\sigma}^2_{t(\text{lin}):g:c}\right)$$

$$= \frac{2}{mg}\left(\frac{\hat{\sigma}^2_{m(y)}(1-\hat{r}_{yy(m)})\hat{\theta}_{m(y\cdot xt)}}{\hat{\sigma}^2_{m(t)}\hat{\theta}_{m(t\cdot x)}(t-f-1)} + \hat{\sigma}^2_{mt(\text{lin}):g:c}\hat{\theta}_{mt(\text{lin}):g:c\cdot x} + m\hat{\sigma}^2_{t(\text{lin})g:c}\hat{\theta}_{t(\text{lin})g:c\cdot x}\right)$$

$$(9.73)$$

This estimated variance is expressed in terms of a single unit change in time. Cast in terms of a period equal to t-1 units of time, the variance is $(t-1)^2\hat{\sigma}^2_{\Delta}$. Any of these expressions for $\hat{\sigma}^2_{\Delta}$ can be used in the power analysis and the choice will depend on which estimates are available.

To illustrate the calculation of this variance, consider the example from Chapter 8 that presented the analysis of an Extended Design in which time was treated as a continuous variable and scaled in months from the onset of the intervention program. The intervention effect was modeled as the difference between the two conditions in their mean linear slope. Each mean slope was based on three group-specific mean slopes and each group-specific mean slope was based on m member-specific slopes.

Table 9.18 presents the covariance-parameter estimates from the full random-coefficients analysis presented originally in Chapter 8. Table 9.18 also presents the covariance-parameter estimates from a reduced analysis of the same data with no fixed effects.

Based on the results from the reduced analysis,

$$\hat{\sigma}_m^2 = \hat{\sigma}_{m:g:c}^2 + \hat{\sigma}_{mt:g:c}^2 + \hat{\sigma}_e^2 = 66.6 + 45.3 = 112$$

Similarly,

$$\hat{r}_{yy(m)} = \frac{\hat{\sigma}_{m:g:c}^2}{\hat{\sigma}_{m:g:c}^2 + \hat{\sigma}_{mt:g:c}^2 + \hat{\sigma}_e^2} = \frac{66.6}{66.6 + 45.3} = 0.595$$

The value for $\hat{\theta}_{m(y\cdot xt)}$ is taken as the ratio of the $\hat{\sigma}_m^2$ estimates from the full and reduced analyses:

$$\hat{\theta}_{m(y\cdot xt)} = \frac{112}{112} = 1.0$$

Table 9.18. Covariance-Parameter Estimates From the Random-Coefficients Analysis of Diastolic Blood Pressure From the Extended Design Example in Chapter 8, as Well as From an Analysis of Those Data With No Fixed Effects

RANDOM COEFFICIENTS ANALYSIS		
Cov Parm		Estimate
INTERCEPT	UN(1,1)	1.9893211
	UN(2,1)	−0.0485726
	UN(2,2)	0.0013556
INTERCEPT	UN(1,1)	66.5786506
	UN(2,1)	−0.1720691
	UN(2,2)	0.0028881
Residual		45.3501345
NO FIXED EFFECTS		
Cov Parm		Estimate
INTERCEPT	UN(1,1)	1.7390160
	UN(2,1)	−0.0368306
	UN(2,2)	0.0009586
INTERCEPT	UN(1,1)	66.5961629
	UN(2,1)	−0.1722064
	UN(2,2)	0.0028904
Residual		45.3434601

The value for $\hat{\sigma}^2_{mt(\text{lin}):g:c}$ from the full analysis is 0.00289. The value from the reduced analysis is 0.00289. The value for $\hat{\theta}_{mt(\text{lin}):g:c \cdot x}$ is taken as the ratio of the $\hat{\sigma}^2_{mt(\text{lin}):g:c}$ from the full and reduced analyses:

$$\hat{\theta}_{mt(\text{lin}):g:c \cdot x} = \frac{0.00289}{0.00289} = 1.0$$

The value for $\hat{\sigma}^2_{t(\text{lin})g:c}$ from the full analysis is 0.001356. The value from the reduced analysis is 0.000959. The value for $\hat{\theta}_{t(\text{lin})g:c \cdot x}$ is taken as the ratio of the $\hat{\sigma}^2_{t(\text{lin})g:c}$ from the full and reduced analyses:

$$\hat{\theta}_{t(\text{lin})g:c \cdot x} = \frac{0.001356}{0.000959} = 1.41$$

In this example, time is represented as a continuous variable scaled in months and the intervention effect is represented as a difference in mean linear slopes. Then the expression $\hat{\sigma}^2_{m(t)}\hat{\theta}_{m(t \cdot x)}$ in Equation 9.73 becomes $\hat{\sigma}^2_{m(t(\text{lin}))}\hat{\theta}_{m(t(\text{lin}) \cdot x)}$. Required is an estimate of the component of variance in the linear term that is attributed to the members, $\hat{\sigma}^2_{m(t(\text{lin}))}$, and an estimate of the reduction in that component that is due to the inclusion of the other terms in the analysis, $\hat{\theta}_{m(t(\text{lin}) \cdot x)}$. To get those estimates, two additional analyses are required, following the scheme used in the previous section.

Table 9.19 presents the covariance-parameter estimates from the full

Table 9.19. Covariance-Parameter Estimates for the Intervention Effect From the Random-Coefficients Analysis of Diastolic Blood Pressure in the Extended Design Example in Chapter 8 and From an Analysis of Those Data With no Fixed Effects

RANDOM COEFFICIENTS ANALYSIS	
Cov Parm	Estimate
INTERCEPT	2.52835
INTERCEPT	0.00000
Residual	373.85088
NO FIXED EFFECTS	
Cov Parm	Estimate
INTERCEPT	268.40182
INTERCEPT	−0.00000
Residual	745.83091

random-coefficients analysis of imonth. Table 9.19 also presents the covariance-parameter estimates from a reduced analysis with no fixed effects. The value for $\hat{\theta}_{m(t(\text{lin})\cdot x)}$ is taken as the ratio of the $\hat{\sigma}^2_{m(t(\text{lin}))}$ estimates from the full and reduced analyses:

$$\hat{\theta}_{m(t(\text{lin})\cdot x)} = \frac{374}{746} = 0.501$$

Cast in terms of the $MS_{t(\text{lin})g:c}$, the standard error of the intervention effect was estimated in Chapter 8 as shown in the upper panel of Table 9.20. Cast in terms of the underlying variance components and other parameters developed here, the standard error is estimated as shown in the lower panel of Table 9.20.

Examples

This section illustrates the methods presented in this chapter. Each example begins with a statement of the research question, as it is the research question that dictates the design and the analysis plan and so provides the context for the power analysis. Following the research question, each example moves se-

Table 9.20. Standard Error of the Intervention Effect From the Random-Coefficients Analysis of Diastolic Blood Pressure in the Extended Design Example From Chapter 8

AS ESTIMATED IN CHAPTER 8

$$\hat{\sigma}_\Delta = \sqrt{2\left(\frac{\hat{MS}_{t(\text{lin})g:c}}{mg}\right)} = \sqrt{\frac{\dfrac{\hat{\sigma}^2_{e(y)}}{\hat{\sigma}^2_{e(t)}(t-f-1)} + \hat{\sigma}^2_{mt(\text{lin}):g:c} + m\hat{\sigma}^2_{t(\text{lin})g:c}}{mg}}$$

$$= \sqrt{2\left(\frac{0.2348}{163.5*3}\right)}$$

$$= 0.0309$$

AS ESTIMATED IN CHAPTER 9

$$\hat{\sigma}_\Delta = \sqrt{\frac{2}{mg}\left(\frac{\hat{\sigma}^2_{m(y)}(1-\hat{r}_{yy(m)})\hat{\theta}_{m(y\cdot xt)}}{\hat{\sigma}^2_{m(t)}\hat{\theta}_{m(t\cdot x)}(t-f-1)} + \hat{\sigma}^2_{mt(\text{lin}):g:c}\hat{\theta}_{mt(\text{lin}):g:c\cdot x} + m\hat{\sigma}^2_{t(\text{lin})g:c}\hat{\theta}_{t(\text{lin})g:c\cdot x}\right)}$$

$$\sqrt{\frac{2}{163.5*3}\left(\frac{112(1-0.595)(1.0)}{746(0.501)(15.83-3-1)} + 0.00289(1.0) + 163.5(0.000959)(1.41)\right)}$$

$$= 0.0309$$

---

quentially through the seven steps of a power analysis that are identified earlier in this chapter.

Investigators should conduct a power analysis for the design and analysis that they intend to employ. However, as it becomes difficult to obtain good estimates of parameters required for that power analysis, the prudent course is to simplify the structure of Δ and employ conservative estimates. It is best to have Δ defined as a single *df* contrast among simple condition-level statistics. This limits the number of parameters that must be estimated and allows the research team to have greater confidence in the results of that analysis. At the same time, simplifying Δ may give a conservative result and lead to a larger study. As long as the increased size does not make the study too difficult or expensive to do, the larger study will have more power to answer the research question.

Example 1: School-Based Smoking Prevention

The Research Question

Will a seventh-grade smoking-prevention program be effective in reducing the ninth-grade incidence of weekly smoking among students who are nonsmokers in the seventh grade?

The Research Design and Plan for the Analysis

To examine the incidence of weekly smoking, a cohort design is proposed. The endpoint will be assessed in a school survey by asking ninth-graders whether they are currently smoking at least once a week. The analysis will be restricted to those students who indicated during a baseline survey at the beginning of the seventh grade that they had never smoked even part of a cigarette. The intervention program will be delivered after the baseline survey and during the seventh grade. In this example, the groups are the schools and the members are the students within those schools.

Several analysis plans are possible for this study. For example, the data could be analyzed via an unadjusted or adjusted time $\times$ condition analysis. However, because the research question is focused on the difference between the two study conditions at the end of the study, it is appropriate to employ an analysis of posttest data with regression adjustment for baseline values.

Step 1: Define Δ

The intervention effect for this design and analytic plan was defined in Equation 6.8 as:

$$\Delta = (\bar{Y}_{..I} - \bar{Y}_{..C}) - \sum_{o=1}^{x} \beta_o (\bar{X}_{o..I} - \bar{X}_{o..C})$$

Step 2: Select a Test Statistic

Given this single df contrast, the t-statistic can be used to evaluate the significance of the observed intervention effect.

Step 3: Determine the Test Statistic's Distribution

The distribution of the t-statistic is determined entirely by the df available for the test of the intervention effect. Those df are $c(g-1) - x_g = 2(g-1) - x_g$.

Step 4: Select Critical Values

The nominal values for the Type I and II error rates will be employed—5% and 20%, respectively. The test will be two-tailed.

Step 5: Develop an Expression for $\hat{\sigma}_{\Delta}^2$

For any design and analytic plan presented in Chapter 5 or 6, readers can turn to the appropriate section to obtain a formula for the variance of the intervention effect. For this design and analysis plan, the variance of that intervention effect was defined in Equation 6.9 as:

$$\sigma_{\Delta}^2 = 2\left(\frac{MS_{g:c}}{mg}\right)$$

That expression is easily expanded to reflect the components of variance, working from the expected mean squares given in Table 6.3:

$$\sigma_{\Delta}^2 = \frac{2(\sigma_e^2 + m\sigma_{g:c}^2)}{mg}$$

Table 6.3 also indicates that σ_e^2 and $\sigma_{g:c}^2$ are the only sources of random variation in this model, as it does not include repeat observations on groups or members, matching or stratification.

From Equation 9.36, recall that regression adjustment for covariates in the context of mixed-model regression is well summarized as:

$$\sigma_y^2(1 - R_{yx}^2) = \sigma_m^2 \theta_m + \sigma_g^2 \theta_g$$

As a result, $\sigma_e^2 = \sigma_m^2 \theta_m$, $\sigma_{g:c}^2 = \sigma_g^2 \theta_g$, and the variance of the intervention effect can be estimated as shown in Equation 9.38:

$$\hat{\sigma}_\Delta^2 = \frac{2(\hat{\sigma}_m^2 \hat{\theta}_m + m \hat{\sigma}_g^2 \hat{\theta}_g)}{mg}$$

Step 6. Estimate the Components of $\hat{\sigma}_\Delta^2$

In this case, the investigators need to obtain values for $\hat{\sigma}_m^2$, $\hat{\theta}_m$, $\hat{\sigma}_g^2$, and $\hat{\theta}_g$. Values for all four parameters can be obtained from an analysis of existing data simply by applying the proposed analysis to those data. However, it is common that such data are not available. In that case, $\hat{\sigma}_m^2$ and $\hat{\sigma}_g^2$ can be obtained with a little manipulation of Equations 1.4 and 1.5 as:

$$\hat{\sigma}_m^2 = \hat{\sigma}_y^2(1 - I\hat{C}C_{m:g:c}) \qquad (9.74)$$

and

$$\hat{\sigma}_g^2 = \hat{\sigma}_y^2(I\hat{C}C_{m:g:c}) \qquad (9.75)$$

where $\hat{\sigma}_y^2$ is the estimate of the total variance in the endpoint and $I\hat{C}C_{m:g:c}$ is the estimate of correlation for that endpoint among members in the same group.

In this case, the endpoint is smoking status in the ninth grade, coded 1 for smokers and 0 for nonsmokers. The total variance of a dichotomous endpoint is estimated as pq, where p is the average incidence rate and $q = 1-p$. Using data from other sources, the average incidence rate in the absence of intervention is estimated at 9%. Then the total variance in the endpoint under the null hypothesis is estimated as:

$$\hat{\sigma}_y^2 = pq = (0.09)(0.91) = 0.0819$$

The $ICC_{m:g:c}$ represents the fraction of that total variation attributable to the groups. Absent better information, it is estimated simply as the fraction of the total variation in the data that the investigators expect to be explained by the groups, here the schools. The investigators might draw on the experience of other investigators who have worked with similar endpoints, populations, and groups, or on their own experience in other studies.

If pilot data are available, a $ICC_{m:g:c}$ is estimated from a simple one-way ANOVA in which the only grouping factor is the group. The $ICC_{m:g:c}$ is estimated as:

$$\frac{MS_{\text{between}} - MS_{\text{within}}}{MS_{\text{between}} + (m-1)MS_{\text{within}}} \tag{9.76}$$

This formula is appropriate for both continuous and dichotomous endpoints (Fleiss, 1981, p. 226; Snedecor and Cochran, 1989, p. 243).

If a published estimate of $ICC_{m:g:c}$ is available and the investigators believe that it is appropriate for the population and circumstances of the proposed study, that value can be used. In this particular case, Murray, Rooney et al. (1994) published estimates of ICCs for several adolescent smoking endpoints based on an analysis of survey data from multiple sources across the United States. Their analysis suggests an average value for $I\hat{C}C_{m:g:c}$ for smoking incidence of 0.00607.

Given this estimate for the $ICC_{m:g:c}$, the two components of variance are estimated as:

$$\hat{\sigma}_m^2 = 0.0819(1 - 0.00607) = 0.0814$$

and

$$\hat{\sigma}_g^2 = 0.0819(0.00607) = 0.000497$$

The ratio $\hat{\theta}_m$ reflects the expected effect of the regression adjustment for covariates on $\hat{\sigma}_m^2$. As noted earlier in this chapter, the member-level variance usually decreases with regression adjustment for covariates, and so $\hat{\theta}_m$ is usually a fraction. The ratio $\hat{\theta}_g$ reflects the expected effect of the regression adjustment for covariates on $\hat{\sigma}_g^2$. The value of $\hat{\theta}_g$ is completely unpredictable in the absence of information for the endpoint, covariates, groups, and members of interest. It may be a fraction, but can be greater than 1.0.

Often, a good approximation for $\hat{\theta}_m$ is $(1 - \hat{R}_{y\cdot x}^2)$. Here $\hat{R}_{y\cdot x}^2$ is an average group-specific squared multiple correlation coefficient that represents the proportion of variance in the endpoint that is accounted for by the covariates.

A conservative approach to selecting values for $\hat{\theta}_m$ and $\hat{\theta}_g$ is to assume that there is no reduction in either component of variance so that both ratios are estimated as 1.0. Where a good estimate for one or the other ratio is available, it can be used while the other ratio is estimated at 1.0. Unfortunately, Murray, Rooney et al. (1994) did not provide estimates for either ratio in their report. Lacking better information, both ratios are estimated as 1.0 for purposes of this example.

Step 7. Apply the Estimates

The generic formula for the detectable difference between two conditions in a Posttest-Only Control Group Design was given in Equation 9.11 as:

$$\hat{\Delta} = \sqrt{\hat{\sigma}_{\Delta}^2 (t_{critical:\ \alpha/2} + t_{critical:\beta})^2}$$

Based on Equation 9.38, $\hat{\sigma}_{\Delta}^2$ in this example is estimated as:

$$\hat{\sigma}_{\Delta}^2 = \frac{2(\hat{\sigma}_m^2\hat{\theta}_m + m\hat{\sigma}_g^2\hat{\theta}_g)}{mg}$$

As a result, the detectable difference in this example is estimated as:

$$\hat{\Delta} = \sqrt{\frac{2(\hat{\sigma}_m^2\hat{\theta}_m + m\hat{\sigma}_g^2\hat{\theta}_g)(t_{critical:\ \alpha/2} + t_{critical:\beta})^2}{mg}} \qquad (9.77)$$

The values selected for $t_{critical:\ \alpha/2}$ and $t_{critical:\beta}$ will depend on the *df* for the *t*-test, computed as $2(g\text{-}1)$.

For an initial estimate, let the average number of seventh-grade nonsmokers per school be $m = 100$. Assume as well that the investigators would like to limit the number of intervention schools to $g = 8$. With these values as starting points, $df = 2(8 - 1) = 14$. The parameter estimates are summarized in Table 9.21.

With these estimates,

$$\hat{\Delta} = \sqrt{\frac{2(0.0814 * 1.0 + 100 * 0.000497 * 1.0)(2.12 + 0.865)^2}{100 * 8}} = 0.0540$$

The analysis would have 80% power to detect an adjusted difference in incidence rates of 5.4% between the intervention and control conditions at posttest. If the control-group incidence rate is 9%, then the incidence rate in the intervention group would have to decline to $9\% - 5.4\% = 3.6\%$.

Using a computer spreadsheet to vary the values of *g* and *m*, detectable differences can be computed across a range of values for *g* and *m* given the other estimates in Table 9.21. The values used for $t_{critical:\ \alpha/2}$ and $t_{critical:\beta}$ depend on $df = 2(g - 1)$, and so vary with *g*. Table 9.22 summarizes the results of such calculations.

Table 9.21. Initial Parameter Estimates for the Smoking-Prevention Example

Parameter or Design Constant	Value
c	2
$\hat{\sigma}_m^2$	0.0814
$\hat{\sigma}_g^2$	0.000497
$\hat{\theta}_m$	1.0
$\hat{\theta}_g$	1.0
m	100
g	8
ddf	14
$t_{\text{critical}:\alpha/2}$	2.15
$t_{\text{critical}:\beta}$	0.865

Three patterns emerge upon close inspection of Table 9.22. First, the detectable difference declines as g increases from 2 toward 32 and as m increases from 25 toward 400. Second, the rate of the decrease in the detectable difference follows a pattern of diminishing returns as m and g increase. Adding a few groups or members to a small study helps quite a bit. Adding a few groups or members to a large study does not help as much. Third, adding groups is much more helpful than adding members. These three patterns will emerge from the power analysis for any group-randomized trial.[7]

Given these results, the investigators can choose the combination of the number of schools per condition (g) and the number of students per school (m) from among those combinations that provide the desired detectable difference. Suppose that the desired detectable difference is a 50% relative reduction in

Table 9.22. Detectable Difference for the Smoking-Prevention Example as a Function of the Number of Schools per Condition *(g)* and the Number of Students Observed in Each School *(m)*

			g		
m	2	4	8	16	32
25	0.3286	0.1453	0.0923	0.0627	0.0436
50	0.2473	0.1093	0.0694	0.0472	0.0328
100	0.1942	0.0859	0.0546	0.0371	0.0258
200	0.1613	0.0713	0.0453	0.0308	0.0214
400	0.1420	0.0628	0.0399	0.0271	0.0188

the incidence rate, which is an absolute detectable difference of 4.5%. Table 9.22 indicates that the study will have 80% power for that effect given 8 schools per condition and 200 students per school, given 16 schools per condition and 100 students per school, or given 32 schools per condition and only 25 students per school. There also will be intermediate combinations that will provide the same level of power, and the investigators can get those combinations by using intermediate values for m and g. The combinations with good power often vary considerably in their cost, and that is an important consideration in any group-randomized trial.

Loss of Groups and Members

Assume that the investigators determine that the assumptions are reasonable and that the combination of $g = 8$ and $m = 200$ is feasible, gives the desired detectable difference, and is affordable. The work is not yet finished, for these figures represent g and m as they must be at the time of the analysis. Some data are likely to be missing, some members and groups may be lost, and some proportion of the schools exposed to the intervention may not comply. The investigators must take expectations around these factors into account in order to ensure that $g = 8$ and $m = 200$ at the time of the analysis.

Let g be the number of groups required for the analysis. Then the number of groups required at the beginning of the study is:

$$g' = \frac{g}{\prod_{i=1}^{n} \left(1 - p(\text{loss due to source}_i)\right)} \tag{9.78}$$

The number of groups required at the beginning of the study, g', is g divided by the cross-product of the one's complement for each of the projected sources of loss $(i = 1 \ldots n)$ for the groups.

In this study, some schools might have a change in administration at some point during the school and refuse to participate in the follow-up survey. Assume that the investigators estimate that the probability of losing a school in a condition is 0.10, or 1 out of every 10 schools. Then, if the investigators want to ensure 80% power for an intervention effect of 4.5% against the threat of 10% of their schools withdrawing from the study, they should begin the study with 9 schools per condition:

$$g' = \frac{g}{\prod_{i=1}^{n} \left(1 - p(\text{loss due to source}_i)\right)} = \frac{8}{(1 - 0.1)} = 8.9 \cong 9$$

Similar calculations should be made for m; here, there are many sources of loss that may arise. Suppose the investigators are concerned that 20% of the students surveyed at baseline may leave the participating schools over the course of the study and not be available for the posttest survey, that 2% of the students surveyed at posttest may have incomplete data, and that 5% of the students eligible for the survey at posttest may be absent. Then, using a parallel formula for m',

$$m' = \frac{m}{\prod_{i=1}^{n}\left(1 - p(\text{loss due to source}_i)\right)} = \frac{200}{(1-0.2)(1-0.02)(1-0.05)}$$

$$= 268.5 \cong 269$$

And if the investigators also anticipate that 2% of the students surveyed at baseline will have incomplete data and 5% of those eligible at baseline will be absent, then the formula must be applied a second time:

$$m' = \frac{m}{\prod_{i=1}^{n}\left(1 - p(\text{loss due to source}_i)\right)} = \frac{269}{(1-0.02)(1-0.05)} = 288.9 \cong 289$$

If the investigators want to ensure 80% power for the intervention effect against all these threats to loss of data, they should begin the study with 9 schools per condition and 289 students per school.

Post Hoc Power Analysis

Another use of the formulae from this chapter is *post hoc* assessment of power. Suppose that the investigators conducted the study with 5 schools in each condition and 100 students in each school. Here, $ddf = 2(5-1) = 8$ and so $t_{\text{critical: } \alpha/2} = 2.31$. Suppose as well that they obtained a nonsignificant result of $\Delta = 5\%$. Suppose now that they want to estimate *post hoc* what their power was to detect an intervention effect of that magnitude.

If the parameter estimates proved accurate, then the power for a difference of 5% is estimated as shown in Table 9.23.

If the investigators did the study with only 5 schools per condition, they would have only 45.3% power to detect an intervention effect of 5% or larger as statistically significant. Given that a 5% intervention effect is quite large when compared to a 9% control-group rate, the study would have been substantially underpowered at $g = 5$.

Table 9.23. Power to Detect an Intervention Effect of 5% Given Only 5 Schools in Each Condition and 100 Students in Each School

$$\text{power} = \text{prob}(\hat{t} \le \hat{t}_\beta), \text{ where } \hat{t}_\beta = \frac{\hat{\Delta}}{\sqrt{\frac{2(\hat{\sigma}_m^2 \hat{\theta}_m + m\hat{\sigma}_g^2 \hat{\theta}_g)}{mg}}} - t_{\text{critical}:\alpha/2}$$

$$\hat{t}_\beta = \frac{0.05}{\sqrt{\frac{2(0.0814*1.0 + 100*0.000497*1.0)}{100*5}}} - 2.31 = -0.123$$

$$\text{power} = \text{prob}(\hat{t} \le -0.123) = 0.453$$

Example 2: Community-Based Binge-Drinking Prevention

The Research Question

Of interest is whether a grassroots community-organization effort can improve enforcement of age-of-sale laws and thereby reduce alcohol consumption among young adults aged 18–20 who live in the participating communities. In particular, the investigators are interested in whether this program can reduce the prevalence of binge drinking in that age group, where binge drinking is defined as the consumption of 5 or more drinks during one occasion.

The Research Design and Analytic Plan

Because repeat observations on the same members might affect their responses, assume that the investigators have decided to employ a nested cross-sectional design. The most common form of the nested cross-sectional design is the Pretest-Posttest Control Group Design, analyzed by the time × condition analysis presented in Chapter 5. This section illustrates the power analysis for that design and analytic plan.

Assume that the endpoint will be assessed in a series of telephone surveys of community residents aged 18–20, with independent samples chosen from each community at each time interval. During the survey, respondents will be asked whether they have consumed 5 or more drinks during a single drinking occasion at any time in the two weeks prior to the survey. The intervention program will begin in the intervention communities after the first survey. The unit of assignment is the community and the unit of observation is the young adult.

For planning purposes, let the time between the pretest and posttest be three years. This will allow three years to develop a grassroots organization and to allow that organization to change the community environment with respect to availability of alcohol for young adults.

Step 1: Define Δ

The intervention effect for this design and analysis plan was defined in Equation 5.11 as:

$$\Delta = (\bar{Y}_{..2I} - \bar{Y}_{..1I}) - (\bar{Y}_{..2C} - \bar{Y}_{o..1C}) - \sum_{o=1}^{x} \beta_o ((\bar{X}_{o..2I} - \bar{X}_{o..1I}) - (\bar{X}_{o..2C} - \bar{X}_{o..1C}))$$

Step 2: Select a Test Statistic

Given this single df contrast, the t-statistic can be used to evaluate the significance of the observed intervention effect.

Step 3: Determine the Test Statistic's Distribution

The distribution of the t-statistic is determined entirely by the df available for the test of the intervention effect. Those df are given in Table 5.4 as $(t-1)c(g-1) = (2-1)2(g-1)$.

Step 4: Select Critical Values

The nominal values for the Type I and II error rates will be employed—5% and 20%, respectively. The test will be two-tailed, as the prevalence rate for binge drinking might increase as a result of the intervention program.

Step 5: Develop an Expression For $\hat{\sigma}^2_\Delta$

For this design and analysis plan, the formula for σ^2_Δ was presented in Equation 5.12 as:

$$\sigma^2_\Delta = 2 * 2 \left(\frac{MS_{tg:c}}{mg} \right)$$

That expression is easily expanded to reflect the components of variance, working from the expected mean squares presented in Table 5.4:

$$\sigma^2_\Delta = \frac{2 * 2(\sigma^2_e + m\sigma^2_{tg:c})}{mg}$$

The table of expected mean squares indicates that σ_e^2 and $\sigma_{tg:c}^2$ are not the only sources of random variation in this analysis, because it provides for repeat observations on the same groups.

Recall from Equation 9.27 that repeat observations on the same groups create two sources of variation among the groups:

$$\sigma_g^2 = \sigma_{g:c}^2 + \sigma_{tg:c}^2$$

Recall from Equations 9.28 and 9.29 that the two components are related through the over-time correlation within groups, $r_{yy(g)}$, as:

$$\sigma_{g:c}^2 = \sigma_g^2(r_{yy(g)}) \quad \text{and} \quad \sigma_{tg:c}^2 = \sigma_g^2(1 - r_{yy(g)})$$

where

$$r_{yy(g)} = \frac{\sigma_{g:c}^2}{\sigma_{g:c}^2 + \sigma_{tg:c}^2}$$

As a result, the variance of the intervention effect is written in terms of the original σ_m^2 and σ_g^2 as shown in Equation 9.30:

$$\sigma_\Delta^2 = \frac{2 * (\sigma_m^2 + m\sigma_g^2(1 - r_{yy(g)}))}{mg}$$

If regression adjustment for covariates is to be employed, that will need to be reflected in the expression for the variance of the intervention effect. Recall from Equation 9.36 that regression adjustment for covariates is reflected as:

$$\sigma_y^2(1 - R_{yx}^2) = \sigma_m^2\theta_m + \sigma_g^2\theta_g$$

As a result, $\sigma_e^2 = \sigma_m^2\theta_m$, $\sigma_{g:c}^2 = \sigma_g^2\theta_g$.

Combining these features, the variance of the intervention effect for this design and analytic plan is estimated as:

$$\hat{\sigma}_\Delta^2 = \frac{2 * 2(\hat{\sigma}_m^2\hat{\theta}_m + m\hat{\sigma}_g^2\hat{\theta}_g(1 - \hat{r}_{yy(g)}))}{mg} \tag{9.79}$$

Step 6. Estimate the Components of $\hat{\sigma}_\Delta^2$

In this case, the investigators need values for $\hat{\sigma}_m^2$, $\hat{\theta}_m$, $\hat{\sigma}_g^2$, $\hat{\theta}_g$, and $\hat{r}_{yy(g)}$. A recent paper by Murray and Short (1995) provides many of the estimates required. They present point estimates for a number of measures related to alcohol consumption in young adults aged 18–20. They also present estimates for residual error and intraclass correlation, both from crude analyses and from analyses that included regression adjustment for group and member characteristics. They report the crude residual error for binge drinking as 0.249 and the adjusted residual error as 0.243. As a result,

$$\hat{\sigma}_m^2 = 0.249 \text{ and } \hat{\theta}_m = \frac{0.243}{0.249} = 0.976$$

In general,

$$\sigma_y^2 = \sigma_m^2 + \sigma_g^2 \tag{9.80}$$

and

$$\text{ICC}_{m:g:c} = \frac{\sigma_g^2}{\sigma_m^2 + \sigma_g^2} \tag{9.81}$$

so that

$$\sigma_g^2 = \frac{\sigma_m^2(ICC_{m:g:c})}{(1 - ICC_{m:g:c})} \tag{9.82}$$

Murray and Short (1995) report the crude $I\hat{C}C$ as 0.00338. As a result, the unadjusted group component of variance is estimated as:

$$\hat{\sigma}_g^2 = \frac{\hat{\sigma}_m^2 \, I\hat{C}C_{m:tg:c}}{1 - I\hat{C}C_{m:tg:c}} = \frac{(0.249)0.00338}{1 - 0.00338} = 0.000844$$

They report the adjusted $I\hat{C}C$ as 0.00087. As a result, the adjusted group component of variance is estimated as:

$$\frac{\hat{\sigma}_m^2 \, I\hat{C}C_{m:tg:c}}{1 - I\hat{C}C_{m:tg:c}} = \frac{(0.249)0.00087}{1 - 0.00087} = 0.000217$$

Given these unadjusted and adjusted values for $\hat{\sigma}_g^2$,

$$\hat{\theta}_g = \frac{0.000217}{0.000844} = 0.257$$

Based on Equation 9.80,

$$\hat{\sigma}_y^2 = \hat{\sigma}_m^2 + \hat{\sigma}_g^2 = 0.249 + 0.000844 = 0.250$$

Murray and Short (1995) do not provide an estimate of $\hat{r}_{yy(g)}$. One approach is to assume that correlation equal to zero, but that is quite conservative given the stability reported nationally for prevalence rates such as this (Johnston et al., 1996). Under these conditions, the investigators might adopt 0.50 as a fair estimate of the correlation.

Step 7. Apply the Estimates

The generic formula for the detectable difference between two conditions was given in Equation 9.11 as:

$$\hat{\Delta} = \sqrt{\hat{\sigma}_{\Delta}^2 (t_{\text{critical: } \alpha/2} + t_{\text{critical}:\beta})^2}$$

Based on Equation 9.79, $\hat{\sigma}_{\Delta}^2$ in this example is estimated as:

$$\hat{\sigma}_{\Delta}^2 = \frac{2*2\left(\hat{\sigma}_m^2 \hat{\theta}_m + m\hat{\sigma}_g^2 \hat{\theta}_g (1 - \hat{r}_{yy(g)})\right)}{mg}$$

As a result, the detectable difference in this example is estimated as:

$$\hat{\Delta} = \sqrt{\frac{2*2(\hat{\sigma}_m^2 \hat{\theta}_m + m\hat{\sigma}_g^2 \hat{\theta}_g (1 - \hat{r}_{yy(g)}))(t_{\text{critical: } \alpha/2} + t_{\text{critical}:\beta})^2}{mg}} \qquad (9.83)$$

The values selected for $t_{\text{critical: } \alpha/2}$ and $t_{\text{critical}:\beta}$ depend on the *df* for the *t*-test, computed as $(t\text{-}1)c(g\text{-}1) = (2\text{-}1)2(g\text{-}1)$.

For an initial estimate, let the average number of young adults per community per survey be fixed at 100. Assume as well that the investigators want to limit the number of intervention communities to $g = 8$. With these values as starting points, $df = (2\text{-}1)2(8\text{-}1) = 14$. The parameter estimates and design constants are summarized in Table 9.24.

With these estimates,

$$\hat{\Delta} = \sqrt{\frac{2*2(0.249(0.976) + 100(0.000844)(0.257)(1 - 0.5))(2.145 + 0.868)^2}{100*8}}$$

$$= 0.107$$

Table 9.24. Initial Parameter Estimates for the Binge-Drinking-Prevention Example

Parameter or Design Constant	Value
c	2
t	2
$\hat{\sigma}_m^2$	0.249
$\hat{\sigma}_g^2$	0.000844
$\hat{\theta}_m$	0.976
$\hat{\theta}_g$	0.257
$\hat{r}_{yy(g)}$	0.50
m	100
g	8
ddf	14
$t_{\text{critical}:\alpha/2}$	2.145
$t_{\text{critical}:\beta}$	0.868

According to this result, the analysis would have 80% power to detect an adjusted net difference in the prevalence of binge drinking of 10.7% between the two conditions over the three years between the pretest and the posttest. If the control-group prevalence rate was 30% and did not change during the study, then the prevalence rate in the intervention group would have to be $30.0\% - 10.7\% = 19.3\%$.

Using a computer spreadsheet to vary the values of g and m, detectable differences were computed across a range of values for g and m given the other estimates in Table 9.23. The values used for $t_{\text{critical}:\ \alpha/2}$ and $t_{\text{critical}:\beta}$ depend on $df = (2-1)2(g-1)$, and so vary with g. Table 9.25 summarizes the results of those calculations.

The three patterns noted in the smoking-prevention example are also apparent here. The detectable difference declines as g increases from 2 toward 32 and as m increases from 25 toward 400. The rate of the decrease in the detectable difference follows a pattern of diminishing returns as m and g increase. Finally, adding groups is much more helpful than adding members.

Assume for a moment that the prevalence rate of binge drinking in the absence of intervention is expected to remain at about 30% and that the investigators want to reduce that figure by one-fourth, to 22.5%. That would be possible given 8 communities per condition and about 200 members per survey, or given 16 communities per condition and just under 100 members per survey, or given 32 communities per condition and about 50 members per survey.

Table 9.25. Detectable Difference for the Binge-Drinking-Prevention Example as a Function of the Number of Communities per Condition (g) and the Number of Young Adults Surveyed in Each Community (m)

			g		
m	2	4	8	16	32
25	0.7521	0.3324	0.2112	0.1436	0.0998
50	0.5347	0.2364	0.1502	0.1021	0.0710
100	0.3822	0.1689	0.1073	0.0730	0.0507
200	0.2760	0.1220	0.0775	0.0527	0.0366
400	0.2030	0.0897	0.0570	0.0387	0.0269

It is important to remember that the detectable differences presented here presume analyzable data from *g* communities in each condition and *m* young adults in each community. Investigators should anticipate sources of loss and inflate the levels of *g* and *m* accordingly, following the procedures included in the previous example.

Extension to Other Examples

These examples provide two applications of the methods presented in this chapter for determination of power, sample size, and detectable difference in the context of group-randomized trials. Equation 9.7 (or 9.8) is readily adapted to other situations for the estimation of power, needing only a structure for $\hat{\sigma}_\Delta^2$. Similarly, Equations 9.11, 9.13, and 9.22 are readily adapted to other situations for the calculation of detectable difference, sample size of members per group, or sample size of groups per condition, needing only a structure for $\hat{\sigma}_\Delta^2$.

Chapters 5 and 6 presented the structure for $\hat{\sigma}_\Delta^2$ for each of the design and analysis plans included in those chapters, including the familiar ANOVA/ANCOVA designs as well as Extended Designs involving trend analyses or random-coefficients analyses. Those structures were written in terms of mean squares but are readily translated to variance components using the table of expected mean squares that was included as part of the presentation for each design and analysis.

If estimates are available for the variance components in those tables of expected mean squares, they may be used directly to compute $\hat{\sigma}_\Delta^2$. Those computations were illustrated in Chapters 7 and 8. The value for $\hat{\sigma}_\Delta^2$ can then be used in Equation 9.7 (or 9.8), 9.11, 9.13, or 9.22.

If estimates are not available for the specific variance components of interest, the generic structure for $\hat{\sigma}_\Delta^2$ given in Equation 9.26 can provide a good starting point. Equation 9.26 is readily adapted to reflect repeat observations on groups or members, regression adjustment for covariates, matching, stratification, trend analysis, or random-coefficients analysis, using the guidelines for those methods provided in this chapter. Indeed, those features can be combined as dictated by the design and analytic plan under consideration.

Summary

This chapter demonstrated how to adapt the familiar formula for the variance of an intervention effect based on a simple difference between two condition means so as to be appropriate for group-randomized trials. It also showed how to extend the basic formula to accommodate repeated measurements on the same groups and members, regression adjustment for covariates, stratification, and matching.

Previous efforts to accommodate these design features have simply assumed that all components of variance are affected in the same way (e.g., Murray and Hannan, 1990). As is now clear, that assumption is not always appropriate, though it may provide a good first-order approximation. While the expressions presented in this chapter are more complex than those published previously, they are also more accurate.

This chapter also showed how to combine several of these elements to develop an expression for the variance of a more complex intervention effect, such as is appropriate given a trend analysis or a random-coefficients analysis. This should make it easier for investigators to plan studies involving such intervention effects.

Endnotes

1. The variance of the members is estimated as the sum of the squared deviations of the observations (y_i) around their mean ($\bar{y}_c$), divided by the number of members observed (m) minus one:

$$\hat{\sigma}_y^2 = \frac{\sum_{i=1}^{m}(y_i - \bar{y}_c)^2}{m-1}$$

2. The choice between these formulae is not made consistently across textbooks. For example, Schlesselman (1982) bases his presentation on β, while Fleiss (1981) bases his on $1 - \beta$.

3. That expression is identical to that given in Chapter 1. Its derivation is shown in Chapter 1, Endnote 2.

4. This value for $\hat{\theta}_{m(t(\text{quad})c\cdot x)}$ is quite small, indicating that the reduction in the member component of variance of the quadratic term for time, `imonth2`, was reduced by just over 96% by the addition of the fixed effects and the random covariate to the analysis. Of course, the fixed effects included both `month` and `imonth`, and both would be expected to be highly correlated with `imonth2`, so that this large reduction is not altogether surprising.

5. In the first line of Equation 9.66, $\hat{\sigma}^2_{t(\text{lin})g:c}$ refers to the adjusted component of variance reflecting any heterogeneity among the group-specific slopes. In the second line of Equation 9.66, $\hat{\sigma}^2_{t(\text{lin})g:c}$ refers to the unadjusted component of variance reflecting any heterogeneity among the group-specific slopes.

6. In the first line of Equation 9.73, $\hat{\sigma}^2_{mt(\text{lin}):g:c}$ refers to the adjusted component of variance reflecting any heterogeneity among the member-specific slopes while $\hat{\sigma}^2_{t(\text{lin})g:c}$ refers to the adjusted component of variance reflecting any heterogeneity among the group-specific slopes. In the second line of Equation 9.73, $\hat{\sigma}^2_{mt(\text{lin}):g:c}$ refers to the unadjusted component of variance reflecting any heterogeneity among the member-specific slopes while $\hat{\sigma}^2_{t(\text{lin})g:c}$ refers to the unadjusted component of variance reflecting any heterogeneity among the group-specific slopes.

7. These patterns were discussed in Chapter 2 and illustrated in Figures 2.1, 2.2, and 2.3.

the net differences were in the expected direction but were modest and not statistically significant. There was some evidence for a favorable effect on projected CHD rates at the peak of the intervention program, but that effect was no longer significant at the end of the study.

Unique Challenges

Every major threat to the validity of the design and analysis of a group-randomized trial is aggravated when there is only a single group allocated to each study condition. Selection is increasingly plausible as an alternative explanation as the number of groups declines, because the assignment rule has less opportunity to balance factors that create selection bias by distributing them among the study conditions. The investigators can limit selection by matching their groups prior to allocation to conditions, but there will always remain some difference among the conditions due to the differences among their groups. Where there is only one group per condition, there is no opportunity to balance differences across conditions.

Local history is particularly plausible when there is only a single group allocated to each condition. The external event related to the outcome need only occur in one group to create a local history effect. To the extent that the exposure to that event is captured in the measurement process and varies among the members, the analyst may be able to make some adjustment for it during the analysis; lacking adequate measurements, there is no way to separate the effect of the external event from the effect of the intervention.

Differential maturation is particularly plausible when there is only a single group allocated to each condition. It requires only that the groups have different maturational patterns. There is some difference in those patterns between any two groups, though the magnitude of the difference varies from situation to situation. If, by chance, the two groups do show measurably different maturational patterns, there is no way to separate those patterns from an intervention effect without assessing those trends carefully before the intervention.

Contamination is particularly plausible when there is only a single group allocated to each condition. The intervention need only contaminate a single comparison site to threaten the validity of the design. The risk of contamination can be reduced by choosing a comparison site at some distance from the intervention site, but that may only increase the risk of selection bias.

The most serious threat to the validity of a study with a single group in each condition concerns its statistical validity. Absent strong assumptions, such a design provides no valid test for the effect of the intervention, as there is no way to separately estimate variation associated with conditions and variation associated with groups. Without at least two groups within each condition, the group and condition components of variance cannot be estimated separately.

This will be true regardless of the number of time intervals included in the design for purposes of data collection.

Critique

The PHHP investigators took a number of steps to enhance the validity of their design and analysis. Their surveys operated at the same time in each of their two communities, so as to avoid confounding due to seasonality effects. Survey staff were rotated between the study communities to avoid confounding due to site-specific staff. As part of each survey, 10% of the respondents were remeasured on key variables to monitor the quality of the original measurements, with corrective action taken as needed. Survey staff were retrained and recertified annually to enhance the reliability of the measures. The sampling protocol was changed after the first year, to break the sample into batches, wherein each batch represented a separate random sample of the community; thereafter, the sampling protocol was unchanged. The survey was presented publicly under a name different from PHHP, so as to limit hypothesis guessing. Effects were measured in terms of several outcomes, each based on a different methodology, so as to limit mono-operation and mono-method bias. Careful records were kept of all contacts with community residents in the intervention community to allow dose-response analyses.

The PHHP investigators tried to address each of the major threats to the validity of group-randomized trials. For example, they tried to deal with selection by the use of a similar community as a comparison site combined with the inclusion of multiple time intervals for data collection in the design. Simple selection biases can distort differences between conditions at a single point in time, but will have no effect on differences in trends in those conditions over time.

The analyses presented in Carleton et al. (1995) provide a good illustration of how selection bias can influence the interpretation of the results. The difference between the two communities at baseline in body-mass index was -0.35 kg/m^2. That difference favored the intervention community and was significant at the 5% level. That finding stands as *de facto* evidence of selection bias in body mass index, though it says nothing about the source of the bias. The investigators also reported comparisons of the two communities at the peak of the intervention and at the end of the intervention as -0.46 and -0.97 kg/m^2, respectively; both differences were highly significant. However, because neither of those differences take the selection bias into account, it would be erroneous to conclude that the true differences were of that magnitude or that the true significance of the differences was so striking. The investigators appropriately reported the net difference between baseline and each follow-up for the two communities, which corrects for the selection bias present in the simple differences. The net differences were as one would expect by simple subtraction, -0.11 and -0.62 kg/m^2; only the latter was reported as significant, and then with a p-value of only 0.042. The apparent difference between the two communities at peak intervention was almost entirely due to the selection bias; similarly, much of the difference observed at post intervention was due to the selection bias.

Local history is a particular threat in a design with only one group in each condition. Unfortunately, the investigators provide no information with which to gauge the presence or absence of external events that might have affected their results in their primary outcome paper. Their report focuses exclusively on risk-factor data and includes no information on population exposure to intervention-like activities, especially in the comparison site. Limited information is provided on the level of contact with residents in the intervention community; however, absent any reference data for the comparison site, it is not possible to know whether the level of exposure to intervention-like activity in the intervention community was more, less, or about the same as that in the comparison community.

It is quite natural to assume that the exposure was greater in the intervention community, but that assumption may not reflect reality. Consider, for example, data published by the sister study in Minnesota, in which exposure was equivalent between the two study conditions at the end of the intervention period (Luepker et al., 1994). The Minnesota investigators had assumed that exposure would be much greater in the intervention communities, and were quite surprised at what the data indicated.

Differential maturation is another threat that cannot be assessed in the PHHP design. The design included only a single baseline survey so that no estimate of baseline trends was possible. Given only a single community allocated to each condition, it is certain that the two communities would differ somewhat in their trends for the outcomes of interest. Absent any indication of the direction and magnitude of that difference prior to intervention, it is not possible to separate effects due to those underlying trends from effects due to the intervention. As the study turned out, the post-intervention trends were quite similar in the two communities. Given that result, it is tempting to conclude that the intervention was not very effective. However, the fair critic must note that it is also possible that the similar trends observed after intervention may in fact reflect a differential change in the two communities, but a change that cannot be measured because no estimates of baseline trends are available.

Contamination was considered as a plausible explanation for the findings by the investigators themselves. The comparison community was within 100 miles of the intervention community, and there were frequent and regular interactions involving residents of the two communities. The investigators chose not to use mass media in part out of concern for contamination, but their reliance on other delivery systems would not preclude contamination. As discussed above for local history, the investigators did not include any data on exposure to intervention-like activities in the comparison community in their main results paper, and so it is not possible to assess the level of any contamination.

The major threat in a community trial with this design is the threat to statistical validity created by violation of the assumptions underlying the statistical analysis. The PHHP investigators were in a particularly good position to consider this threat, as they have taken an active role in the discussion of these issues over the last decade (Feldman, 1988; Feldman and McKinlay, 1994; McKinlay, 1994; McKinlay et al., 1988; McKinlay et al., 1989; Murray, McKinlay et al., 1994; Zucker et al., 1995).

Chapter 4 reviewed the general issue of the unit of assignment vs. the unit of analysis, and that discussion is particularly relevant to the design with a single group in each condition. Here, the investigator has only a few choices in terms of analysis. Any analysis that ignores variation due to the groups has an inflated Type I error rate and should be avoided. The degree of the inflation depends both on the magnitude of the intraclass correlation that indexes the variation of the groups relative to the members, and on the number of members observed in each group. The inflation of the Type I error rate can be substantial (Zucker, 1990). The PHHP investigators recognized the danger inherent in this approach and took steps to avoid it.

Chapter 4 presented an alternative in which the data are analyzed at the level of the subgroup. Chapter 4 presented another alternative in which the data are analyzed ignoring the group but with a *post hoc* correction for variance inflation due to the nested design. Both approaches represent improvements over the analysis in which the group is ignored, and both were employed as part of the PHHP risk-factor analysis.

The use of batches in the PHHP analysis represents a variation on the use of subgroups described in Chapter 4. Indeed, the subgroup analysis presented in Chapter 4 is a derivative of the batch analysis presented in Feldman et al. (1996). The batch analysis was first proposed by Sonja McKinlay in the late 1980s as a compromise solution to the problem of limited *ddf* and inflated variance in group-randomized trials. Dr. McKinlay developed the concept for the PHHP design, which had only a single group in each condition. There have been many discussions between the author and Drs. McKinlay and Feldman about this issue over the years, and those discussions led directly to the subgroup material in Chapter 4.

The rationale for the subgroup analysis is that if most of the variance inflation due to the group is captured in the subgroups, the analysis can be conducted at the subgroup level. This increases the *ddf* available for the test of interest while simultaneously reflecting some or most of the variance inflation due to the nested design. The subgroup analysis stands as a compromise position that may be useful when the number of groups in each condition is limited, but only if the assumptions underlying the subgroup analysis are met.

The validity of the subgroup analysis rests on the assumption that the subgroups capture most of the variance inflation associated with the nested design. A recent simulation study confirmed that the Type I error rate is always inflated with a subgroup analysis, but that the degree of inflation depends on both the magnitude of the extra variation and the fraction of the group variance that is captured by the subgroups (Murray et al., 1996). That simulation study found that the subgroup analysis could not be made to yield a reliably appropriate Type I error rate unless the intraclass correlation was small (≤ 0.005) *and* the subgroup accounted for most of the extra variation ($\geq 80\%$).

When the design includes multiple groups in each condition, it is possible to estimate the group component of variance and determine how well the batch analysis performs. Unfortunately, when the design includes only a single group in each condition, as it did in PHHP, it is not possible to estimate the group component of variance. In that case, the batch analysis must proceed based only on the assumption that the batches account for a large fraction of that variance. Feldman et al. (1996) argue that because each of the PHHP batches represented an independent random sample of the underlying population, that assumption is more likely to apply than in other circumstances. There is certainly merit to that argument, but it remains a strong and untestable assumption.

The use of a *post hoc* correction of standard errors for variance inflation due to the nested design was outlined in Chapter 4. It was presented as a useful approach when the analysts have confidence in the validity of the external estimate employed in the correction. As it turns out, most of the results reported in Carleton et al. (1995) were based primarily on contrasts and estimates that included such a *post hoc* correction for variation due to batch as estimated from their own data, not from an external source. This correction is helpful, in the same way that the subgroup analysis is helpful compared to an analysis at the member level. However, in PHHP, that analysis rests on the same untestable assumption that the batch accounts for most of the variation associated with groups.

Summary

As seen in the PHHP, even very good analysts can struggle to develop a valid analysis plan when faced with a design based on a single group allocated to each condition. For trials early in the evolution of a particular area, such a design may be appropriate; those early trials are designed to develop hypotheses for evaluation in more rigorous trials at a later time. However, for group-randomized trials intended to allow clear causal inference, designs based on only one or even a few groups per condition should be avoided. Investigators and policy makers should not have to rely on strong but untestable assumptions to interpret the results of those trials.

The Healthy Worker Project (HWP)

Background

There are many reasons to consider worksites as a setting for health-promotion and disease-prevention research. Worksites provide convenient access to populations of interest for investigators. The physical environment may also provide facilities that can be used both for intervention and data-collection activities. The social environment may provide social support for behavior change. Employers may view health-promotion and disease-prevention activities as a method to reduce absenteeism and health-care costs, or as a benefit they can provide to their employees. From a design perspective, worksites stand as a good example of communities within a community, and allow the investigator to conduct a much smaller trial with many more groups per condition than would have been possible if whole communities had been allocated to conditions.

Jeffery et al. (1993) presented the results of the Healthy Worker Project (HWP), one of several worksite-based health-promotion studies conducted in the late 1980s and early 1990s. The HWP was chosen as a case study because it illustrates many of the features of a good worksite study.[1]

Description

The HWP focused on obesity and cigarette smoking. Obesity and smoking were common in the population, they were risk factors for multiple disease outcomes, and most persons who were overweight or who smoked were interested in losing weight and/or quitting smoking. In addition, the investigators had conducted a number of preliminary studies to develop and test many of the intervention components and measurement instruments to be used in the HWP.

The HWP began recruitment in 1987. All worksites in the Twin Cities metropolitan area that had between 400 and 900 employees were identified from a commercial listing service. Sites were approached in random order from that list, initially by letter and then with a follow-up telephone call. Interested worksites were visited by project staff and recruited for the study. Of 154 sites contacted, 36 were judged ineligible, 83 declined to participate, and 32 were recruited to the study (27%). There were clear differences between the sites that agreed to participate and those that did not, both in terms of work-force size and stability, and type of business, with smaller, more stable companies agreeing to participate, and with a higher fraction of public-sector companies agreeing to participate than were represented in the total population of companies. Even so, the participating sites were widely distributed in terms of their functions, which included manufacturing, retail, assembly, financial, health care, education, and government.

Participating sites completed a baseline survey of 200 employees selected at random from within each site. Those employees were recruited for a second survey two years later as a cohort. In addition, an independent sample of 200 employees was drawn at random at the two-year posttest, providing a second cross-sectional sample. The balance of this case-study presentation focuses on the two cross-sectional samples and their analysis.

Workers selected for the survey were surveyed at work. Direct measures were taken of weight, height, and expired-air carbon monoxide (CO). A self-administered questionnaire assessed demographic characteristics and other factors related to weight and smoking. Workers who could not be surveyed at work were approached at home by telephone in 29 of the 32 sites. The response rates for the on-site surveys were 75% and 77% for baseline and the 2-year posttest, respectively. The response rates for the telephone surveys were 77% and 87%, respectively. The net response rates combining the on-site and phone methods were 92% and 94% for the baseline and follow-up surveys, respectively.

The primary outcomes were smoking prevalence and average body mass index. The analysis was conducted in two stages. In a first stage, worker-level covariates were used to generate an adjusted mean for each worksite, separately at baseline and follow-up. In a second stage, those adjusted means were used to test for the effect of the intervention program, which was estimated as the net change over time between the two conditions. As such, the HWP analysis illustrates the adjusted time $\times$ condition analysis from Chapter 5, conducted in two stages.

Critique

The HWP investigators took a number of steps to enhance the validity of their design and analysis. By choosing worksites from the community as a whole, they enhanced the external validity of their study. By not assigning groups to study conditions on the basis of baseline scores, they limited the threat of statistical regression. They employed both direct measurement and self-report for the primary outcomes (height, weight, CO) for employees surveyed at work, and so limited mono-operation bias, mono-method bias, hypothesis guessing, and experimenter expectancies. This scheme also allowed them to adjust the self-report height and weight data collected by phone using gender-specific regression equations developed from the data collected on site. This correction further enhanced the construct validity of the height and weight data and improved the reliability of those measures. No such correction was used for smoking, though Jeffery et al. (1993) report that the false-report rate in the on-site participants was only 2% with no difference between the intervention and comparison conditions. That finding also enhanced the construct validity of the smoking data. Workers in both conditions were surveyed on the same schedule using the same instruments, limiting testing and instrumentation as threats to internal validity. As noted above, the participation rates were quite high, over 90% at both baseline and follow-up, limiting the threat of selection. The investigators repeated their primary analyses in subsamples defined by source of data (phone vs. on-site) and duration of employment (short- vs. long-term) and obtained similar estimates of intervention effects in both groups. The parallel results in these two sets of subgroups enhanced the internal and external validity of the study, respectively. Finally, the use of dose-response analyses within the intervention condition further bolstered the study's construct validity.

The investigators addressed each of the major threats to the validity of group-randomized trials. Through random assignment of 16 worksites to each of their two study conditions, they largely eliminated the potential threats of selection and differential maturation and history. It is increasingly unlikely that the average trends or levels of factors related to the outcome are different among the study conditions as the number of groups allocated to each condition increases. Similarly, it becomes increasingly implausible that some external event could influence the groups on one condition more than the groups in the other condition as those groups increase in number and geographic interspersion, as occurs with random assignment of a large number of groups to each condition.

The investigators further reduced the threat of selection bias by adjusting for gender, education, age, occupation, and marital status in their analysis. Greater assurance of baseline comparability could have been obtained by stratifying the worksites on smoking prevalence or average body mass index prior to randomization, but 16 groups per condition provides considerable protection even in the absence of stratification, and an adjusted analysis should take care of most residual confounding. That their approach was effective is confirmed by data presented in their paper showing no differences between the study conditions at baseline (Jeffery et al., 1993).

Contamination was limited through their close control over the intervention materials and instruction. All classes were taught by study staff, who could easily control participation and distribution of intervention materials.

The investigators ensured the statistical validity of their study through their selection of analytic methods. As noted above, their analysis was an example of the adjusted two-stage approach presented in Chapter 4. In a first stage, member-level covariates were used to generate an adjusted mean for each worksite. In a second stage, those adjusted means were used to test for the effect of the intervention program. As a result, the unit of analysis for the intervention effect was the worksite, and the analysis accommodated regression adjustment for member-level covariates as well.

The results published in Jeffery et al. (1993) indicated that the net decline in smoking prevalence rate was significantly greater in the intervention condition than in the comparison condition (-3.0% vs. $+1.0\%$). There was little difference between the two conditions reported for average body mass index.

Dose-response analyses were conducted using the data from the intervention worksites. The correlation between change in smoking and participation in the smoking cessation classes was significant at $r = 0.45$. The correlation between change in body mass index and participation in the weight-loss classes was even higher, $r = 0.55$, and was also significant.

The strong dose-response correlation for body mass index is inconsistent with the absence of a treatment effect for body mass index. Careful reading of the report reveals that the investigators included an additional covariate in their analysis of the body mass index data—smoking status. The reasoning for that adjustment is not given in the paper, but likely stems from the strong association between smoking cessation and weight gain. The investigators may have expected weight gain among quitters and included the adjustment for smoking status to avoid what otherwise might appear as a negative intervention effect on body mass index. This is a very reasonable concern, but the solution unavoidably raises a different concern, that of overadjustment. If the intervention caused a change in smoking status, then adjustment of any other dependent variable for change in smoking status may effectively adjust out a portion of the intervention effect on that dependent variable. That may artificially reduce the association between the new dependent variable and condition toward zero. The parameter estimate for condition in a general linear mixed model is always interpreted as the change in the dependent variable per unit change in condition, with all other variables in the model held constant. If the analyst holds change in smoking status constant, and if change in smoking status represents much of the intervention effect, then the adjusted parameter coefficient for condition is biased toward zero.[2]

Absent any other data, it is not possible to know whether or not an overadjustment occurred in the HWP. Two additional analyses would shed light on the question, but neither was reported by the investigators. First, it would be of interest to look at the body mass index analysis without adjustment for smoking status. Second, it would be of interest to conduct separate analyses of body mass index for participants who quit smoking during the study and those who did not. If the adjustment for smoking reduced the estimate of the intervention effect for body mass index, that estimate would be larger in the unadjusted analysis. Similarly, if change in smoking status explained all of the intervention effect on body mass index, there would be no effect in the stratum comprised of persons who had not quit smoking and a measurable effect in the stratum comprised of persons who had quit smoking. The investigators would still have to wrestle with the adverse effect of smoking cessation on weight as they interpreted the results of these analyses, but they might shed more light on the impact of the intervention.

Summary

The HWP illustrates the many benefits that derive from random assignment of a good number of groups to each condition. The major threats to internal validity, including selection, differential history, and differential maturation, are largely addressed through this act alone. Combined with a valid analysis, this design will allow the investigators to make a fair assessment of the efficacy of their intervention program.

Rapid Early Action for Coronary Treatment (REACT)

Background

In 1994, the National Heart Lung and Blood Institute (NHLBI) funded a collaborative effort designed to reduce patient delay time between onset of symptoms of acute myocardial infarction (AMI) and contact with hospital-based emergency medical care. The steering committee soon adopted the name Rapid Early Action for Coronary Treatment (REACT). This study was chosen as a case study for several reasons. First, it is a multicenter group-randomized trial involving five field centers, a coordinating center, and the NHLBI; the first two case studies were based entirely at one center and did not involve either a coordinating center or the funding agency as a partner in the investigation. Second, REACT was the first community trial to employ continuous surveillance as the primary vehicle for data collection. This approach allowed the REACT investigators to estimate the intervention effect as a difference in the time trends in delay time computed for the two study conditions. Unfortunately, the trial was still in progress at this writing, so it was not possible to review the study in the context of its findings.[3]

Description

Early treatment is critical to survival and recovery for patients with symptoms of AMI, because there is a steep decline in survival as the interval increases between onset of symptoms and treatment. Unfortunately, many persons who experience symptoms do not seek emergency medical care right away, even if they are conscious and able to do so. The goal of the REACT trial was to evaluate the effects of an 18-month community-based intervention program designed to reduce delay time for patients experiencing symptoms of AMI. The intervention was designed to educate potential patients about the benefits of seeking early care and to educate others who might observe an AMI victim and be in a position to seek emergency care on their behalf.

REACT was a multicenter randomized community trial, with 10 matched pairs of communities selected and recruited by the five field centers; each field center was responsible for two pairs (Simons-Morton et al., under review). Communities were selected to be large enough (total population 56,000 to 170,000) to provide a sufficient number of persons hospitalized with symptoms of AMI. Communities were selected to have local media channels for the intervention and to have 911 service and emergency medical services. Communities were selected to be far enough apart to limit overlap of media channels. Finally, communities were selected to represent the total U.S. population in terms of sex distribution, race/ethnicity distribution, and geography. Selected communities were pair-matched within their field centers on population size and on selected sociodemographic characteristics. Within each pair, one community was assigned at random by the coordinating center to the intervention condition and the other to the comparison condition.

The REACT intervention program included four components: community organization, professional education, patient education, and community education. Process-evaluation methods were used to monitor each component, but the design of the main trial focused on the combined effect of the components, not on their individual effects.

The primary outcome for the REACT trial was delay time, defined as the interval between onset of AMI symptoms and arrival at the hospital. All hospitals that provide care to community residents with acute ischemic heart disease participated in the trial; pediatric, psychiatric, rehabilitation, and convalescent hospitals, as well as hospitals without emergency departments, were excluded. Emergency department staff at the participating hospitals identified all patients presenting with chest pain or a related symptom. The project staff then inquired as to the time of onset of those symptoms and recorded that information in the patient's chart. At weekly intervals, REACT staff reviewed the emergency department records for all visits in the previous week. Chart abstraction was completed for all patients who reported chest pain or a synonymous symptom such as chest discomfort. The abstracted data became part of the REACT database, maintained by the coordinating center. Critical among the data entered into that database were the patient's age, zip code, delay time, admission status, and discharge code. To be included in the outcome analysis, patients must have been over age 30, a resident in the study community, reported chest pain or a synonymous symptom upon arrival at the emergency department, been admitted for possible acute CHD (possible acute MI or unstable angina), and have a discharge code indicating a problem of cardiac-related origin. Additional information on potential confounders and effect modifiers was also included in the database.

Exposure to the REACT intervention program and to intervention-like activities was assessed as part of the process evaluation. In both intervention and comparison communities, three surveys gathered the process-evaluation data: (1) a telephone survey of patients hospitalized with a diagnosis of acute ischemia, (2) a telephone survey of a sample of patients who reported chest pain at the emergency department but who were not hospitalized, and (3) a series of population surveys based on random digit dialing. These efforts were supplemented in the intervention communities by detailed logs of activities related to community organization, professional education, patient education, and community education.

The primary analysis will compare the intervention and comparison conditions in terms of their difference in mean slope in log delay time among patients meeting the eligibility criteria (Feldman et al., under review). A two-stage analysis is planned. In the first stage, community slopes for log delay time will be estimated, with adjustment for individual-level covariates. In a second stage, the intervention effect will be estimated as the difference in the mean slopes observed for the two study conditions. The variation in the condition mean slopes will be assessed against the variation of the community-specific slopes; as such, this analysis is an application of the random-coefficients model described in Chapter 5.

Critique

The REACT design has many of the strengths presented above for the Healthy Worker Project. By choosing field centers and communities from the several sections of the country (Minnesota, Washington and Oregon, Texas, Alabama, and Massachusetts), the investigators enhanced the external validity of their study. By not assigning communities to study conditions on the basis of baseline scores, they limited the threat of statistical regression. The systematic surveillance of emergency departments was designed to capture as large a fraction of patients experiencing chest pain as possible, thereby limiting selec-

tion bias. Surveillance in all sites was conducted according to a common protocol and used the same instruments, limiting testing and instrumentation as
threats to internal validity. Regular quality-control visits were built into the
protocol. The standardization and regular quality control limited the threats of
experimenter expectancies and hypothesis guessing, though observers could
not be blinded as to the condition of the communities. The primary outcome
and analytic plan were well defined in the protocol. Secondary outcomes and
secondary analyses were also defined in the protocol. In addition, secondary
definitions were proposed for the primary outcomes, based on different measurement methods; this served to limit mono-method and mono-operation bias
in the measurements.

The REACT investigators addressed each of the major threats to the validity
of group-randomized trials. Through random assignment of 10 communities
from within matched pairs to each of their two study conditions, they largely
eliminated the potential threats of selection and differential maturation and
history. It is increasingly unlikely that the average trends or levels of factors
related to the outcome could be different among the study conditions as the
number of groups allocated to each condition increases. Similarly, it becomes
increasingly implausible that some external event could influence the groups
in one condition more than the groups in the other condition as those groups
increase in number and geographic interspersion, as occurs with random assignment of a number of groups to each condition. Matching further reduced
these threats.

The investigators will further reduce the threats of selection bias by adjusting for individual covariates in their analysis. The matching and randomization should take care of most selection issues, and the regression adjustment
should limit residual confounding.

Contamination was a threat to the REACT study. It was not possible to fully
contain an intervention when much of the intervention occurred publicly and
through the mass media. The communities were selected to limit overlap of
media channels, but that only makes it more difficult for the intervention messages to cross the condition lines, not impossible. The investigators put in
place a process-evaluation system that includes several exposure measures.
This allowed them to assess the degree of contamination and to conduct dose-
response analyses within conditions. While these measures do nothing to prevent contamination, they do permit the investigators to determine the extent to
which it occurs.

The investigators ensured the statistical validity of their study through their
selection of analysis methods. As noted above, their analysis is an example of
an adjusted random-coefficients analysis. An adjusted slope will be estimated
for each community, and then those slopes treated as the raw data in a second-

stage analysis for intervention effects. The unit of analysis will be the community, with *df* based on the number of communities, not the number of patients.

The investigators were careful to anticipate that delay time in its original scale is quite skewed, with a long right tail. As a result, they will apply a log transform. Based on data from previous studies, that transform is expected to yield a nearly normal distribution. The transformed variable will be the dependent variable in the primary analysis.

Summary

The REACT design and analysis plan carried all the strengths described above for the HWP. In addition, because it is a multicenter trial, it has the advantage of replication at multiple sites in varied populations around the country. As a result, the generalizability of the results is enhanced compared to results from a similar trial conducted in only a single center.

Nested Cohort Designs

The Vermont School and Mass Media Study

Background

There have been approximately one hundred group-randomized trials for smoking prevention published in the last twenty years (Rooney and Murray, 1996). Flynn et al. (1992) reported the results of one of those trials, a five-year program designed to prevent cigarette smoking among children and adolescents. A follow-up paper provided results based on measures taken two years after the end of the prevention program (Flynn et al., 1994). The Vermont School and Mass Media Study was chosen as a case study because it illustrates several of the design features that have been recommended for nested-cohort designs and because it illustrates many of the problems that are common to long-term follow-up in school-based studies.

Description

Four communities participated in the study, with two from the northeastern United States and two from the western United States. The four communities were chosen as best matches among standard metropolitan statistical areas from those states, with one pair of communities chosen from Vermont and one from Montana. To be eligible, communities had to have a media market that did not overlap another study community; had to have a population less than

400,000 but more than 50,000; and had to meet the study's matching criteria for demographic variables, including education, income, and education. Within the SMSAs chosen for the study, specific school districts and schools were chosen to provide good matches on the demographic characteristics based on census data for educational attainment and household income. Consent was obtained from school districts, from parents, and from individual students.

Two conditions were included in the study. The intensive intervention condition included both a school-based smoking-prevention program and a television and radio campaign. The comparison condition received only the school-based program. As such, both conditions involved active intervention to prevent smoking. The contrast between the two can be considered as a school-and-media vs. school-only contrast.

Assignment to study conditions was not random. In one pair, one community was selected for the school-only condition in order to avoid media contamination of nearby communities that were participating in other health-promotion research projects. In the other pair, the school-and-media condition was assigned to the community that had more limited media reach and lower media costs.

Students enrolled in the fourth through sixth grades in the participating schools were surveyed at baseline in the spring of 1985. The intervention programs were introduced in the fall of the next school year and continued for a total of four school years. Four additional surveys were conducted annually each spring through 1989, when the students were in the eighth through tenth grades. After missing one year, an additional survey was conducted in the spring of 1991, when the students were in the tenth through twelfth grades.

The primary outcome in the 1992 report was a smoking-behavior index, computed as the average of three smoking self-report items weighted to reflect the number of cigarettes smoked per week (Pechacek et al., 1984). A saliva sample was also obtained from each student as part of the school surveys, for assessment of thiocyanate in order to obtain an objective measure of smoking. At the last follow-up survey, the primary outcome was weekly smoking prevalence; those students no longer in the participating schools were surveyed by telephone and no saliva sample was collected from those students.

The analyses presented in the 1992 report were restricted to the fraction of the cohort that had completed all five surveys. Forty-three percent of the students in the school-only condition and 50% of the students in the school-and-media condition met that requirement. The 1994 report included analyses restricted to the fraction that had completed all six surveys and separate analyses restricted to those that had completed the baseline and last follow-up survey. Thirty-eight percent of the students participated in all six surveys, while fully 86% participated in the baseline and the last follow-up survey.

Both reports presented analyses at two levels. The primary analysis was conducted at the level of the student, ignoring community. Secondary analyses were conducted at the level of the community. Adjustment for covariates was not mentioned as a part of either analysis in the 1992 report. Adjustment for baseline values on selected covariates was part of the student-level analysis in the 1994 report but not of the community-level analysis.

The results published in 1992 indicated a significantly lower level of smoking in the school-and-media condition, both in the primary and secondary analyses. The results published in 1994 supported that pattern, both in the primary and secondary analyses, but only in the full-exposure cohort. When the analysis was based on the more complete sample of students who completed both the first and sixth survey, the school-and-media condition had a significantly lower level of smoking in the primary analysis but not in the secondary analysis.

Critique

The procedures employed in the study provided good protection against many of the threats to validity. The testing schedule and measurement methods were the same in both conditions, thereby limiting the risk of differential testing and instrumentation. Communities were not assigned to conditions on the basis of baseline levels, thereby limiting the risk of regression. The primary outcome, smoking, was assessed in several different ways, with both self-report and biochemical measures, thereby limiting mono-method and mono-operation bias. Both conditions received an intervention, thereby limiting the risk of hypothesis guessing in one condition alone. The use of the biochemical validation has been shown to improve the reliability of smoking self-report measures (Murray and Perry, 1987; Murray et al., 1987). The media intervention was under substantial control of the investigators, thereby limiting the risk of unreliable treatment implementation.

The investigators also took steps to address the major threats to the validity of their trial. Indeed, they were unusually complete in their review of potential threats to the interpretation of their results in their 1992 report and provided evidence on most of the major issues.

Assignment of communities to conditions was not random and instead was based on logistical and political considerations. This is not uncommon in group-randomized trials involving only a few groups in each condition, but does raise the threat of selection bias. The best strategy is to use random assignment, as only random assignment gives each group an equal opportunity to be assigned to each condition. Equal opportunity is quite important in the absence of matching, particularly if the groups are heterogeneous with respect to factors related to the outcome. The same statement would hold if the communities were matched but the matching was ineffective. Even given effective matching, random assignment is still preferred. This is because the investigators will never have information on all possible confounders, and it is always possible that their matching was incomplete. Randomization of only a few groups to each condition provides little protection against uneven distribution of such factors, however, so careful matching can be an important adjunct to randomization.

Based on data published in the 1992 report, the matching was effective in establishing comparability of the conditions in terms of demographic characteristics such as adult educational attainment and household income. However, these variables are only mildly related to adolescent smoking levels, and so that finding cannot remove entirely the concern about selection bias. The investigators also presented data in their 1992 report for baseline levels of several more proximal risk factors. The school-and-media–condition students were at lower risk than the school-only students on several of these factors and at higher risk on others. It is difficult to determine whether the net effect would favor either condition. The analyses presented in the 1994 report provide the best evidence against selection bias. That report indicated that the lower smoking rates in the school-and-media condition remained even after adjustment for multiple risk factors.

Absent any information about the trends in adolescent smoking in the study communities, and particularly given only two communities per condition, there is also concern over differential maturation or secular trends. With only a small number of communities, it is plausible that the one or both communities in one condition might have been following a higher trajectory for adolescent smoking than the communities in the other condition. However, the fact that the intervention effect remained even after adjustment for baseline risk factors reduces this threat.

The investigators reported data on exposure to the school-based program in their 1992 report. Those data indicate similar exposure in three communities, but 10%–20% lower reported exposure in the fourth community. That same community also had the highest scores on several of the smoking risk factors. Because that community received the less intensive intervention, a critical reader might wonder whether the combination of higher risk and lower exposure might have resulted in higher smoking rates in that community and biased upward the estimate of the intervention effect. That concern is resolved by examination of the community-specific results, which clearly indicate quite similar smoking patterns over time in the communities assigned to the same condition.

The threat of differential history is not likely in this instance, even though there are only two communities in each condition, because the two communities in each condition were separated by several thousand miles. However, an external event in only one community, if it had a substantial effect on adolescent smoking, could more easily affect the condition mean when there are only two communities in a condition than when there are many. Once again, the similarity of the results for the communities in the same condition argues against such an effect.

Mortality and differential mortality are substantial threats in the analyses restricted to those students present for all surveys. In the 1992 report, the cohort was reduced to just under 50% of the original sample. By 1994, the cohort was down to 38% of the original sample. Such attrition levels are not uncommon in school-based studies, but create a serious threat to interpretation. If the type of students lost from the two conditions was different, or if the type of students lost was different from the type of students who remained, the estimate of the intervention effect would be biased. The first pattern is a threat to the internal validity of the study; the second is a threat to the external validity of the study. Data from the 1992 report make it clear that those who left the study schools were at higher risk of smoking. Findings in the 1994 report indicate that the intervention effect estimated from the full-exposure cohort was stronger ($OR = 0.62$) than the effect estimated from the complete-follow-up sample ($OR = 0.79$). Taken together, those findings suggest that the school-and-media program was less effective in the high-risk students and illustrate the bias that attrition can introduce.

The authors note in their reports that "the study design was based on the individual as the unit of analysis" (Flynn et al., 1994, p. 1149) and that "a supplemental analysis is presented in which the community is the unit" (Flynn, 1992, p. 828). These statements reflect a common misconception that study design is based on the intentions of the investigators rather than on their actions. In fact, it is always the actions that define the design, sometimes in spite of the investigators' intentions. In this case, the investigators allocated whole communities to their study conditions. Perforce, the proper unit of analysis was the community, intentions notwithstanding.

Given their design, all analyses that failed to reflect the extra variation expected from the nested design would be expected to have an inflated Type I error rate. This would be the case for all analyses based only on the individual students, with no consideration given to the nested communities. Only the analyses based on the communities would be expected to have a nominal Type I error rate, and then only if properly executed. The details provided for the community-level analyses are limited, both in the 1992 and in the 1994 reports, but follow-up conversations with the investigators confirmed the validity of the community-level analyses.[4] Those analyses supported a reduction in smoking in the school-and-media condition, but only in the full-exposure cohort. The odds ratio of 0.79 in the complete-follow-up sample was not significant in the community-level analysis. Given 4 *ddf* for the reported community-level analysis, the power of that analysis was quite limited.

Taken together, the results from this study indicate that the school-and-media intervention was more effective in reducing smoking levels among adolescents than was the school program alone. The effect appears stronger among students who remained in the participating schools through high school, students shown in other studies to be at lower risk of becoming addicted smokers. The intervention effect was reduced, and no longer statistically significant, when measured in the full follow-up sample.

Summary

With only two groups allocated to each condition, the Vermont School and Mass Media Study design was subject to serious threats to validity. However, the investigators were very thorough in their consideration of the threats to their design and provided information to address most of them. As a result, their report provides useful evidence that their school-and-media intervention was effective.

The Sydney Ambulance Service Trial

Background

Gomel et al. (1993) reported the results of a community trial designed to reduce cardiovascular risk among employees of the Ambulance Service in Sydney, Australia. This study was chosen because of its use of a large number of small, identifiable groups as units of assignment. This strategy limited the total cost of intervention and evaluation but allowed for a strong design with good power. It is a strategy that has much to recommend it.

Description

Twenty-eight Ambulance Service stations were selected at random from among the stations located in the metropolitan Sydney area. The only criterion was that each station had to have at least 12 employees. Selection was stratified by region, so that seven stations were selected from each of the four regions of Sydney. All employees in those stations were invited to participate. Exclusions were limited to those who expected to be absent from work for more than one-third of the initial three-month intervention period, those who were pending transfer to a different station, and those who had serious health problems. Over 88% of the 488 eligible workers agreed to participate.

Stations were assigned at random to one of four conditions. Because some conditions were more expensive than others, fewer stations were randomized to the intensive intervention conditions than to the less intensive conditions.

All staff at a station then received the same intervention, appropriate for the assigned condition. Recruitment occurred in five waves over an 18-month period; intervention began immediately after recruitment and continued for up to six months, depending on the condition.

All conditions involved some level of intervention. The simplest provided a basic health-risk assessment with referral of high-risk cases to their physician. The most complex involved a combination of personalized counseling to reduce risk and incentives for achieving risk-reduction goals over a six-month period. Intermediate conditions provided health-risk assessment plus general health education or personalized counseling without the incentives.

Measurements were taken at baseline and again at 3, 6, and 12 months after the baseline survey. All measures were taken following a standardized protocol implemented by trained staff. The major outcomes were body mass index, percentage of body fat estimated from skinfold measures, blood pressure, serum cholesterol, smoking status validated by cotinine, and aerobic capacity assessed during an ergometer test.

Some data were lost, due primarily to equipment failure or loss to follow-up. Imputation methods were used to replace the missing data, and those methods varied according to the reason for the missing data and the type of data. For data lost due to equipment failure, values were inputted using age- and sex-specific means from all other participants. For continuous variables, missing data were replaced by the mean value for that participant's previous observations. For smoking status, participants lost to follow-up were treated as smokers for purposes of analysis.

Several of the variables were subject to log or square-root transformations prior to analysis to normalize the data. These included body mass index, cholesterol, and aerobic capacity.

Repeated-measures ANOVA was used to assess intervention effects for all variables except smoking status. The nested design was reflected in the analysis, as "variability between stations within interventions was used as the denominator in testing for differences between interventions" (Gomel et al., 1993, p. 1233). That description matches the adjusted time $\times$ condition analysis presented in Chapter 6. A priori contrasts assessed the effect of risk-factor education alone, the effect of incentives, and the effect of behavioral counseling. Other contrasts examined trends. The analysis of smoking status "did not test for differences between stations within interventions because of the small number of smokers at each station" (Gomel et al., 1993, p. 1234). Instead, conditions were compared by ordinary chi-square tests for differences in the proportion of baseline smokers whose cessation was confirmed by the cotinine test.

In general, there was no difference between the health-risk-assessment condition and the general risk factor education condition, or between the behavioral counseling with incentives condition and the behavioral counseling without incentives conditions. However, the behavioral counseling approach had significant and beneficial effects over the less intensive approaches for body mass index, percent body fat, systolic blood pressure (SBP), and smoking cessation, at least in the short term. The behavioral-counseling effects held through the end of the study for body mass index and continuous abstinence.

Critique

The investigators employed a number of strategies to enhance the validity of their design and analysis. They employed a common protocol and sequence for measurements in each station to limit testing and instrumentation and to enhance the reliability of the measurements. They did not assign stations to conditions on the basis of pretest scores, and so avoided regression effects. They had remarkably low mortality after recruitment; this both enhanced the generalizability of their findings and limited the bias in the estimate of the intervention effect that might result from recruitment of a more select population. All conditions received an intervention, limiting the risk of compensatory equalization, compensatory rivalry, or resentful demoralization. Physical and biochemical measures were taken, in addition to self-report measures; this served to reduce mono-method bias and to enhance the reliability and validity of the outcome measures. The ambulance stations provided a much more homogeneous pool of assignment units than has been the case in many other worksite studies; this served to improve power by limiting random heterogeneity of respondents.

The investigators also addressed the major threats to validity in their study. Random assignment of a moderate number of ambulance stations to most of the conditions served to limit selection bias. Because the stations were quite homogeneous to begin with and were distributed in the same geographic area, the random assignment also served to limit the threats of differential maturation and differential history, respectively. The randomization was not entirely effective, however, in part because only a limited number of stations was randomized to the behavioral counseling conditions because of their high cost. Only 4 and 6 stations were randomized to those conditions, compared to 8 and 10 in the other two. By chance, there was much greater variability in SBP among the stations assigned to the two behavioral counseling conditions than to the less intensive conditions. There also was a notable difference in the job-classification distribution in the behavioral counselling plus incentives condition, which had the smallest number of stations. This pattern underscores the limitations of randomization without matching when only a few units are allocated to each condition.

Contamination was a threat from the beginning of the study, because all the stations were in the same metropolitan area. That provided opportunities for staff from stations assigned to different conditions to interact and exchange information about their programs. Transfers of staff among stations assigned to different conditions also occurred. These forces would tend to reduce the intervention effects observed in the study.

The investigators did a good job of thinking through the constructs of interest, both in the measurements and in the interventions. Their use of four intervention conditions allowed them to look systematically at efficacy of incentives, behavioral counseling, and risk-factor education in isolation from other components. Their measurement of multiple risk factors allowed them to examine the differential effect of the intervention on those multiple risk factors. Their use of different strength interventions allowed them to determine whether increasing dose was related to increasing effect, with potential confounders controlled via randomization rather than only through analysis techniques. Their combination of intervention components allowed for some limited examination of the interaction of those components relative to the individual components.

The analysis plan accounted for the allocation of identifiable groups to study conditions. They reported that variation among conditions was assessed against variation among stations and reported *ddf* for their tests that were consistent with evaluation at the level of the group.[5] The investigators are also to be commended for the use of *a priori* contrasts to focus the analysis.

The analyses of the smoking results were based on the members and ignored the groups. This strategy generally inflates the Type I error rate, often badly. In this study, the behavioral counseling conditions had a 3-month cessation rate of 18%, compared to 3% in the less intensive conditions. The usual chi-square was 8.27, which had a *p*-value of 0.004 with 1 *df.* Suppose, however, that the intraclass correlation for cessation had been 0.10. With 15 participants per station on average, the DEFF would be estimated as $1+(15-1)*0.10 = 2.4$, and the corrected chi-square would be estimated as $8.27/2.4 = 3.44$, a nonsignificant result. Absent further information from the study, it is not possible to know what the intraclass correlation for cessation was in the data. Estimates published from the Minnesota Heart Health Program (Hannan et al., 1994) suggest that at the community level, the $\hat{ICC}$ for smoking is approximately 0.001. If the value obtained in the ambulance service study was in that range, then the Type I error rate in the member-level analysis would not be greatly inflated (Murray et al, 1996).

Summary

On balance, this was a strong design and an appropriate analysis plan for all the variables, except perhaps smoking status. The results are consistent with a

significant and beneficial effect on several cardiovascular risk factors as a result of a behavioral counseling intervention that required about 2.5 hours contact with each participant over six months. The authors note that their effect
estimate was likely deflated by the participation in the surveys of many ambulance service workers who made only modest attempts at change. However,
while this may have diluted their effect estimate, it simultaneously provided a
more valid estimate of the effect in the whole population of ambulance service
workers. That estimate will prove more useful than one limited only to highly
motivated workers.

The Child and Adolescent Trial for Cardiovascular Health (CATCH)

Background

Luepker, Perry et al. (1996) reported the major outcome results for the Child
and Adolescent Trial for Cardiovascular Health (CATCH). CATCH was selected as a case study because it is the largest and most rigorous school-based
group-randomized trial published to date, and because of the role that it played
in my understanding of the design and analysis issues in group-randomized
trials.[6]

Description

CATCH was a multicenter group-randomized trial, with field centers in San
Diego, Houston, New Orleans, and Minneapolis. The coordinating center was
in Watertown, Massachusetts, and the project office was at the National Heart
Lung and Blood Institute in Bethesda. The project was funded as a collaborative agreement, so there was close cooperation among the field centers, the
coordinating center, and the NHLBI and joint planning for all elements of the
design, implementation, and analysis.

Each field center recruited 24 schools that met the eligibility requirements
for the study (Lytle et al., 1994). Schools had to commit to participate in the
three-year Phase II trial, including all measurement and intervention activities.
Schools also had to accept random assignment of schools to study conditions
after the baseline survey was completed.

Schools were randomized to intervention (56 schools) and control conditions (40 schools). The intervention schools were randomized into two equal
groups of 28 schools each. One intervention group received a school-based
program that included intervention components directed at the school food
service, the physical education curriculum, and the classroom curriculum. The
second intervention group received all these components, and in addition, a
component aimed at the third-grader's family. The control group received their

usual programs related to health, but none of the CATCH programs or materials until the end of the study.

As first proposed, CATCH had one primary endpoint, serum cholesterol measured in individual students (Zucker et al., 1995). However, at the end of the planning period, the CATCH Steering Committee expanded the focus of the study to address three primary endpoints, two that were at the school level (fat and sodium in the school lunch and time spent in vigorous physical activity) and one that was individual level (serum cholesterol). Secondary outcomes included psychosocial variables related to diet, 24-hour recall measures of dietary intake, a self-administered physical-activity checklist, blood pressure, skinfold thickness, height, weight, and aerobic fitness.

The baseline student survey was conducted in the fall of 1991. All third-grade students enrolled in the 96 participating schools were eligible to participate in the baseline survey. Just over 5000 students completed that survey, accounting for 60.4% of those eligible. Baseline measures of the school lunch and the physical education program were also taken in the fall of 1991. The student survey was repeated at the end of the third, fourth, and fifth grades. The school lunch measures were repeated at the end of fourth and fifth grades. Assessment of the physical education program was repeated during each of the six semesters of the third-, fourth-, and fifth-grade school years.

The options for analysis that were considered for the CATCH trial are described in detail in Zucker et al. (1995). In the end, the analyses were conducted using mixed-model regression procedures. The individual-level data were analyzed with regression adjustment for the baseline values on the endpoint and other individual-level covariates. To examine possible interactions between condition and field site, sex, and race, separate stratified analyses were conducted for each stratification factor. School-level data were analyzed using repeated-measures ANCOVA; compound symmetry was assumed for the repeat measures on the same schools over time. The repeated-measures analyses were also repeated with stratification on field site. The repeated-measures analyses were based on school-level measures.

For percent of calories as fat in the school lunch, there was a significant net decline over time favoring the pooled intervention conditions. For time spent in moderate or vigorous physical activity during the physical education classes, there was a significant net increase over time favoring the pooled intervention conditions. For serum cholesterol, there was a nonsignificant decline over time favoring the pooled intervention conditions.

Critique

The CATCH trial was quite strong in its defenses against threats to validity. All students and schools were measured using the same standardized protocols in both the intervention and control conditions, limiting the risk of testing and instrumentation effects. Schools were not assigned to conditions on the basis of pretest scores, thereby limiting the threat of statistical regression. None of the schools dropped out of the study, eliminating mortality as a threat at the school level. Almost 80% of the students measured at baseline were also measured at the end of the study, limiting mortality as a threat at the individual level. There were no differences in the primary and secondary outcomes between continuing participants and those lost to follow-up, or between conditions or sex groups, limiting the threat of differential mortality. There was some greater loss at follow-up among African-American students and students from California, however, and this may limit generalizability to these groups. No data were provided with which to assess the potential threats of compensatory equalization, compensatory rivalry, and resentful demoralization. Mono-operation and mono-method bias were essentially eliminated in the design of the study, as multiple approaches to both measurement and intervention were included. The self-report measures were subject to hypothesis guessing and evaluation apprehension, but the school-level and physiological measures were not. Experimenter expectancies pose a threat to some of the measures, such as the 24-hour dietary recalls and the school physical-activity observations, but they pose no risk for the serum cholesterol analyses and menu analyses, which were conducted with the staff blind to the study condition. The use of standardized measurement protocols, and the extensive development and testing of measures that took place during Phase I of the CATCH trial, helped ensure adequate reliability of measures. The extensive process evaluation and feedback provided during Phase II helped ensure reliable and consistent implementation of the intervention programs. Generalizability of the findings is greatly enhanced by the efforts of the investigators to include schools and students from African American and Hispanic populations and to represent boys and girls equally. Generalizability is further enhanced by the finding of no significant differences in program results with respect to site, sex, or ethnic group for all primary and secondary outcomes.

The CATCH investigators also took steps to guard against the major threats to validity in a group-randomized trial. They limited selection, differential history, and differential maturation by random assignment of 96 schools to study conditions from within four field centers in different parts of the country. Those threats become increasingly implausible as the number of groups increases and as their geographic interspersion increases. The effectiveness of their randomization of a large number of groups from within several field centers is demonstrated by the absence of any baseline differences among the study conditions for any of the primary or secondary outcomes.

Contamination was discussed as a threat by the investigators (Luepker, Perry et al., 1996). Because schools were randomized to study conditions from within field centers, each field center had both intervention and control schools from the same school districts. This is quite typical in school-based studies, but does pose a risk for contamination. Teachers and other officials as well as students change schools within a district over time, and this creates an opportunity for intermingling of students and staff exposed to different conditions. Any such intermingling would likely bias the estimate of the intervention effect toward zero. The Luepker, Perry et al. (1996) paper reports that contamination was not detected by CATCH staff.

The investigators point to weak interventions as a possible threat to their study. They are well aware of the limited time and resources that can be used for health-promotion activities in public schools. They are also aware that their parent intervention was not as strong as they might have liked. That the parent program did not generate any better results on primary or secondary outcomes is consistent with a weak parent intervention.

The threats to statistical validity were well addressed in CATCH. The analytic plan addressed the nested design and the expected positive intraclass correlation among measures taken from students in the same school (Zucker et al., 1995). All analyses reported in the Luepker, Perry et al. (1996) paper employed the school as the unit of analysis, with adjustment for student- and school-level covariates. There appears little threat from violated assumptions of statistical tests. The investigators do report the results for a number of analyses, and this can raise the threat of an inflated Type I error rate. However, the CATCH investigators were careful to delineate primary and secondary endpoints and to specify *a priori* hypotheses for each measure.

One minor concern in the CATCH analyses as reported was the apparent reliance on the compound-symmetry assumption for the repeated-measures analyses of several of the school-level outcomes. As noted in Chapter 6, patterns of declining correlation over time are common, and patterns of constant correlation over time are less common. As it turns out, the CATCH investigators did examine alternative structures for the within-member covariance matrix, though the results of those analyses didn't make it into the final paper. They considered both a Toeplitz structure and an unstructured form for the matrix and determined that the compound-symmetry structure was adequate.

Careful readers may note in Chapter 6 that field center is treated as a random effect in the presentation of the analysis of data from a multicenter group-randomized trial. In contrast, the CATCH investigators treated field center as a fixed effect in their analyses. The analysis employed in CATCH and that recommended in Chapter 6 are actually more similar than this observation might suggest. In both cases, a preliminary test is made for the interaction between condition and field center, with school(condition × field center) as the error term. If that interaction is not significant, as happened in CATCH, the interaction term is removed from the model. In that case, the correct error term for condition is school(condition $\times$ field center); that is exactly how the *F*-test is constructed whether field center is treated as a fixed or as a random effect. In other words, once the condition $\times$ field center interaction is removed, the designation of field center as fixed or random has no effect on the calculation of the *F*-test.

Summary

CATCH was well designed to guard against the threats to validity in a group-randomized trial. The positive effects for many of the school-level measures speak to the adequacy of the intervention to generate change in those measures. The failure to demonstrate effects in serum cholesterol and other individual-level risk factors suggests that the intervention was not strong enough to create measurable effects in those variables. Whether such school-level effects eventually translate into individual-level effects requires long-term follow-up, and such follow-up is now under way for the CATCH cohort.

Summary

These case studies illustrate the wide variety of designs and analyses that are employed in group-randomized trials. They also illustrate the wide variety of research questions for which group-randomized trials are appropriate. With thoughtful consideration of the special issues of design and analysis that face group-randomized trials, creative investigators can design trials that will provide valid answers for these important questions.

Endnotes

1. Though HWP was conducted in the author's home Division, the author had no involvement with either the design or the analysis of the study. Responsibility for the design and analysis fell largely to Drs. Jeffery, Jacobs, and McGovern.
2. Overadjustment of this type is quite similar in its effect to adjustment for a mediating variable. In any three-variable situation where the third variable mediates the effect of the first variable on the second, addition of the third variable to the analysis inevitably reduces the strength of the association between the first and second. There may be little association left between the first and second when the mediating variable is held constant.
3. The author is one of the investigators for the University of Minnesota field center in the REACT trial. He serves on the Design and Analysis Committee for the national study.
4. Correspondence with the investigators confirmed that the community-level analysis was a variation of the trend analysis for the time $\times$ condition ANCOVA described in Chapter 5. In the present case, the analysis was conducted in two stages, computing time $\times$ community means in a first stage and then fitting the trend analysis to those means in

the second stage. The reported analysis differed from that presented in Chapter 5 in that the investigators did not pool the *df* for higher-order polynomials involving time with the residual error at the community level.

5. *ddf* often provide a good indication of whether the unit of analysis was at the group or member level, as *ddf* based on the latter will often be quite large, approaching the total sample size, while *ddf* based on the former will often be quite limited, approaching the product of the number of surveys and the number of groups.

6. CATCH was funded in two phases beginning in 1987. During the planning period, the CATCH investigators met regularly to discuss issues related to the design, implementation, and analysis of the CATCH project. I served as a member of the Design and Analysis Committee during that phase and participated in numerous discussions with David Zucker, a statistician then on the staff at the National Heart Lung and Blood Institute. Those conversations proved critical both in elucidating the implications of the nested design (Zucker, 1990) and in establishing my continuing interest in the design and analysis of group-randomized trials (Murray, Hannan and Zucker, 1989). My active involvement in CATCH ended once the design and analysis plans were established in 1991, though I did help to prepare the paper on the statistical aspects of the CATCH design (Zucker et al., 1995). I played no role in the analysis or interpretation of the data published in Luepker, Perry et al. (1996).

References

Addelman, S. (1970) Variability of treatments and experimental units in the design and analysis of experiments. *Journal of the American Statistical Association, 65*(331), 1095–1109.

Baranowski, T., Lin, L. S., Wetter, D. W., Resnicow, K., and Hearn, M.D. (1997) Theory as mediating variables: Why aren't community interventions working as desired? *Annals of Epidemiology, 7*(S7), 89–95.

Berger, J. O., and Pericchi, L. R. (1996) The intrinsic Bayes factor for model selection and prediction. *Journal of the American Statistical Association, 91*(433), 109–122.

Blair, R. C., and Higgins, J. J. (1986) Comment on "Statistical power with group mean as the unit of analysis." *Journal of Educational Statistics, 11*(2), 161–169.

Braithwaite, R. L. (1994) Challenges to evaluation in rural coalitions. *Journal of Community Psychology,* CSAP Special Issue, 188–200.

Breslow, N. E., and Clayton, D.G. (1993) Approximate inference in generalized linear mixed models. *Journal of the American Statistical Association, 88*(421), 9–25.

Bryk, A. S., and Raudenbush, S. W. (1992) *Hierarchical Linear Models: Applications and Data Analysis Methods.* Newbury Park, CA: Sage Publications, Inc.

Carleton, R. A., Lasater, T. M., Assaf, A. R., Feldman, H. A., McKinlay, S., and the Pawtucket Heart Health Program Writing Group (1995) The Pawtucket Heart Health Program: Community changes in cardiovascular risk factors and projected disease risk. *American Journal of Public Health, 85*(6), 777–785.

Cheung, K. C., Keeves, J. P., Sellin, N., and Tsoi, S. C. (1990) The analysis of multilevel data in educational research: Studies of problems and their solutions. *International Journal of Educational Research, 14,* 215–319.

Cohen, J. (1988) *Statistical Power Analysis for the Behavioral Sciences,* 2nd ed. New York: Academic Press.

Cohen, J., and Cohen, P. (1983) *Applied Multiple Regression/Correlation Analysis for the Behavioral Sciences,* 2nd ed. Hillsdale, NJ: Lawrence Erlbaum Associates.

Cohen, S. B., Xanthopoulos, J. A., and Jones, G. K. (1988) An evaluation of statistical software procedures appropriate for the regression analysis of complex survey data. *Journal of Official Statistics, 4*(1),17–34.

COMMIT Research Group (1995a) Community intervention trial for smoking cessation (COMMIT): I. Cohort results from a four-year community intervention. *American Journal of Public Health, 85*(2), 183–192.

COMMIT Research Group (1995b) Community intervention trial for smoking cessation (COMMIT): II. Changes in adult cigarette smoking prevalence. *American Journal of Public Health, 85*(2), 193–200.

Cook, T. D., and Campbell, D. T. (1979) *Quasi-experimentation: Design and Analysis Issues for Field Settings*. Chicago: Rand-McNally College Publishing Company.

Cook, R., Roehl, J., Oros, C., and Trudeau, J. (1994) Conceptual and methodological issues in the evaluation of community-based substance abuse prevention coalitions: Lessons learned from the national evaluation of the community partnership program. *Journal of Community Psychology*, CSAP Special Issue, 155–169.

Cornfield, J. (1978) Randomization by group: A formal analysis. *American Journal of Epidemiology, 108*(2), 100–102.

Davis, C. E., Hunsberger, S., Murray, D. M., Fabsitz, R., Himes, J. H., and Stephenson, L. K. Design and statistical analysis for Pathways. (under review).

DeLeeuw, J., and Kreft, I. G. G. (1986) Random coefficient models for multilevel analysis. *Journal of Educational Statistics, 11*(1), 57–85.

DeLeeuw, J., and Kreft, I. G. G. (1995) Questioning multilevel models. *Journal of Educational and Behavioral Statistics, 20*(2), 171–189.

Diehr, P., Martin, D. C., Koepsell, T., and Cheadle, A. (1995a) Breaking the matches in a paired t-test for community interventions when the number of pairs is small. *Statistics in Medicine, 14*, 1491–1504.

Diehr, P., Martin, D. C., Koepsell, T., Cheadle, A., Psaty, B. M., and Wagern, E. H. (1995b) Optimal survey design for community intervention evaluations: Cohort or cross-sectional? *Journal of Clinical Epidemiology, 48*(12), 1461–1472.

Diggle, P. J., Liang, K. Y., and Zeger, S. L. (1994) *Analysis of Longitudinal Data*. New York: Oxford University Press.

Dixon, W. J. (ed.) (1992) *BMDP Statistical Software Manual, Release 7*. Berkeley, CA: University of California Press.

Donner, A. (1984a) Linear regression analysis with repeated measurements. *Journal of Chronic Disease, 37*(6), 441–448.

Donner, A. (1984b) Approaches to sample size estimation in the design of clinical trials—a review. *Statistics in Medicine, 3*, 199–214.

Donner, A. (1985) A regression approach to the analysis of data arising from cluster randomization. *International Journal of Epidemiology, 14*(2), 322–326.

Donner, A. (1992) Sample size requirements for stratified cluster randomization designs. *Statistics in Medicine, 11*, 743–750.

Donner, A. (1995) Symposium on community intervention trials. *American Journal of Epidemiology, 142*(6), 567–568.

Donner, A., Birkett, N., and Buck, C. (1981) Randomization by cluster: Sample size requirements and analysis. *American Journal of Epidemiology, 114*(6), 906–914.

Donner, A., Brown, K. S., and Brasher, P. (1990) A methodological review of nontherapeutic intervention trials employing cluster randomization, 1979–1989. *International Journal of Epidemiology, 19*, 795–800.

Donner, A., and Klar, N. (1996) Statistical considerations in the design and analysis of community intervention trials. *Journal of Clinical Epidemiology, 49*(4), 435–439.

Draper, D. (1995) Inference and hierarchical modeling in the social sciences. *Journal of Educational and Behavioral Statistics, 20*(2), 115–147.

Dwyer, J. H., Feinleib, M., Lippert, P., and Hoffmeister, H. (1992) *Statistical Models for Longitudinal Studies of Health*. New York: Oxford University Press.

Dwyer, J. H., MacKinnon, D. P., Pentz, M. A., Flay, B. R., Hansen, W. B., Wang, E. Y. I., and Johnson, C. A. (1989) Estimating intervention effects in longitudinal studies. *American Journal of Epidemiology, 130*(4), 781–795.

Ellickson, P. L. (1994) Getting and keeping schools and kids for evaluation studies. *Journal of Community Psychology*, CSAP Special Issue, 102–116.

Efron, B. (1982) *The Jackknife, the Bootstrap and Other Resampling Plans*. Philadelphia, PA: Society for Industrial and Applied Mathematics.

Farquhar, J. W., Fortmann, S. P., Flora, J. A., Taylor, B., Haskell, W. L., Williams, P. T., Maccoby, N., and Wood, P. D. (1990) Effects of communitywide education on cardiovascular disease risk factors: The Stanford Five-City Project. *Journal of the American Medical Association, 264*(3), 359–365.

Feldman, H. A. (1988) Families of lines: Random effects in linear regression analysis. *Journal of Applied Physiology, 64*(4), 1721–1732.

Feldman, H. A. (1997) Selecting endpoint variables for a community intervention trial. *Annals of Epidemiology, 7*(S7), 78–88.

Feldman, H. A., and McKinlay, S. M. (1994) Cohort versus cross-sectional design in large field trials: Precision, sample size, and a unifying model. *Statistics in Medicine, 13*, 61–78.

Feldman, H. A., McKinlay, S. M., and Niknian, M. (1996) Batch sampling to improve power in a community trial: Experience from the Pawtucket Heart Health Program. *Evaluation Review, 20*(3), 244–274.

Feldman, H. A., Proschan, M., Murray, D. M., Goff, D., Stylianou, M., Dulberg, E., McGovern, P. G., Chan, W., Mann, C., and Bittner, V., for the REACT Study Group. Statistical design of REACT (Rapid Early Action for Coronary Treatment), a multisite community trial with continual data collection. *Controlled Clinical Trials* (under review).

Feng, Z., and Grizzle, J.E. (1992) Correlated binomial variates: Properties of estimator of intraclass correlation and its effect on sample size calculation. *Statistics in Medicine, 11*, 1607–1614.

Flay, B. R. (1985) Psychosocial approaches to smoking prevention: A review of findings. *Health Psychology, 4*(5), 449–488.

Fleiss, J. L. (1981) *Statistical Methods for Rates and Proportions,* 2nd ed. New York: John Wiley and Sons.

Flora, J. A., Lefebvre, C., Murray, D. M., Stone, E. J., Assaf, A., Mittelmark, M., and Finnegan, J. R. (1993) A community education monitoring system: Methods from the Stanford Five-City Project, the Minnesota Heart Health Program, and the Pawtucket Heart Health Program. *Health Education Research, 8*(1), 81–95.

Flora, J. A., and Saphir, M. N., Schooler, C., and Rimal, R. N. (1997) Toward a framework for intervention channels: Reach, involvement, and impact. *Annals of Epidemiology, 7*(S7), 104–112

Flynn, B. S., Worden, J. K., Secker-Walker, R. H., Badger, G. J., Geller, B. M., and Costanza, M. C. (1992) Prevention of cigarette smoking through mass media intervention and school programs. *American Journal of Public Health, 82*(6) 827–834.

Flynn, B. S., Worden, J. K., Secker-Walker, R. H., Pirie, P. L., Badger, G. J., Carpenter, J. H., and Geller, B. M. (1994) Mass media and school interventions for cigarette smoking prevention: Effects 2 years after completion. *American Journal of Public Health, 84*(7), 1148–1150.

Fortmann, S. P., Flora, J. A., Winkleby, M. A., Schooler, C., Taylor, C. B., and Farquhar, J. W. (1995) Community intervention trials: Reflections on the Stanford Five-City Project experience. *American Journal of Epidemiology, 142*(6), 576–586.

Freedman, L. S., Green, S. B., and Byar, D. P. (1990) Assessing the gain in efficiency due to matching in a community intervention study. *Statistics in Medicine, 9,* 943–952.

Gail, M., Byar, D., Pechacek, T., and Corle, D. (1992) Aspects of statistical design for the community intervention trial for smoking cessation (COMMIT). *Controlled Clinical Trials, 13,* 6–21.

Gail, M. H., Mark, S. D., Carroll, R. J., Green, S. B., and Pee, D. (1996) On design considerations and randomization-based inference for community intervention trials. *Statistics in Medicine,* 15, 1069–1092.

Glynn, T. J. (1989) Essential elements of school-based smoking prevention programs. *Journal of School Health, 59*(5), 181–188.

Goldstein, H. (1987) *Multilevel Models in Educational and Social Research.* New York: Oxford University Press.

Goldstein, H. (1994) Multilevel cross-classified models. *Sociological Methods and Research, 22*(3), 364–375.

Goldstein, H. (1995) Hierarchical data modeling in the social sciences. *Journal of Educational and Behavioral Statistics, 20*(2), 201–204.

Gomel, M., Oldenburg, B., Simpson, J. M., and Owen, N. (1993) Work-site cardiovascular risk reduction: A randomized trial of health risk assessment, education, counseling, and incentives. *American Journal of Public Health, 83*(9), 1231–1238.

Goodman, R. M., and Wandersman, A. (1994) FORECAST: A formative approach to evaluating community coalitions and community-based initiatives. *Journal of Community Psychology,* CSAP Special Issue, 6–25.

Green, S. B., Corle, D. K., Gail, M. H., Mark, S. D., Pee, D., Freedman, L. S., Graubard, B. I., and Lynn, W. R. (1995) Interplay between design and analysis for behavioral intervention trials with community as the unit of randomization. *American Journal of Epidemiology, 142*(6), 587–593.

Hannan, P. J., and Murray, D. M. (1996) Gauss or Bernoulli? A Monte Carlo comparison of the performance of the linear mixed model and the logistic mixed model analyses in simulated community trials with a dichotomous outcome variable at the individual level. *Evaluation Review, 20*(3), 338–352.

Hannan, P. J., Murray, D. M., Jacobs, D. R., and McGovern, P. G. (1994) Parameters to aid in the design and analysis of community trials: Intraclass correlations from the Minnesota Heart Health Program. *Epidemiology, 5*(1), 88–95.

Hansen, W. B., and Kaftarian, S. J. (1994) Strategies for comparing multiple-site evaluations under nonequivalent design conditions. *Journal of Community Psychology,* CSAP Special Issue, 170–187.

Harper, P. G., and Murray, D. M. (1994) An organizational strategy to improve adolescent measles-mumps-rubella (MMR) vaccination in a low socioeconomic population: A method to reduce missed opportunities. *Archives of Family Medicine, 3,* 257–262.

Harrow, B. S., Lasater, T. M., Gans, K. M. (1996) A strategy for accurate collection of incremental cost data for cost-effectiveness analyses in field trials: Pawtucket's Minimal Contact Cholesterol Education Intervention. *Evaluation Review, 20*(3), 275–290.

Harville, D. A. (1977) Maximum likelihood approaches to variance component estimation and to related problems. *Journal of the American Statistical Association, 72,* 320–338.

Hedeker, D., Gibbons, R. D., and Flay, B. R. (1994) Random-effects regression models for clustered data with an example from smoking prevention research. *Journal of Consulting and Clinical Psychology, 62*(4), 757–765.

Hopkins, K. D. (1982) The unit of analysis: Group means versus individual observations. *American Education Research Journal, 19*(1), 5–18.

Hopkins, K. D. (1983) A strategy for analyzing ANOVA designs having one or more random factors. *Educational and Psychological Measurement, 43,* 107–113.

Hox, J. J. (1994) Hierarchical regression models for interviewer and respondent effects. *Sociological Methods and Research, 22*(3), 300–318.

Hox, J. J., and Kreft, I. G. G. (1994) Multilevel analysis methods. *Sociological Methods and Research, 22*(3), 283–299.

Hsieh, F. Y. (1988) Sample size formulae for intervention studies with the cluster as unit of randomization. *Statistics in Medicine, 8,* 1195–1201.

Hunt, G. P. (1994) Ethnography and the pursuit of culture: The use of ethnography in evaluating the Community Partnership Program. *Journal of Community Psychology,* CSAP Special Issue, 52–60.

Jacobs, D. R., Luepker, R. V., Mittelmark, M., Folsom, A. R., Pirie, P. L., Mascioli, S. R., Hannan, P. J., Pechacek, T. F., Bracht, N. F., Carlaw, R. W., Kline, F. G., and Blackburn, H. (1986) Community-wide prevention strategies: Evaluation design of the Minnesota Heart Health Program. *Journal of Chronic Diseases, 39*(10), 775–788.

Jeffery, R. W., Forster, J. L., French, S. A., Kelder, S. H., Lando, H. A., McGovern, P. G., Jacobs, D. R., and Baxter, J. E. (1993) The healthy worker project: A worksite intervention for weight control and smoking cessation. *American Journal of Public Health, 83*(3), 395–401.

Johnston, L. D., O'Malley, P. M., and Bachman, J. G. (1996) *National Survey Results on Drug Use from the Monitoring the Future Study, 1975–1994, Volume II, College Students and Young Adults.* (NIH Publication No. 96–4027). Rockville, MD: National Institute on Drug Abuse.

Kaftarian, S. J., and Hansen, W. B. (1994) Improving methodologies for the evaluation of community-based substance abuse prevention programs. *Journal of Community Psychology,* CSAP Special Issue, 3–5.

Kandel, D. B., and Logan, J. A. (1984) Patterns of drug use from adolescence to young adulthood: I. Periods of risk for initiation, continued use, and discontinuation. *American Journal of Public Health, 74*(7), 660–666.

Kass, R. E., and Raftery, A. E. (1995). Bayes factors. *Journal of the American Statistical Association, 90*(430), 773–795.

Kass, R. E., and Wasserman, L. (1995) A reference Bayesian test for nested hypotheses and its relationship to the Schwarz criterion. *Journal of the American Statistical Association, 90*(431), 928–934.

Kelsey, J. L., Thompson, W. D., and Evans, A. S. (1996) *Methods in Observational Epidemiology,* 2nd ed. New York: Oxford University Press.

Kempthorne, O. (1952) *The Design and Analysis of Experiments.* New York: John Wiley and Sons.

Keselman, H. J., and Keselman, J. C. (1993) Analysis of repeated measurements. In L.K. Edwards (ed.), *Applied Analysis of Variance in Behavioral Science* (pp. 105–145). New York: Marcel Dekker, Inc.

Kim, S., Crutchfield, C., Williams, C., and Hepler, N. (1994) An innovative and unconventional approach to program evaluation in the field of substance abuse prevention: A threshold-gating approach using single system evaluation designs. *Journal of Community Psychology,* CSAP Special Issue, 61–78.

Kirk, R. E. (1982) *Experimental Design: Procedures for the Behavioral Sciences,* 2nd ed. Belmont, CA: Brooks/Cole Publishing Co.

Kish, L. (1965) *Survey Sampling.* New York: John Wiley and Sons.

Kish, L. (1987) *Statistical Design for Research.* New York: John Wiley and Sons.

Koepsell, T. D., Diehr, P. H., Cheadle, A., and Kristal, A. (1995) Invited commentary: Symposium on community intervention trials. *American Journal of Epidemiology, 142*(6), 594–599.

Koepsell, T. D., Martin, D. C., Diehr, P. H., Psaty, B. M., Wagner, E. H., Perrin, E. B., Cheadle, A. (1991) Data analysis and sample size issues in evaluations of community-based health promotion and disease prevention programs: A mixed-model analysis of variance approach. *Journal of Clinical Epidemiology, 44*(7), 701–713.

Koepsell, T. D., Wagner, E. H., Cheadle A. C., Patrick, D. L., Martin, D. C., Diehr, P. H., and Perrin, E. B. (1992) Selected methodological issues in evaluating community-based health promotion and disease prevention programs. *Annual Review of Public Health, 13,* 31–57.

Kreft, I. G. G. (1995) Guest editor's introduction. *Journal of Educational and Behavioral Statistics, 20*(2), 109–113.

Kreft, I. G. G., and DeLeeuw, J. (1994) The gender gap in earnings: A two-way nested multiple regression analysis with random effects. *Sociological Methods and Research, 22*(3), 319–341.

Kreft, I. G. G., DeLeeuw, J., and Van der Leeden, R. (1994) Review of five multilevel analysis programs: BMDP-5V, GENMOD, HLM, ML3, VARCL. *The American Statistician, 48*(4), 324–335.

Laird, N. M., and Ware, J. H. (1982) Random effects models for longitudinal data. *Biometrics, 38,* 963–974.

Laird, N., Lange, N., and Stram, D. (1987) Maximum likelihood computations with repeated measures: Application of the EM algorithm. *Journal of the American Statistical Association, 82*(397), 97–105.

Lasater, T. M., Becker, D. M., Hill M. N., and Gans, K. M. (1997) Synthesis of findings and issues from religious-based CVD prevention trials. *Annals of Epidemiology, 7*(S2), 46–53.

Liang, K. Y. and Zeger, S. L. (1986) Longitudinal data analysis using generalized linear models. *Biometrika, 73,* 13–22.

Lilienfeld, D. E. and Stolley, P. D. (1994) *Foundations of Epidemiology,* 3rd ed. New York: Oxford University Press, Inc.

Littell, R. C., Milliken, G. A., Stroup, W. W., and Wolfinger, R. D. (1996) *SAS System for MIXED Models.* Cary, NC: SAS Institute, Inc.

Lohman, T. G., Caballero, B., Himes, J. H., Hunsberger, S., Houtkooper, L. B., Going, S. B., Weber, J., Reid, R., Davis, C. E., Stewart, D., and Stephenson, L. Estimation of body fat from anthropometry and bioelectric impedance in Native American children. (under review).

Longford, N. T. (1995) Hierarchical models and social sciences. *Journal of Educational and Behavioral Statistics, 20*(2), 205–209.

Luepker, R. V., Murray, D. M., Jacobs, D. R., Mittelmark, M. B., Bracht, N., Carlaw, R., Crow, R., Elmer, P., Finnegan, J., Folsom, A. R., Grimm, R., Hannan, P. J., Jeffery, R., Lando, H., McGovern, P., Mullis, R., Perry, C. L., Pechacek, T., Pirie, P., Sprafka, M., Weisbrod, R., Blackburn, H. (1994) Community education for cardiovascular disease prevention: Risk factor changes in the Minnesota Heart Health Program. *American Journal of Public Health, 84*(9), 1383–1393.

Luepker, R. V., Perry, C. L., McKinlay, S. M., Nader, P. R., Parcel, G. S., Stone, E. J., Webber, L. S., Elder, J. P., Feldman, H. A., Johnson, C. C., Kelder, S. H., and Wu, M.

(1996) Outcomes of a field trial to improve children's dietary patterns and physical activity: The Child and Adolescent Trial for Cardiovascular Health (CATCH). *Journal of the American Medical Association, 275*(10), 768–776.

Luepker, R. V., Råstam, L., Hannan, P. J., Murray, D. M., Gray, C., Baker, W. L., Crow, R., Jacobs, D. R., Jr., Pirie, P. L., Mascioli, S. R., Mittelmark, M. B., and Blackburn, H. (1996) Community education for cardiovascular disease prevention: Morbidity and mortality results from the Minnesota Heart Health Program. *American Journal of Epidemiology, 144*(4), 351–362.

Lytle, L. A., Johnson, C. C., Bachman, K. , Wambsgans, K., Perry, C. L., Stone, E. J., and Budman, S. (1994) Successful recruitment strategies for school-based health promotion: Experiences from CATCH. *Journal of School Health, 64*(10), 405–409.

Lytle, L. A., Nichaman, M. Z., Obarzanek, E., Glovsky, E., Montgomery, D., Nicklas, T., Zive, M., and Feldman, H. (1993) Validation of 24-hour recalls assisted by food records in third-grade children. *Journal of the American Dietetic Association, 93*(12), 1431–1436.

Martin, D. C., Diehr, P., Perrin, E. B., and Koepsell, T. D. (1993) The effect of matching on the power of randomized community intervention studies. *Statistics in Medicine, 12,* 329–338.

Mason, W. M., Wong, G. M., and Entwistle, B. (1983) Contextual analysis through the multilevel linear model. In S. Leinhardt (ed.), *Sociological Methodology* (pp. 72–103). San Francisco: Jossey-Bass.

McCullagh, P., and Nelder, J. A. (1983) *Generalized Linear Models,* 1st ed. London: Chapman and Hall.

McCullagh, P., and Nelder, J. A. (1989) *Generalized Linear Models,* 2nd ed. London: Chapman and Hall.

McDonald, R. P. (1994) The bilevel reticular action model for path analysis with latent variables. *Sociological Methods and Research, 22*(3), 399–413.

McGraw, S. A., Sellers, D. E., Stone, E. J., Bebchuk, J., Edmundson, E. W., Johnson, C. C., Bachman, K. J., and Luepker, R. V. (1996) Using process data to explain outcomes: An illustration from the Child and Adolescent Trial for Cardiovascular Health (CATCH). *Evaluation Review, 20*(3), 291–312.

McKinlay, J. B. (1996) More appropriate evaluation methods for community-level health interventions: Introduction to the special issue. *Evaluation Review, 20*(3), 237–243.

McKinlay, S. M. (1994) Cost-efficient designs of cluster unit trials. *Preventive Medicine, 23,* 606–611.

McKinlay, S. M., McGraw, S. A., Kipp, D. M., Assaf, A. R., and Carleton, R. A. (1988) An innovative approach to the evaluation of large community programs. In W. A. Gordon, J. A. Herd, and A. Baum (ed.), *Perspectives on Behavioral Medicine,* Vol. 3, *Prevention and Rehabilitation* (pp. 89–107). New York: Academic Press.

McKinlay, S. M., Stone, E. J., and Zucker, D. M. (1989) Research design and analysis issues. *Health Education Quarterly, 16*(2), 307–313.

Meinert, C. (1986) *Clinical Trials: Design, Conduct, and Analysis.* New York: Oxford University Press.

Morris, C. N. (1995) Hierarchical models for educational data: An overview. *Journal of Educational and Behavioral Statistics, 20*(2), 190–200.

Murray, D. M. (1995) Design and analysis of community trials: Lessons from the Minnesota Heart Health Program. *American Journal of Epidemiology, 142*(6), 569–575.

Murray, D. M. (1997) Design and analysis of group-randomized trials: A review of recent developments. *Annals of Epidemiology, 7*(S7), 69–77.

Murray, D. M., and Hannan, P. J. (1990) Planning for the appropriate analysis in school-based drug-use prevention studies. *Journal of Consulting and Clinical Psychology, 58*(4), 458–468.

Murray, D. M., Hannan, P. J., and Baker, W. L. (1996) A Monte Carlo study of alternative responses to intraclass correlation in community trials: Is it ever possible to avoid Cornfield's penalties? *Evaluation Review, 20*(3), 313–337.

Murray, D. M., Hannan, P., Jacobs, D., McGovern, P. J., Schmid, L., Baker, W. L., and Gray, C. (1994) Assessing intervention effects in the Minnesota Heart Health Program. *American Journal of Epidemiology, 139*(1), 91–103.

Murray, D. M., Hannan, P. J., Wolfinger, R. D., Baker, W. L., and Dwyer, J. H. Analysis of data from group-randomized trials with repeat observations on the same groups. *Statistics in Medicine* (in press).

Murray, D. M., Hannan, P. J., and Zucker, D. (1989) Analysis issues in school-based health promotion studies. *Health Education Quarterly, 16*(2), 315–320.

Murray, D. M., McKinlay, S. M., Martin, D., Donner, A. P., Dwyer, J. H., Raudenbush, S. W., Graubard, B. I. (1994) Design and analysis issues in community trials. *Evaluation Review, 18*(4), 493–514.

Murray, D. M., O'Connell, C., Schmid, L., and Perry, C. L. (1987) The validity of smoking self-reports by adolescents: A reexamination of the bogus pipeline procedure. *Addictive Behaviors, 12,* 7–15.

Murray, D. M., and Perry, C. L. (1987) The measurement of substance use among adolescents: When is the "bogus pipeline" method needed? *Addictive Behaviors, 12,* 225–233.

Murray, D. M., Rooney, B. L., Hannan, P. J., Peterson, A. V., Ary, D. V., Futterman, R., Biglan, A., Botvin, G. J., Evans, R. I., Flay, B. R., Getz, J. G., Marek, P. M., Orlandi, M., Pentz, M. A., Perry, C. L., and Schinke, S. P. (1994) Intraclass correlation among common measures of adolescent smoking: Estimates, correlates and applications in smoking prevention studies. *American Journal of Epidemiology, 140*(11), 1038–1050.

Murray, D. M., and Short, B. (1995) Intraclass correlation among measures related to alcohol use by young adults: Estimates, correlates and applications in intervention studies. *Journal of Studies on Alcohol, 56*(6), 681–694.

Murray, D. M., and Short, B. (1996) Intraclass correlation among measures related to alcohol use by school-aged adolescents: Estimates, correlates and applications in intervention studies. *Journal of Drug Education, 26*(3), 207–230.

Murray, D. M., and Short, B. (1997) Intraclass correlation among measures related to tobacco use by adolescents: Estimates, correlates and applications in intervention studies. *Addictive Behaviors, 22*(1), 1–12.

Murray, D. M., and Wolfinger, R. D. (1994) Analysis issues in the evaluation of community trials: Progress toward solutions in SAS/STAT MIXED. *Journal of Community Psychology,* CSAP Special Issue, 140–154.

Muthén, B. O. (1994) Multilevel covariance structure analysis. *Sociological Methods and Research, 22*(3), 376–398.

Nelder, J. A. (1994) The statistics of linear models: Back to basics. *Statistics and Computing, 4,* 221–234.

Ockene, J. K., McBride, P. E., Sallis, J. F., Bonollo, D. P., and Ockene, I. S. (1997) Synthesis of lessons learned from cardiopulmonary preventive interventions in healthcare practice settings. *Annals of Epidemiology, 7*(S7) 32–45.

Pechacek, T. F., Murray, D. M., Luepker, R. V., Mittelmark, M. B., Johnson, C. A., and Schultz, J. M. (1984) Measurement of adolescent smoking behavior: Rationale and methods. *Journal of Behavioral Medicine, 7*(1), 123–140.

Pentz, M. A. (1994) Adaptive evaluation strategies for estimating effects of community-based drug abuse prevention programs. *Journal of Community Psychology,* CSAP Special Issue, 26–51.

Perry, C. L., Kelder, S. H., Murray, D. M., and Klepp, K. I. (1992) Community-wide smoking prevention: Long-term outcomes of the Minnesota Heart Health Program and the class of 1989 study. *American Journal of Public Health, 82*(9), 1210–1216.

Puska, P., Salonen, J. T., Nissinen, A., Tuomilehto, J., Vartiainen, E., Korhonen, H., Tanskanen, A., Ronnqvist, P., Koskela, K., Huttunen, J. (1983) Change in risk factors for coronary heart disease during 10 years of community intervention programme (North Karelia Project). *British Medical Journal Clinical Research Edition, 287,*(6408) 1840–1844.

Raudenbush, S. W. (1995) Reexamining, reaffirming, and improving application of hierarchical models. *Journal of Educational and Behavioral Statistics, 20*(2), 210–220.

Raudenbush, S. W. (1997) Statistical analysis and optimal design in cluster randomized trials. *Psychological Methods, 2*(2), 173–185.

Resnicow, K., and Robinson, T. (1997) School-based cardiovascular prevention studies: Review and synthesis. *Annals of Epidemiology, 7*(S7), 14–31.

Rodriguez, G., and Goldman, N. (1995) An assessment of estimation procedures for multilevel models with binary responses. *Journal of the Royal Statistical Society, 158* (Part 1), 73–89.

Rodriguez, R., Tobias, R., and Wolfinger, R. W. (1995) Comments on J. A. Nelder, 'The statistics of linear models: Back to basics.' *Statistics and Computing, 5,* 97–101.

Rogosa, D., and Saner, H. (1995) Longitudinal data analysis examples with random coefficient. *Journal of Educational and Behavioral Statistics, 20*(2), 149–170.

Rooney, B. L., and Murray, D. M. (1996) A meta-analysis of smoking prevention programs after adjustment for errors in the unit of analysis. *Health Education Quarterly, 23*(1), 48–64.

Rutter, C. M., and Elashoff, R. M. (1994) Analysis of longitudinal data: Random coefficient regression modelling. *Statistics in Medicine, 13,* 1211–1231.

SAS Institute, Inc. (1989) *SAS/STAT User's Guide, Version 6,* Fourth Edition, Volume 2. Cary, NC: SAS Institute, Inc.

SAS Institute, Inc. (1992) *SAS Technical Report P-229, SAS/STAT Software: Changes and Enhancements, Release 6.07* (pp. 287–368). Cary, NC: SAS Institute, Inc.

SAS Institute, Inc. (1996) *SAS/STAT Software: Changes and Enhancements, through Release 6.11.* Cary, NC: SAS Institute, Inc.

Satterthwaite, F. E. (1946) An approximate distribution of estimates of variance components. *Biometrics Bulletin, 2,* 110–114.

Schlesselman, J. J. (1982) *Case-control Studies: Design, Conduct, Analysis.* New York: Oxford University Press.

Schooler, C., Farquhar, J. W., Fortmann, S. P., and Flora, J. A. (1997) Synthesis of findings and issues from community prevention trials. *Annals of Epidemiology, 7*(S2), 54–68.

Searle, S. R. (1971) *Linear Models.* New York: John Wiley and Sons.

Self, S. G., and Liang, K.Y. (1987) Asymptotic properties of maximum likelihood estimators and likelihood ratio tests under nonstandard conditions. *Journal of the American Statistical Association, 82,* 605–610.

Shah, B. V., Barnwell, B. G., and Bieler, G. S. (1995) *SUDAAN: Software for Analysis of Correlated Data, User's Manual, Release 6.40.* Research Triangle Park, NC: Research Triangle Institute.

Siddiqui, O., Hedeker, D., Flay, B., and Hu, F. (1996) Intraclass correlation estimates in a school-based smoking prevention study—Outcome and mediating variables, by sex and ethnicity. *American Journal of Epidemiology, 144*(4), 425–433.

Simons-Morton, D. G., Goff, D., Luepker, R. V., Osganian, S., Goldberg, R., Raczynski, J. M., Eisenberg, M., Zapka, J., Proschan, M., Feldman, H., and Hedges, J. for the REACT study group. Rapid Early Action for Coronary Treatment (REACT): Rationale, design, and community characteristics. (under review).

Simpson, J. M., Klar, N., and Donner, A. (1995) Accounting for cluster randomization: A review of primary prevention trials, 1990 through 1993. *American Journal of Public Health, 85*(10), 1378–1383.

Skinner, C. J., Holt, D., and Smith, T. M. F. (1989) *Analysis of Complex Surveys.* New York: John Wiley and Sons.

Snedecor, G. W., and Cochran, W. M. (1989) *Statistical Methods,* 8th ed. Ames, IA: The Iowa State University Press.

Snijders, T. A. B., and Bosker, R. J. (1994) Modeled variance in two-level models. *Sociological Methods and Research, 22*(3), 342–363.

Springer, J. F., and Phillips, J. L. (1994) Policy learning and evaluation design: Lessons from the Community Partnership Demonstration Program. *Journal of Community Psychology,* CSAP Special Issue, 117–139.

Statistical Sciences, Inc. (1993) *S-Plus, Version 3.1.* Seattle: Statistical Sciences, Inc.

Stiratelli, R., Laird, N., and Ware, J. H. (1984) Random-effects models for serial observations with binary response. *Biometrics, 40,* 961–971.

Susser, M. (1995). Editorial: The tribulations of trials—interventions in communities. *American Journal of Public Health, 85*(2), 156–158.

Swallow, W. H., and Monahan, J. F. (1984) Monte Carlo comparison of ANOVA, MIVQUE, REML, and ML estimators of variance components. *Technometrics, 26*(1), 47–57.

Thornquist, M. D., and Anderson, G. L. (1992, November) Small sample properties of generalized estimating equations in group-randomized designs with Gaussian response. Paper presented at the 120th Annual Meeting of the American Public Health Association. Washington, D.C.

U.S. Department of Health and Human Services (1994) *Preventing Tobacco Use Among Young People: A Report of the Surgeon General.* Atlanta, GA: U.S. Department of Health and Human Services, Public Health Service, Centers for Disease Control and Prevention, National Center for Chronic Disease Prevention and Health Promotion, Office on Smoking and Health. (DHHS Publication No. S/N-017-001-00491-0). Washington, D.C.: U.S. Government Printing Office.

Wagenaar, A. C., Murray, D. M., Wolfson, M., Forster, J. L., and Finnegan, J. R. (1994) Communities Mobilizing for Change on Alcohol: Design of a randomized community trial. *Journal of Community Psychology,* CSAP Special Issue, 79–101.

Ware, J. H. (1985) Linear models for the analysis of longitudinal studies. *The American Statistician, 39*(2), 95–101.

Wedderburn, R. W. M. (1974) Quasi-likelihood functions, generalized linear models and the Gauss-Newton method. *Biometrika, 61,* 439–447.

The WESREG SAS Procedure, Version 1.3 for SAS 6.08. (1994). Bethesda, MD: WESTAT, Inc.

Winer, B. J. (1971) *Statistical Principles in Experimental Design,* 2nd ed. New York: McGraw-Hill.

Winer, B. J., Brown, D. R., and Michels, K. (1991) *Statistical Principles in Experimental Design.* New York: McGraw-Hill.

Winkleby, M. A. (1997) Accelerating cardiovascular risk factor change in minority and low socioeconomic groups. *Annals of Epidemiology, 7*(S7), 96–104.

Winkleby, M. A., Feldman, H., and Murray, D. M. (1997) Joint analysis of three community intervention trials for reduction of cardiovascular disease risk. *Journal of Clinical Epidemiology, 50,* 645–658.

Wolfinger, R. D. (1992) *A Tutorial on Mixed Models.* Cary, NC: SAS Institute.

Wolfinger, R. D. (1993) Covariance structure selection in general mixed models. *Community Statistics, 22*(4), 1079–1106.

Wolfinger, R. D. (1996) Heterogeneous variance-covariance structures for repeated measures. *Journal of Agricultural, Biological, and Environmental Statistics, 1*(2), 205–230.

Wolfinger, R., and O'Connell, M. (1993) Generalized linear mixed models: A pseudo-likelihood approach. *Journal of Statistical Computation and Simulation, 48,* 233–243.

Wolter, K. M. (1985) *Introduction to Variance Estimation.* New York: Springer-Verlag.

Zeger, S. L., and Liang, K. Y. (1986) Longitudinal data analysis for discrete and continuous outcomes. *Biometrics, 42,* 121–130.

Zeger, S. L., Liang, K., and Albert, P. S. (1988) Models for longitudinal data: A generalized estimating equation approach. *Biometrics, 44,* 1049–1060.

Zucker, D. M. (1990) An analysis of variance pitfall: The fixed effects analysis in a nested design. *Educational and Psychological Measurement, 50,* 731–738.

Zucker, D. M., Lakatos, E., Webber, L. S., Murray, D. M., McKinlay, S. M., Feldman, H. A., Kelder, S. H., and Nader, P. R. (1995) Statistical design of the Child and Adolescent Trial for Cardiovascular Health (CATCH): Implication of cluster randomization. *Controlled Clinical Trials, 16,* 96–118.

Author Index

Addelman, S., 77

Baranowski, T., 16
Berger, J.O., 129 n. 2
Blair, R.C., 103
Braithwaite, R.L., 16
Breslow, N.E., 90, 95–96, 120, 124
Bryk, A.S., 10, 101, 122, 172

Carleton, R.A., 11, 15, 109, 130 n. 10, 415–422
Cheung, K.C., 122
Cohen, J., 353, 381
Cohen, S.B., 119
Cook, R., 16, 33
Cook, T.D., vi, 11, 21–23, 64 n. 2, 67
Cornfield, J., 3, 13, 14, 291 n. 8

Davis, C.E., 73, 206, 210
DeLeeuw, J., 16, 122
Diehr, P., 43, 70, 72, 74
Diggle, P.J., 87, 99, 100, 124, 183
Dixon, W.J., 120, 121
Donner, A., v, 8, 10, 16, 88, 91, 120, 354, 366
Draper, D., 16
Dwyer, J.H., 45, 172

Ellickson, P.L., 16
Efron, B., 98

Farquhar, J.W., 11, 15
Feldman, H.A., 16, 70, 73, 109, 111, 113, 130 n. 10, 172, 354, 366, 416, 420, 421, 428

Feng, Z., 354
Flay, B.R., 13
Fleiss, J.L., 353, 400, 412 n. 2
Flora, J.A., 16, 416
Flynn, B.S., 430–435
Fortmann, S.P., 16, 49
Freedman, L.S., 354

Gail, M.H., 14, 17, 70, 73, 115–117, 3\[
Glynn, T.J., 4
Goldstein, H., 10, 16, 94, 122
Gomel, M., 435, 436
Goodman, R.M., 16
Green, S.B., 16, 115

Hannan, P.J., 16, 39, 92, 103, 353, 354, 363, 438, 444 n. 6
Hansen, W.B., 16
Harper, P.G., 24
Harrow, B.S., 16
Harville, D.A., 88
Hedeker, D., 120, 123
Hopkins, K.D., 106, 108, 112
Hox, J.J., 16, 122, 172
Hsieh, F.Y., 354, 366
Hunt, G.P., 16

Jacobs, D.R., 223, 295
Jeffery, R.W., 422–426
Johnston, L.D., 409

Kaftarian, S.J., 16
Kandel, D.B., 25
Kass, R.E., 129 n. 2, 214, 336
Kelsey, J.L., vi, 12, 19, 353

Subject Index

Printed in the United States
153577LV00001B/16/P